Evidence-Based Public Health

Evidence-Based Public Health

THIRD EDITION

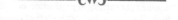

Ross C. Brownson, PhD

*Bernard Becker Professor of Public Health and Director, Prevention
Research Center in St. Louis, Brown School and School of Medicine,
Washington University in St. Louis*

Elizabeth A. Baker, PhD, MPH

*Professor of Behavioral Science and Health Education, College for
Public Health and Social Justice, Saint Louis University*

Anjali D. Deshpande, PhD, MPH

*Clinical Associate Professor in the Department of Epidemiology,
and Director of the MPH Program, University of Iowa College of
Public Health*

Kathleen N. Gillespie, PhD

*Associate Professor of Health Management and Policy, College for
Public Health and Social Justice, Saint Louis University*

OXFORD
UNIVERSITY PRESS

OXFORD
UNIVERSITY PRESS

Oxford University Press is a department of the University of Oxford. It furthers
the University's objective of excellence in research, scholarship, and education
by publishing worldwide. Oxford is a registered trade mark of Oxford University
Press in the UK and certain other countries.

Published in the United States of America by Oxford University Press
198 Madison Avenue, New York, NY 10016, United States of America.

© Oxford University Press 2018
First Edition published in 2003
Second Edition published in 2010
Third Edition published in 2018

Library of Congress Cataloging-in-Publication Data
Names: Brownson, Ross C., author | Baker, Elizabeth A. (Elizabeth Anne),
author. | Deshpande, Anjali D., author. | Gillespie, Kathleen N., author.
Title: Evidence-based public health / Ross C. Brownson, Elizabeth A. Baker,
Anjali D. Deshpande, Kathleen N. Gillespie.
Description: Third edition. | Oxford ; New York : Oxford University Press,
[2017] | Preceded by Evidence-based public health / Ross C. Brownson ...
[et al.]. 2nd ed. 2011. | Includes bibliographical references and index.
Identifiers: LCCN 2016055380 (print) | LCCN 2016055959 (ebook) |
ISBN 9780190620936 (pbk. : alk. paper) | ISBN 9780190620943 (e-book) |
ISBN 9780190620950 (e-book)
Subjects: | MESH: Public Health | Evidence-Based Practice | Public Health
Administration
Classification: LCC RA427 (print) | LCC RA427 (ebook) | NLM WA 100 |
DDC 362.1—dc23
LC record available at https://lccn.loc.gov/2016055380

7 9 8
Printed by Marquis, Canada

We dedicate this book to our close colleague and friend, Terry Leet. He was one of the original contributors to our training program in Evidence-Based Public Health and an author on previous editions of this book. Terry was an outstanding scholar and teacher, and we miss him every day.

CONTENTS

FOREWORD

Evidence-based public health has become an often-used phrase by both practitioners and policymakers. However, its meaning and proper place in the development, conduct, and evaluation of public health programs and policies are often misunderstood. When we hear the word *evidence,* most of us conjure up the mental picture of a courtroom, with opposing lawyers presenting their evidence, or of law enforcement personnel sifting through a crime scene for evidence to be used in judicial proceedings.

Evidence, so central to our notion of justice, is equally central to public health. It should inform all of our judgments about what policies, programs, and system changes to implement, in what populations, and what will be the expected result. For example, "Is the goal to improve the health and well-being of the target population equally, or to also reduce health inequities, because the distribution of ill-health and injuries is so skewed in virtually all geopolitical units?"

In public health, there are four principal user groups for evidence. Public health practitioners with executive and managerial responsibilities and their many public and private partners want to know the evidence for alternative strategies, whether they are policies, programs, or other activities. Too infrequently do busy practitioners find the time to ask the fundamental question, "What are the most important things I can do to improve the public's health?" In pursuit of answers, population-based data are the first prerequisite, covering health status, health risks, and health problems for the overall population and sociodemographic subsegments. Also important are the population's attitudes and beliefs about various major health problems.

The second prerequisite is data on potential interventions. What is the range of alternatives? What do we know about each? What is their individual and conjoint effectiveness in improving health in the populations we are serving? And what is the relative health impact per dollar invested for single or combined interventions? This marriage of information can lead to a rational prioritization of opportunities, constrained only by resources and feasibility.

More often, public health practitioners and their partners have a narrower set of options. Funds from national, state, or local governments are earmarked for a specific purpose, such as surveillance and treatment of sexually transmitted infections, inspection of retail food establishments, or treatment for substance abusers. Still, practitioners have the opportunity, even the obligation, to survey the evidence carefully for alternative ways to achieve the desired health goals be they population wide or more narrowly focused.

The next user group includes policymakers at local, regional, state, national, and international levels. As elected public stewards, they are faced with macro-level decisions on how to allocate the public resources. These responsibilities often include making policies on controversial public issues. Under what conditions should private gun ownership be allowed? How much tax should be levied on traditional cigarettes, and how should these tax revenues be used? Should e-cigarettes be taxed the same as combustibles? Should needle exchange programs be legal for intravenous drug addicts? Should treatment be the required alternative for perpetrators of nonviolent offenses who committed crimes while abusing alcohol or other drugs? What are the best strategies to reverse the obesity epidemic? Good politicians want to know the evidence for the effects of options they are being asked to consider or may want to propose.

Key nongovernmental stakeholders are a third user group for evidence. This group includes many organizations whose missions focus on or include improving health, directly or through enhancing the social and physical environments that are key population health determinants. Other stakeholders include the public, especially those who vote, as well as interest groups formed to support or oppose specific policies or programs. Issues abound, ranging from the legality and accessibility of abortion, to what foods should be served at public schools, or whether home visiting for the families of neonates should be a required health care benefit. Although passion on these issues can run high, evidence can temper views or suggest a feasible range for compromise. Sometimes voters are asked to weigh in on proposed policies through local or state initiative processes. Many of these, from clear indoor air ordinances to water and air regulatory changes or legalizing marijuana, can greatly affect the health of the public.

The final user group is composed of researchers on population health issues. They seek to evaluate the impact of specific policies or programs. Part of their critical role is to both develop and use evidence to explore research hypotheses. Some are primarily interested in the methods used to determine the quality and implications of research on population-based interventions. They frequently ask, "Was the study design appropriate?" and "What are the criteria for determining the adequacy of the study methods?" Others look at the factors that facilitate or retard progress in translating evidence into practice, or in what range of situations an evidence-based intervention can be applied with confidence as to its effectiveness. And an increasing number of researchers are looking at how to model the effects and relative cost-effectiveness to a particular population, and how to determine the likely impacts over time.

This volume should be sweet music to all of these groups. Anyone needing to be convinced of the benefit of systematic development and synthesis of evidence for various public health purposes will quickly be won over. A step-by-step approach to compiling and assessing evidence of what works and what does not is well explicated. In a logical sequence, the reader is guided in how to use the results of his or her search for evidence in developing program or policy options, including the weighing of benefits versus barriers, and then in developing an action plan. To complete the cycle of science, the book describes how to evaluate whatever action is taken. Using this volume does not require extensive formal training in the key disciplines of epidemiology, biostatistics, or behavioral science, but those with strong disciplinary skills will also find much to learn from and put to practical use here.

If every public health practitioner absorbed and applied the key lessons in this volume, public health would enjoy a higher health and financial return on the taxpayer's investment Armed with strong evidence of what works, public health practitioners could be more successful in competing for limited public dollars because they would have strong evidence of what works that is easy to support and difficult to refute. The same standard of difficult-to-refute evidence is much less common in competing requests for scarce public resources.

Jonathan E. Fielding, MD, MPH, MBA
Distinguished Professor of Health Policy and Management,
Fielding School of Public Health, and Distinguished Professor of Pediatrics,
Geffen School of Medicine, School of Public Health,
University of California, Los Angeles

PREFACE

As we finish this third edition of *Evidence-Based Public Health,* we reflect on the promise and challenges for public health. There are tangible examples where the gap between research and practice has been shortened. This may be best illustrated over the twentieth century in the United States, where life expectancy rose from 49 years in 1900 to 77 years in 2000. In large part, this increasing longevity was due to the application of public health advances on a population level (e.g., vaccinations, cleaner air and water, tobacco control policies). Yet for every victory, there is a parallel example of progress yet to be realized. For example, effective treatment for tuberculosis has been available since the 1950s, yet globally tuberculosis still accounts for 2 million annual deaths, with 2 billion people infected. In many ways, the chapters in this book draw on successes (e.g., what works in tobacco control) and remaining challenges (e.g., how to achieve health equity for populations lacking in basic needs of food, shelter, and safety).

Although there are many underlying reasons for these health challenges, our lack of progress on certain public health issues illustrates gaps in applying principles of evidence-based public health. There are at least four ways in which a public health program or policy may fall short in applying these principles:

1. Choosing an intervention approach whose effectiveness is not established in the scientific literature
2. Selecting a potentially effective program or policy, yet achieving only weak, incomplete implementation or "reach," thereby failing to attain objectives (some call this Type III error)
3. Conducting an inadequate or incorrect evaluation that results in a lack of generalizable knowledge on the effectiveness of a program or policy
4. Paying inadequate attention to adapting an intervention to the population and context of interest

To enhance evidence-based decision making, this book addresses all four possibilities and attempts to provide practical guidance on how to choose, adapt, carry out, and evaluate evidence-based programs and policies in public health settings. It also begins to address a fifth, overarching need for a highly trained public health workforce.

Progress will require us to answer questions such as the following:

- Are we applying the evidence that is well established in scientific studies?
- Are there ways to take the lessons learned from successful interventions and apply them to other issues and settings?
- How do we foster greater leadership and stronger political will that supports evidence-based decision making?
- How do we develop and apply incentives so that practitioners will make better use of evidence?
- What lessons from one region of the globe can be applied in a different country?

The original need for this book was recognized during the authors' experiences in public health and health care organizations, legislatures, experiences in the classroom, and discussions with colleagues about the major issues and challenges in finding and using evidence in public health practice. This edition retains our "real-world" orientation, in which we recognize that evidence-based decision making is a complex, iterative, and nuanced *process*. It is not simply a need to use only science-tested, evidence-based interventions. In some cases, the intervention evidence base is developing in light of an epidemic (e.g., control of Zika virus)—hence the need to base decisions on the best *available* evidence, not the best *possible* evidence. It also requires practitioners to remember that public health decisions are shaped by the range of evidence (e.g., experience, political will, resources, values), not solely on science.

Our book deals not only with finding and using *existing* scientific evidence but also with implementation and evaluation of interventions that *generate* new evidence on effectiveness. Because all these topics are broad and require multidisciplinary skills and perspectives, each chapter covers the basic issues and provides multiple examples to illustrate important concepts. In addition, each chapter provides linkages to diverse literature and selected websites for readers wanting more detailed information. Readers should note that websites are volatile, and when a link changes, a search engine may be useful in locating the new web address.

Much of our book's material originated from several courses that we have taught over the past 15 years. One that we offer with the Missouri Department of Health and Senior Services, "Evidence-Based Decision-Making in Public Health," is designed for midlevel managers in state health agencies and leaders of city and county health agencies. We developed a national version of this course with the National Association of Chronic Disease Directors and the Centers for Disease Control and Prevention (CDC). The same course has been adapted for use in many other US states. To conduct international trainings, primarily for practitioners in Central and Eastern Europe, we have collaborated with the CDC, the World Health Organization/Pan American Health Organization, and the CINDI (Countrywide Integrated Noncommunicable Diseases Intervention) Programme. This extensive engagement with practitioners has taught us many fundamental principles, gaps in the evidence-based decision-making process, reasons for these gaps, and solutions.

The format for this third edition is very similar to the approach taken in the course and the second edition. Chapter 1 provides the rationale for evidence-based approaches to decision making in public health. In a new chapter (chapter 2), we describe approaches for building capacity in evidence-based decision making. Chapter 3 presents concepts of causality that help in determining when scientific evidence is sufficient for public health action. Chapter 4 describes economic evaluation and some related analytic tools that help determine whether an effective intervention is worth doing based on its benefits and costs. The next seven chapters lay out a sequential framework for the following:

1. Conducting a community assessment
2. Developing an initial statement of the issue
3. Quantifying the issue
4. Searching the scientific literature and using systematic reviews
5. Developing and prioritizing intervention options
6. Developing an action plan and implementing interventions
7. Evaluating the program or policy

Although an evidence-based process is far from linear, these seven steps are described in some detail to illustrate their importance in making scientifically based decisions about public health programs and policies. We conclude with a chapter on future opportunities for enhancing evidence-based public health.

This book has been written for public health professionals without extensive formal training in the public health sciences (i.e., behavioral science, biostatistics, environmental and occupational health, epidemiology, and health management and policy) and for students in public health and preventive medicine. It can be used in graduate training or for the many emerging undergraduate public health programs. We hope the book will be useful for state and local health agencies, nonprofit organizations, academic institutions, health care organizations, and national public health agencies. Although the book is intended primarily for a North American audience, this third edition draws more heavily on examples from many parts of the world, and we believe that although contextual conditions will vary, the key principles and skills outlined are applicable in both developed and developing countries. Earlier editions of *Evidence-Based Public Health* were translated into Chinese and Japanese and have been used in training programs for practitioners in Latin America, Europe, and the Middle East. Training-related materials are available at: http://www.evidencebasedpublichealth.org/.

The future of public health holds enormous potential, and public health professionals have more tools at their fingertips than ever before to meet a wide range of challenges. We hope this book will be a useful resource for bridging research with the policies and the practice of public health. With focused study, leadership, teamwork, persistence, and good timing, the promise of evidence-based decision making can be achieved.

R. C. B.

E. A. B.

A. D. D.

K. N. G.

ACKNOWLEDGMENTS

We are grateful to numerous individuals who contributed to the development of the third edition of this book.

We particularly wish to thank Garland Land, who co-chaired the original work group that developed the concept for our course, "Evidence-Based Decision Making in Public Health." A number of outstanding graduate students have helped us with the course, including Laura Caisley, Mariah Dreisinger, Wes Gibbert, Carolyn Harris, Lori Hattan, Julie Jacobs, Shannon Keating, and Leslie McIntosh. We are grateful for support from the Centers for Disease Control and Prevention: Ginny Bales, Wayne Giles, Kurt Greenlund, and Mike Waller; to leaders within the National Association of Chronic Disease Directors: Marti Macchi and John Robitscher; and to leaders in the CINDI and CARMEN networks: Gunter Diem, Vilius Grabauskas, Branka Legetic, and Aushra Shatchkute. Many other course instructors and collaborators contributed to this work: Mary Adams, Carsten Baumann, Carol Brownson, Claudia Campbell, Nilza de Assis, Linda Dix, Paul Erwin, Ellen Jones, Terry Leet, Aulikki Nissinen, Shoba Ramanadhan, Darcy Scharff, Paul Siegel, Eduardo Simoes, Sylvie Stachenko, Bill True, Erkki Vartiainen, Fran Wheeler, Cheryl Valko, and Jozica Zakotnik. Several colleagues reviewed chapters or sections: Rebecca Armstrong, Carol Brownson, Gabriel Kaplan, Maggie Padek, Tahna Pettman, Natalicio Serrano, John Troidl, and Hayfaa Wahbi.

Perhaps most important, we thank the thousands of dedicated public health practitioners who have taken our courses and have added many critical ideas to the discourse on evidence-based decision making in public health.

Finally, we are indebted to Chad Zimmerman, Oxford University Press, who provided valuable advice and support throughout the production of this third edition.

CHAPTER 1

✃

The Need for Evidence-Based
Public Health

Public health workers . . . deserve to get somewhere by design, not just by perseverance.
McKinlay and Marceau

Public health research and practice are credited with many notable achievements, including much of the 30-year gain in life expectancy in the United
States over the twentieth century.[1] A large part of this increase can be attributed to provision of safe water and food, sewage treatment and disposal,
tobacco use prevention and cessation, injury prevention, control of infectious
diseases through immunization and other means, and other population-based
interventions.

Despite these successes, many additional challenges and opportunities to
improve the public's health remain. To achieve state and national objectives
for improved public health, more widespread adoption of evidence-based
strategies has been recommended.[2-6] Increased focus on evidence-based public health (EBPH) has numerous direct and indirect benefits, including access
to more and higher quality information on what works, a higher likelihood of
successful programs and policies being implemented, greater workforce productivity, and more efficient use of public and private resources.[4, 7]

Ideally, public health practitioners should always incorporate scientific
evidence in selecting and implementing programs, developing policies, and
evaluating progress. Society pays a high opportunity cost when interventions
that yield the highest health return on an investment are not implemented
(i.e., in light of limited resources, the benefit given up by implementing less
effective interventions).[8] In practice, decisions are often based on perceived
short-term opportunities, lacking systematic planning and review of the best

evidence regarding effective approaches. Still apparent today,[9] these concerns were noted nearly three decades ago when the Institute of Medicine determined that decision making in public health is too often driven by "... crises, hot issues, and concerns of organized interest groups" (p. 4).[10] Barriers to implementing EBPH include the political environment (including lack of political will) and deficits in relevant and timely research, information systems, resources, leadership, organizational culture, and the ability to connect research with policy.[11–15]

Nearly every public health problem is complex,[16] requiring attention at multiple levels and among many different disciplines. Part of the complexity is that populations are affected disproportionately, creating inequities in health and access to resources. Partnerships that bring together diverse people and organizations have the potential for developing new and creative ways of addressing public health issues.[17] Transdisciplinary research provides valuable opportunities to collaborate on interventions to improve the health and well-being of both individuals and communities.[18,19] For example, tobacco research efforts have been successful in facilitating cooperation among disciplines such as advertising, policy, business, medical science, and behavioral science. Research activities within these tobacco networks try to fill the gaps between scientific discovery and research translation by engaging a wide range of stakeholders.[20,21] A transdisciplinary approach has also shown some evidence of effectiveness in obesity prevention by engaging numerous sectors, including food production, urban planning, transportation, schools, and health.[22]

As these disciplines converge, several concepts are fundamental to achieving a more evidence-based approach to public health practice. First, we need scientific information on the programs and policies that are most likely to be effective in promoting health (i.e., undertake evaluation research to generate sound evidence).[4] An array of effective interventions is now available from numerous sources, including the *Guide to Community Preventive Services*,[23] the *Guide to Clinical Preventive Services*,[24] Cancer Control PLANET,[25] the Cochrane Reviews,[26] and the National Registry of Evidence-based Programs and Practices.[27] Second, to translate science to practice, we need to marry information on evidence-based interventions from the peer-reviewed literature with the realities of a specific real-world environment.[28,29] To do so, we need to better define processes that lead to evidence-based decision making.[30] Third, wide-scale dissemination of interventions of proven effectiveness must occur more consistently at state and local levels.[31] And finally, we need to more effectively build collaborations and networks that cross sectors and disciplines.

This chapter includes three major sections that describe (1) relevant background issues, including a brief history, definitions, an overview of evidence-based medicine, and other concepts underlying EBPH; (2) several key characteristics of an evidenced-based process that crosses numerous disciplines; and (3) analytic tools to enhance the uptake of EBPH and the disciplines responsible. A major goal of this chapter is to move the process of decision making toward a proactive approach that incorporates effective use of scientific evidence and data, while engaging numerous sectors and partners for transdisciplinary problem solving.

BACKGROUND

Formal discourse on the nature and scope of EBPH originated about two decades ago. Several authors have attempted to define EBPH. In 1997, Jenicek defined EBPH as the "... conscientious, explicit, and judicious use of current best evidence in making decisions about the care of communities and populations in the domain of health protection, disease prevention, health maintenance and improvement (health promotion)."[32] In 1999, scholars and practitioners in Australia[5] and the United States[33] elaborated further on the concept of EBPH. Glasziou and colleagues posed a series of questions to enhance uptake of EBPH (e.g., "Does this intervention help alleviate this problem?") and identified 14 sources of high-quality evidence.[5] Brownson and colleagues described a multistage process by which practitioners are able to take a more evidence-based approach to decision making.[4,33] Kohatsu and colleagues broadened earlier definitions of EBPH to include the perspectives of community members, fostering a more population-centered approach.[28] Rychetnik and colleagues summarized many key concepts in a glossary for EBPH.[34] There appears to be a consensus that a combination of scientific evidence, as well as values, resources, and context should enter into decision making (Figure 1.1).[2,4,34,35] A concise definition emerged from Kohatsu: "Evidence-based public

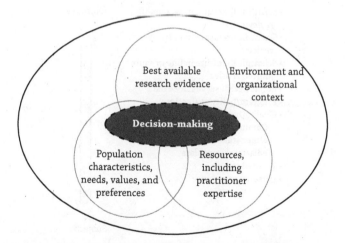

Figure 1.1: Domains that influence evidence-based decision making.
Source: From Satterfeld et al.[35]

health is the process of integrating science-based interventions with community preferences to improve the health of populations" (p. 419).[28] Particularly in Canada and Australia, the term "evidence-informed decision making" is commonly used.[36,37] In part, the "evidence-informed" description seeks to emphasize that public health decisions are not based *only* on research.[38]

In addition, Satterfield and colleagues examined evidence-based practice across five disciplines (public health, social work, medicine, nursing, and psychology) and found many common challenges, including (1) how evidence should be defined; (2) how and when the patient's and/or other contextual factors should enter the decision-making process; (3) the definition and role of the experts or key stakeholders; and (4) what other variables should be considered when selecting an evidence-based practice (e.g., age, social class).[35]

Defining Evidence

At the most basic level, evidence involves "the available body of facts or information indicating whether a belief or proposition is true or valid."[39] The idea of evidence often derives from legal settings in Western societies. In law, evidence comes in the form of stories, witness accounts, police testimony, expert opinions, and forensic science.[40] Our notions of evidence are defined in large part by our professional training and experience. For a public health professional, evidence is some form of data—including epidemiologic (quantitative) data, results of program or policy evaluations, and qualitative data—that is used in making judgments or decisions (Figure 1.2).[41] Public

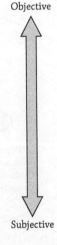

Objective

- Scientific literature in systematic reviews
- Scientific literature in narrative reviews
- Scientific literature in one or more journal articles
- Public health surveillance data
- Program/policy evaluations
- Qualitative data
  - Community members
  - Other stakeholders
- Media/marketing data
- Word of mouth
- Personal experience

Subjective

Figure 1.2: Different forms of evidence.
Source: Adapted from Chambers and Kerner.[41]

health evidence is usually the result of a complex cycle of observation, theory, and experiment.[42] However, the value of evidence is in the eye of the beholder (e.g., usefulness of evidence may vary by discipline or sector).[43] Medical evidence includes not only research but also characteristics of the patient, a patient's readiness to undergo a therapy, and society's values.[44] Policy makers seek out distributional consequences (i.e., who has to pay, how much, and who benefits)[45]; and in practice settings, anecdotes sometimes trump empirical data.[46] Evidence is usually imperfect and, as noted by Muir Gray: "The absence of excellent evidence does not make evidence-based decision making impossible; what is required is the best evidence available not the best evidence possible."[2]

Several authors have defined types of scientific evidence for public health practice (Table 1.1).[4,33,34] Type 1 evidence defines the causes of diseases and the magnitude, severity, and preventability of risk factors and diseases. It suggests that "*something* should be done" about a particular disease or risk factor. Type 2 evidence describes the relative impact of specific interventions to affect health, adding "*specifically*, this should be done."[4] There is likely to be even less published research on type 3 evidence—which shows how and under what contextual conditions interventions were implemented and how they were received, thus informing "*how* something should (or could) be done."[34] This contextual evidence is highly valued by practitioners.[47] A literature review from Milat and colleagues[48] showed the relative lack of dissemination research (Type 3) compared with descriptive/epidemiologic research (Type 1). In the most recent time period (2008–2009), between 3% and 7% of published studies were dissemination studies. Experience from Australia indicates that stakeholders can be engaged to assess the usefulness of evidence in public health practice along with the gaps in the EBPH process (Box 1.1).[36, 49]

Studies to date have tended to overemphasize internal validity (e.g., well-controlled efficacy trials such as randomized trials), while giving sparse attention to external validity (e.g., the translation of science to the various circumstances of practice).[50,51] The evidence framework proposed by Spencer and colleagues is useful because it provides four categories of evidence (best, leading, promising, emerging) and takes into account elements of external validity (reach, feasibility, sustainability, and transferability) (Figure 1.3).[52] This broader framing of evidence is addressed in some tools for rating the quality of intervention effectiveness (e.g., *Using What Works for Health*[53]).

Particularly for policy-related evidence, research hierarchies that favor the randomized trial have serious limitations.[38,46,54] It has been noted that adherence to a strict hierarchy of study designs may reinforce an "inverse evidence law" by which interventions most likely to influence whole populations (e.g., policy change) are least valued in an evidence matrix emphasizing randomized designs.[55, 56]

Table 1.1. COMPARISON OF THE TYPES OF SCIENTIFIC EVIDENCE

Characteristic	Type One	Type Two	Type Three
Goal/action	Identify a problem or priority (something should be done)	Identify what works (what should be done)	Identify how to implement (what works for whom, in what context, and why)
Typical data/relationship	Size and strength of preventable risk—disease relationship (measures of burden, descriptive data, etiologic research)	Relative effectiveness of public health intervention	Information on the adaptation and implementation of an effective intervention
Common setting	Clinic or controlled community setting	Socially intact groups or community-wide	Socially intact groups or community-wide
Example 1 questions	Does smoking cause lung cancer?	Will price increases with a targeted media campaign reduce smoking rates?	What are the political challenges of price increases in different geographic settings?
Example 2 questions	Is the density of fast-food outlets linked with obesity?	Do policies that restrict fast-food outlets change caloric intake?	How do community attitudes about fast-food policies influence policy change?
Quantity	Most	Moderate	Least

Understanding the Context for Evidence

Type 3 evidence derives from the context of an intervention.[34] Although numerous authors have written about the role of context in informing evidence-based practice,[34,57–60] there is little consensus on its definition. When moving from clinical interventions to population-level and policy interventions, context becomes more uncertain, variable, and complex.[61] For example, we know that social and economic factors can result in inequities in health and access to health care resources.[62] One useful definition of context highlights information needed to adapt and implement an evidence-based intervention in a particular setting or population.[34] The context for type 3 evidence specifies five overlapping domains (see Table 1.2).[63] First, there are characteristics of the target population for an intervention such as education level and health history. Next, interpersonal variables provide important context. For example, a person with family support to seek screening because of a family history of cancer might be more likely to undergo cancer screening. Third, organizational variables should be considered when

---

Box 1.1

DEVELOPING A PRACTICAL UNDERSTANDING OF AN EVIDENCE TYPOLOGY IN AUSTRALIA

In Australia, as in other parts of the globe, there are numerous taxonomies, typologies, and frameworks (hereafter referred to as "typologies") to guide evidence-informed decision making (EIDM) for public health. Relatively little is known about the practical utility and application of these various typologies. To be useful, they must acknowledge that the process of EIDM includes not only research evidence but also of several other types of information. The many other inputs include political and organizational factors, such as politics, habits and traditions, pragmatics, resources, and values and ethics. The *Public Health Insight* group, based in Australia,[49] tested the relevance of the typology described in this chapter: data (Type 1), intervention effectiveness (Type 2), and implementation evidence (Type 3). The team triangulated relevant findings from three applied research and evaluation projects. Practitioners were perceived to be highly competent at finding and using Type 1 data for priority setting (describing the problem). They were less effective at finding and using Type 2 (impact) and Type 3 (implementation) evidence. Organizational processes for using Types 2 and 3 evidence were almost nonexistent. The findings suggest that a typology for EIDM is useful for defining key concepts, identifying gaps, and determining the needs in organizational cultures and the broader public health system.

---

considering context for a specific intervention. For example, whether an agency is successful in carrying out an evidence-based program will be influenced by its capacity (e.g., a trained workforce, agency leadership).[64,65] The important role of capacity building (e.g., more training toward prevention, increasing the skills of professionals) has been noted as a "grand challenge" for public health efforts.[66] Fourth, social norms and culture are known to shape many health behaviors. Finally, larger political and economic forces affect context. For example, a high rate for a certain disease may influence a state's political will to address the issue in a meaningful and systematic way. Particularly for high-risk and understudied populations, there is a pressing need for evidence on contextual variables and ways of adapting programs and policies across settings and population subgroups. This is particularly important in a range of public health efforts to address health equity and health disparities, in which certain challenges are pronounced (e.g., collecting the wrong data, sample size issues, lack of resources allocated for health equity).[67,68] Contextual issues are being addressed more fully in the new "realist review," which is a systematic review process that seeks to examine not

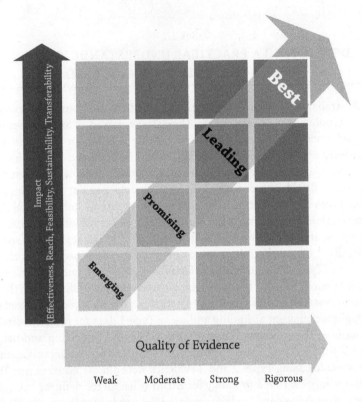

Figure 1.3: Typology of scientific evidence.
Source: From Spencer et al.[52]

only whether an intervention works but also *how* interventions work in real world settings.[69]

Challenges Related to Public Health Evidence

Evidence for public health has been described as underpopulated, dispersed, and different.[70,71] It is underpopulated because there are relatively few well-done evaluations of how well evidence-based interventions apply across different social groups (type 3 evidence). Information for public health decision making is also more dispersed than evidence for clinical interventions. For example, evidence on the health effects of the built environment might be found in transportation or planning journals. Finally, public health evidence is different, in part because much of the science base for interventions is derived from nonrandomized designs or so-called natural experiments (i.e., generally takes the form of an observational study in which the researcher cannot control or withhold the allocation of an intervention to particular areas or communities, but where natural or predetermined variation in allocation occurs.[72])

Table 1.2. CONTEXTUAL VARIABLES FOR INTERVENTION
DESIGN, IMPLEMENTATION, AND ADAPTATION

Category	Examples
Individual	Education level
	Basic human needs[a]
	Personal health history
Interpersonal	Family health history
	Support from peers
	Social capital
Organizational	Staff composition
	Staff expertise
	Physical infrastructure
	Organizational culture
Sociocultural	Social norms
	Values
	Cultural traditions
	Health equity
	History
Political and economic	Political will
	Political ideology
	Lobbying and special interests
	Costs and benefits

[a]Basic human needs include food, shelter, warmth, safety.[63]

Triangulating Evidence

Triangulation involves the accumulation and analyses of evidence from a variety of sources to gain insight into a particular topic[73] and often combines quantitative and qualitative data.[4] It generally involves the use of multiple methods of data collection and/or analysis (i.e., mixed methods that combines quantitative and qualitative approaches) to determine points of commonality or disagreement. Triangulation is often beneficial because of the complementary nature of information from different sources. Though quantitative data provide an excellent opportunity to determine *how* variables are related for large numbers of people, these data provide little in the way of understanding *why* these relationships exist. Qualitative data, on the other hand, can help provide information to explain quantitative findings, or what has been called "illuminating meaning."[74] There are many examples of the use of triangulation of qualitative and quantitative data to evaluate health programs and policies, including HIV prevention programs,[75] family planning programs,[76] obesity prevention interventions,[77] smoking cessation programs,[78] and physical activity promotion.[79] These examples also illustrate the roles of numerous disciplines in addressing pressing public health problems.

Cultural and Geographic Differences

The tenets of EBPH have largely been developed in a Western, European-American context.[80] The conceptual approach arises from the epistemological underpinnings of logical positivism,[81] which finds meaning through rigorous observation and measurement. This is reflected in a professional preference among clinicians for research designs such as the randomized controlled trial. In addition, most studies in the EBPH literature are academic-based research, usually with external funding for well-established investigators. In contrast, in developing countries and in impoverished areas of developed countries, the evidence base for how best to address common public health problems is often limited, even though the scope of the problem may be enormous.[6] Cavill compared evidence-based interventions across countries in Europe, showing that much of the evidence base in several areas is limited to empirical observations.[82] In China, the application of EBPH concepts is at an early stage, suggesting considerable room for growth.[83] Even in more developed countries (including the United States), information published in peer-reviewed journals or data available through websites and official organizations may not adequately represent all populations of interest.

Key Role of EBPH in Accreditation Efforts

A national voluntary accreditation program for public health agencies was established through the Public Health Accreditation Board (PHAB) in 2007.[84] As an effort to improve both the quality and performance of public health agencies at all levels, the accreditation process is structured around 12 domains that roughly coincide with the 10 Essential Public Health Services, with additional domains on management and administration (domain 11) and governance (domain 12).[85] The accreditation process intersects with EBPH on at least three levels. First, the entire process is based on the predication that if a public health agency meets certain standards and measures, quality and performance will be enhanced. The evidence for such a predication, however, is incomplete at best, and often relies on the type of best evidence available that can only be described as sound judgment, based on experience in practice. Second, domain 10 of the PHAB process is "Contribute to and Apply the Evidence Base of Public Health." Successfully accomplishing the standards and measures under domain 10 involves using EBPH from such sources as the *Guide to Community Preventive Services*, having access to research expertise, and communicating the facts and implications of research to appropriate audiences. Third, the prerequisites for accreditation—a community health assessment, a community health improvement plan, and an agency strategic plan—are key elements of EBPH, as will be described later in this chapter.

A critical aspect of the early implementation of PHAB is the development of an evaluation and research agenda, based on a logic model for accreditation, which can serve as a guide for strengthening the evidence base for accreditation. In many ways the accreditation process is parallel to the development of EBPH: the actual use of standards and measures presents opportunities to strengthen the evidence base for accreditation, and, as EBPH evolves, new findings will help inform the refinement of standards and measures over time.

Audiences for Evidence-Based Public Health

There are four overlapping user groups for EBPH as defined by Fielding.[86] The first includes public health practitioners with executive and managerial responsibilities who want to know the scope and quality of evidence for alternative strategies (e.g., programs, policies). In practice, however, public health practitioners frequently have a relatively narrow set of options. Funds from federal, state, or local sources are most often earmarked for a specific purpose (e.g., surveillance and treatment of sexually transmitted diseases, inspection of retail food establishments). Still, the public health practitioner has the opportunity, even the obligation, to carefully review the evidence for alternative ways to achieve the desired health goals. The next user group is policy makers at local, regional, state, national, and international levels. They are faced with macro-level decisions on how to allocate the public resources for which they are stewards. This group has the additional responsibility of making policies on controversial public issues. The third group is composed of stakeholders who will be affected by any intervention. This includes the public, especially those who vote, as well as interest groups formed to support or oppose specific policies, such as the legality of abortion, whether the community water supply should be fluoridated, or whether adults must be issued handgun licenses if they pass background checks. The final user group is composed of researchers on population health issues, such as those who evaluate the impact of a specific policy or programs. They both develop and use evidence to answer research questions.

Similarities and Differences Between Evidence-Based Public Health and Evidence-Based Medicine

The concept of evidence-based practice is well established in numerous disciplines, including psychology,[87] social work,[88,89] and nursing.[90] It is probably best established in medicine. The doctrine of evidence-based medicine (EBM) was formally introduced in 1992.[91] Its origins can be traced back to the seminal work of Cochrane, who noted that many medical treatments lacked scientific effectiveness.[92] A basic tenet of EBM is to de-emphasize unsystematic clinical experience and place greater emphasis on evidence from clinical research. This approach requires new skills, such as efficient literature searching and an understanding of types of evidence in evaluating the clinical literature.[93] There has been a rapid growth in the literature on EBM, contributing to its formal recognition. Using the search term "evidence-based medicine," there were 255 citations in PubMed in 1990, rising to 2,898 in 2000, to 8,348 citations in 2010, and to 13,798 in 2015. Even though the formal terminology of EBM is relatively recent, its concepts are embedded in earlier efforts, such as the Canadian Task Force on the Periodic Health Examination[94] and the *Guide to Clinical Preventive Services*.[24]

There are important distinctions between evidence-based approaches in medicine and public health. First, the type and volume of evidence differ. Medical studies of pharmaceuticals and procedures often rely on randomized controlled trials of individuals, the most scientifically rigorous of epidemiologic studies. In contrast, public health interventions usually rely on cross-sectional studies, quasi-experimental designs, and time-series analyses. These studies sometimes lack a comparison group and require more caveats in interpretation of results. Over the past 50 years, there have been more than one million randomized controlled trials of medical treatments. There are many fewer studies of the effectiveness of public health interventions[4] because they are difficult to design and their results often derive from natural experiments (e.g., a state adopting a new policy compared with other states). EBPH has borrowed the term "intervention" from clinical disciplines, insinuating specificity and discreteness. However, in public health, we seldom have a single "intervention," but rather a program that involves a blending of several interventions within a community. Large community-based trials can be more expensive to conduct than randomized experiments in a clinic. Population-based studies generally require a longer time period between intervention and outcome. For example, a study on the effects of smoking cessation on lung cancer mortality would require decades of data collection and analysis. Contrast that with treatment of a medical condition (e.g., an antibiotic for symptoms of pneumonia), which is likely to produce effects in days or weeks, or even a surgical trial for cancer with endpoints of mortality within a few years.

The formal training of persons working in public health is much more variable than that in medicine or other clinical disciplines.[95] Unlike medicine, public health relies on a variety of disciplines, and there is not a single academic credential that "certifies" a public health practitioner, although efforts to establish credentials (via an exam) are now in place for those with formal public health training (e.g., the National Board of Public Health Examiners Certified in Public Health exam).[96] This higher level of heterogeneity means that multiple perspectives are involved in a more complicated decision-making process. It also suggests that effective public health practice places a premium on routine, on-the-job training.

KEY CHARACTERISTICS OF EVIDENCE-BASED DECISION MAKING

It is useful to consider several overarching, common characteristics of evidence-based approaches to public health practice. These notions are expanded on in other chapters. Described subsequently, these various attributes of EBPH and key characteristics include the following:

- Making decisions based on the best available peer-reviewed evidence (both quantitative and qualitative research)
- Using data and information systems systematically
- Applying program planning frameworks (that often have a foundation in behavioral science theory)
- Engaging the community of focus in assessment and decision making
- Conducting sound evaluation
- Disseminating what is learned to key stakeholders and decision makers

Accomplishing these activities in EBPH is likely to require a synthesis of scientific skills, enhanced communication, common sense, and political acumen.

Decisions Are Based on the Best Possible Evidence

As one evaluates evidence, it is useful to understand where to turn for the best available scientific evidence. A starting point is the scientific literature and guidelines developed by expert panels. In addition, preliminary findings from researchers and practitioners are often presented at regional, national, and international professional meetings.

Data and Information Systems Are Used

A tried and true public health adage is, "what gets measured, gets done."[97] This has typically been applied to long-term endpoints (e.g., rates of mortality), and data for many public health endpoints and populations are not readily available at one's fingertips. Data are being developed more for local-level issues (e.g., the Selected Metropolitan/Micropolitan Area Risk Trends of the Behavioral Risk Factor Surveillance System [SMART BRFSS]), and a few early efforts are underway to develop public health policy surveillance systems.

Systematic Planning Approaches Are Used

When a program or policy approach is decided on, a variety of planning frameworks and models can be applied (e.g., ecological[98,99] and systems dynamic models[100]). These models point to the importance of addressing problems at multiple levels and stress the interaction and integration of factors within and across all levels—individual, interpersonal, community, organizational, and governmental. The goal is to create healthy community environments that support the health and well-being of all people. That may involve a combination of programs and policies designed to enable people to live healthier lifestyles.[101] Effective interventions are most often grounded in health-behavior theory.[42, 102]

Community Engagement Occurs

Community-based approaches involve community members across multiple sectors in research and intervention projects and show progress in improving population health and addressing health disparities.[103,104] As a critical step in transdisciplinary problem solving, practitioners, academicians, and community members collaboratively define issues of concern, develop strategies for intervention, and evaluate the outcomes. This approach relies on stakeholder input, builds on existing resources, facilitates collaboration among all parties, and integrates knowledge and action that seek to lead to a fair distribution of the benefits of an intervention for all partners.[104–106]

Sound Evaluation Principles Are Followed

Too often in public health, programs and policies are implemented without much attention to systematic evaluation. In addition, even when programs are ineffective, they are sometimes continued because of historical or political considerations. Evaluation plans must be laid early in program development and should include both formative and outcome evaluation (as further described in chapter 11).

Results Are Disseminated to Others Who Need to Know

When a program or policy has been implemented, or when final results are known, others in public health—as well as community members themselves—can rely on findings to enhance their own use of evidence in decision making. Dissemination may occur to health professionals via the scientific literature, to the general public via the media, to communities of focus via reports and meetings, to policy makers through personal meetings, and to public health professionals through training courses. It is important to identify appropriate channels for dissemination[107] because public health professionals differ in where they seek information (e.g., public health practitioners prefer peer leaders in practice, whereas academicians prefer peer-reviewed journals).[108]

ANALYTIC TOOLS AND APPROACHES TO ENHANCE THE UPTAKE OF EVIDENCE-BASED PUBLIC HEALTH

Several analytic tools and planning approaches can help practitioners in answering questions such as the following:

- What is the size of the public health problem?
- Are there effective interventions for addressing the problem?
- What information about the local context and this particular intervention is helpful in deciding its potential use in the situation at hand?
- Is a particular program or policy worth doing (i.e., is it better than alternatives) and will it provide a satisfactory return on investment, measured in monetary terms, health impacts, or impacts on health disparities?
- How can we understand the effect of a program or policy on health equity?

In this section, we briefly introduce a series of important tools and analytic methods—many of these are covered in detail in later chapters.

Public Health Surveillance

Public health surveillance is a critical tool for those using EBPH (as will be described in much more detail in chapter 7). It involves the ongoing systematic collection, analysis, and interpretation of specific health data, closely integrated with the timely dissemination of these data to those responsible for preventing and controlling disease or injury.[109] Public health surveillance systems should have the capacity to collect and analyze data, disseminate data to public health programs, and regularly evaluate the effectiveness of the use of the disseminated data.[110]

Systematic Reviews and Evidence-Based Guidelines

Systematic reviews are syntheses of comprehensive collections of information on a particular topic. Reading a good review can be one of the most efficient ways to become familiar with state-of-the-art research and practice on many specific topics in public health. The use of explicit, systematic methods (i.e., decision rules) in reviews limits bias and reduces chance effects, thus providing more reliable results on which to make decisions.[111] One of the most useful sets of reviews for public health interventions is the *Guide to Community Preventive Services* (the *Community Guide*),[23] which provides an overview of current scientific literature through a well-defined, rigorous method in which available studies themselves are the units of analysis. The *Community Guide* seeks to answer, (1) "What interventions have been evaluated and what have been their effects?" (2) "What aspects of interventions can help *Community Guide* users select from among the set of interventions of proven effectiveness?" and (3) "What might this intervention cost and how do these compare with the likely health impacts?" A good systematic review should allow the practitioner to understand the local contextual conditions necessary for successful implementation.[112]

Economic Evaluation

Economic evaluation is an important component of evidence-based practice.[113] It can provide information to help assess the relative value of alternative expenditures on public health programs and policies. In cost-benefit analysis, all of the costs and consequences of the decision options are valued in monetary terms. More often, the economic investment associated with an intervention is compared with the health impacts, such as cases of disease prevented or years of life saved. This technique, cost-effectiveness analysis, can suggest the relative value of alternative interventions (i.e., health return on dollars invested).[113] Cost-effectiveness analysis has become an increasingly important tool for researchers, practitioners, and policy makers. However, relevant data to support this type of analysis are not always available, especially for possible public policies designed to improve health.[46,114] Additional information on economic evaluation is provided in chapter 4.

Health Impact Assessment

Health impact assessment (HIA) is a relatively new method that seeks to estimate the probable impact of a policy or intervention in nonhealth sectors (such as agriculture, transportation, and economic development) on the health of the population.[115] Some HIAs have focused on ensuring the involvement of relevant stakeholders in the development of a specific project. This is essential for an environmental impact assessment required by law for many large place-based projects. Overall, HIA has been gaining acceptance as a tool because of mounting evidence that social and physical environments are important determinants of health and health disparities in populations. It is now being used to help assess the potential effects of many policies and programs on health status and outcomes.[116-118] This approach dovetails with the conceptualization and application of "health in all policies."[119]

Participatory Approaches

Participatory approaches that actively involve community members in research and intervention projects[103,104,120] show promise in engaging communities in EBPH.[28] Practitioners, academicians, and community members collaboratively define issues of concern, develop strategies for intervention, and evaluate the outcomes. This approach relies on stakeholder input,[121] builds on existing resources, facilitates collaboration among all parties, and integrates knowledge and action that hopefully will lead to a fair distribution of the benefits of an intervention or project for all partners.[104,105] Stakeholders, or key players, are individuals or agencies that have a vested interest in the issue at hand. In the development of health policies, for example, policy makers are especially important stakeholders. Stakeholders should include those who would potentially receive, use, and benefit from the program or policy being considered. Three groups of stakeholders are relevant: people developing programs, those affected by interventions, and those who use results of program evaluations. Participatory approaches may also present challenges in adhering to EBPH principles, especially in reaching agreement on which approaches are most appropriate for addressing a particular health problem.[122]

SUMMARY

The successful implementation of EBPH in public health practice is both a science and an art. The science is built on epidemiologic, behavioral, and policy research showing the size and scope of a public health problem and which interventions are likely to be effective in addressing the problem. The art of decision making often involves knowing what information is important to a particular stakeholder at the right time. Unlike solving a math problem, significant decisions in public health must balance science and art because rational, evidence-based decision making often involves choosing one alternative from among a set of rational choices. By applying the concepts of EBPH outlined in this chapter, decision making and, ultimately, public health practice can be improved.

KEY CHAPTER POINTS

- To achieve state and national objectives for improved population health, more widespread adoption of evidence-based strategies is recommended.
- There are several important distinctions between EBPH and clinical disciplines, including the volume of evidence, study designs used to inform research and practice, the setting or context where the intervention is applied, and the training and certification of professionals.
- Key components of EBPH include making decisions based on the best available, peer-reviewed evidence; using data and information systems systematically; applying program-planning frameworks; engaging the community in decision making; conducting sound evaluation; and disseminating what is learned.
- Numerous analytic tools and approaches that can enhance the greater use of EBPH include public health surveillance, systematic reviews, economic evaluation, health impact assessment, and participatory approaches.

SUGGESTED READINGS AND SELECTED WEBSITES

Suggested Readings

Brownson, RC, Fielding JE, Maylahn CM. Evidence-based public health: a fundamental concept for public health practice. *Annu Rev Public Health.* 2009;30:175–201.

Frieden TR. Six components necessary for effective public health program implementation. *Am J Public Health.* Jan 2013;104(1):17–22.

Glasziou P, Longbottom H. Evidence-based public health practice. *Aust N Z J Public Health.* 1999;23(4):436–440.

Green LW, Ottoson JM, Garcia C, Hiatt RA. Diffusion theory and knowledge dissemination, utilization, and integration in public health. *Annu Rev Public Health.* 2009;30:151–174.

Guyatt G, Rennie D, Meade M, Cook D, eds. *Users' Guides to the Medical Literature. A Manual for Evidence-Based Clinical Practice.* 3rd ed. Chicago, IL: American Medical Association Press; 2015.

Muir Gray JA. *Evidence-Based Healthcare: How to Make Decisions about Health Services and Public Health.* 3rd ed. New York and Edinburgh: Churchill Livingstone Elsevier; 2009.

Oliver K, Innvar S, Lorenc T, Woodman J, Thomas J. A systematic review of barriers to and facilitators of the use of evidence by policymakers. *BMC Health Serv Res.* 2014;14:2.

Rychetnik L, Hawe P, Waters E, Barratt A, Frommer M. A glossary for evidence based public health. *J Epidemiol Community Health.* Jul 2004;58(7):538–545.

Selected Websites

American Public Health Association (APHA) <http://www.apha.org>. The APHA is the oldest and most diverse organization of public health professionals in the world, representing more than 50,000 members. The Association and its members have been influencing policies and setting priorities in public health since 1872. The APHA site provides links to many other useful websites.

Canadian Task Force on Preventive Health Care < http://canadiantaskforce.ca/>. This website is designed to serve as a practical guide to health care providers, planners, and consumers for determining the inclusion or exclusion, content, and frequency of a wide variety of preventive health interventions, using the evidence-based recommendations of the Canadian Task Force on Preventive Health Care.

Cancer Control P.L.A.N.E.T. <https://ccplanet.cancer.gov/>. Cancer Control P.L.A.N.E.T. acts as a portal to provide access to data and resources for designing, implementing, and evaluating evidence-based cancer control programs. The site provides five steps (with links) for developing a comprehensive cancer control plan or program.

Center for Prevention—Altarum Institute (CFP) <http://altarum.org/research-centers/center-for-prevention>. Working to emphasize disease prevention and health promotion in national policy and practice, the CFP is one of the research centers of the Altarum Institute. The site includes action guides that translate several of the *Community Guide* recommendations into easy-to-follow implementation guidelines on priority health topics such as sexual health, tobacco control, aspirin, and chlamydia.

Centers for Disease Control and Prevention (CDC) Community Health Resources <http://www.cdc.gov/nccdphp/dch/online-resource/index.htm>. This searchable site provides access to the CDC's best resources for planning, implementing, and evaluating community health interventions and programs to address chronic disease and health disparities issues. The site links to hundreds of useful planning guides, evaluation frameworks, communication materials, behavioral and risk factor data, fact sheets, scientific articles, key reports, and state and local program contacts.

Guide to Community Preventive Services (the *Community Guide*) <http://www.the-communityguide.org/index.html>. The *Guide* provides guidance in choosing evidence-based programs and policies to improve health and prevent disease at the community level. The Task Force on Community Preventive Services, an independent, nonfederal, volunteer body of public health and prevention experts appointed by the director of the Centers for Disease Control and Prevention, has systematically reviewed more than 200 interventions to produce the recommendations and findings available at this site. The topics covered in the *Guide* currently include adolescent health, alcohol-excessive consumption, asthma, birth defects, cancer, cardiovascular disease, diabetes, emergency preparedness, health communication, health equity, HIV/AIDS, sexually transmitted infections and pregnancy, mental health, motor vehicle injury, nutrition, obesity, oral health, physical activity, social environment, tobacco, vaccination, violence, and worksite.

Health Evidence <http://www.healthevidence.org/>. Health Evidence allows visitors to search and access systematic reviews evaluating the effectiveness of public health interventions. The portal provides support in interpreting evidence and applying it to program and policy decision making.

Intervention Mapping www.interventionmapping.com. The Intervention Mapping protocol describes the iterative path from problem identification to problem solving or mitigation. Each of the six steps comprises several tasks, each of which integrates theory and evidence. The completion of the tasks in a step creates a product that is the guide for the subsequent step. The completion of all the steps serves as a blueprint for designing, implementing, and evaluating an intervention based on a foundation of theoretical, empirical, and practical information.

Johns Hopkins Center for Global Health <http://www.hopkinsglobalhealth.org/>. The Johns Hopkins Center for Global Health site maintains an extensive list of links to global health organizations and resources. This site includes health-related statistics by country, including background information on the country and basic health statistics.

National Registry of Evidence-based Programs and Practices (NREPP) <http://www.nrepp.samhsa.gov/>. Developed by the Substance Abuse and Mental Health Services Administration, NREPP is a searchable database of interventions for the prevention and treatment of mental and substance use disorders. The interventions have been reviewed and rated by independent reviewers.

Public Health Agency of Canada: Canadian Best Practices Portal http://cbpp-pcpe.phac-aspc.gc.ca/. This portal provides a consolidated one-stop shop for busy health professionals and public health decision makers. It is a compilation of multiple sources of trusted and credible information. The portal links to resources and solutions to plan programs for promoting health and preventing diseases for populations and communities.

US Preventive Services Task Force (USPSTF) <http://www.ahrq.gov/professionals/clinicians-providers/guidelines-recommendations/index.html>. The USPSTF conducts standardized reviews of scientific evidence for the effectiveness of a broad range of clinical preventive services, including screening, counseling, and preventive medications. Its recommendations are considered the gold standard for clinical preventive services in the United States. Available at this site are USPSTF clinical recommendations by topic and a pocket *Guide to Clinical Preventive Services* (2014).

University of California Los Angeles Health Impact Assessment Clearinghouse Learning and Information Center <http://www.hiaguide.org>. This site contains summaries of health impact assessments (HIAs) conducted in the United States, HIA-related news, and information about HIA methods and tools. An online training manual is provided.

Using What Works: Adapting Evidence-Based Programs to Fit Your Needs <http://cancercontrol.cancer.gov/use_what_works/start.htm>. The National Cancer Institute (NCI) provides modules on evidence-based Programs, including information on finding evidence-based programs as well as having them fit your needs.

What Works for Health http://www.countyhealthrankings.org/roadmaps/what-works-for-health. This site includes systematic reviews, individual peer-reviewed studies, private organizations, and gray literature to find evidence. It is useful for finding intervention evidence for topic areas that have not undergone extensive systematic review. For each included topic area, there are implementation examples and resources that communities can use to move forward with their chosen strategies.

World Health Organization (WHO) Health Impact Assessments <http://www.who.int/hia/en/>. The WHO provides health impact assessment (HIA) guides and examples from several countries. Many links are provided to assist in understanding and conducting HIAs.

REFERENCES

1. National Center for Health Statistics. *Health, United States, 2000 With Adolescent Health Chartbook*. Hyattsville, MD: Centers for Disease Control and Prevention, National Center for Health Statistics; 2000.
2. Muir Gray JA. *Evidence-Based Healthcare: How to Make Decisions About Health Services and Public Health*. 3rd ed. New York and Edinburgh: Churchill Livingstone Elsevier; 2009.
3. Brownson RC, Fielding JE, Maylahn CM. Evidence-based public health: a fundamental concept for public health practice. *Annu Rev Public Health*. Apr 21 2009;30:175–201.
4. Brownson RC, Baker EA, Leet TL, Gillespie KN, True WR. *Evidence-Based Public Health*. 2nd ed. New York, NY: Oxford University Press; 2011.
5. Glasziou P, Longbottom H. Evidence-based public health practice. *Aust N Z J Public Health*. 1999;23(4):436–440.
6. McMichael C, Waters E, Volmink J. Evidence-based public health: what does it offer developing countries? *J Public Health (Oxf)*. Jun 2005;27(2):215–221.
7. Kohatsu ND, Melton RJ. A health department perspective on the Guide to Community Preventive Services. *Am J Prev Med*. Jan 2000;18(1 Suppl):3–4.
8. Fielding JE. Where is the evidence? *Annu Rev Public Health*. 2001;22:v–vi.
9. Committee on Public Health Strategies to Improve Health. *For the Public's Health: Investing in a Healthier Future*. Washington, DC: Institute of Medicine of The National Academies; 2012.
10. Institute of Medicine. Committee for the Study of the Future of Public Health. *The Future of Public Health*. Washington, DC: National Academy Press; 1988.
11. Dobbins M, Cockerill R, Barnsley J, Ciliska D. Factors of the innovation, organization, environment, and individual that predict the influence five systematic reviews had on public health decisions. *Int J Technol Assess Health Care*. Fall 2001;17(4):467–478.
12. Dodson EA, Baker EA, Brownson RC. Use of evidence-based interventions in state health departments: a qualitative assessment of barriers and solutions. *J Public Health Manag Pract*. Nov-Dec 2010;16(6):E9–E15.
13. Jacob RR, Baker EA, Allen P, et al. Training needs and supports for evidence-based decision making among the public health workforce in the United States. *BMC Health Serv Res*. Nov 14 2014;14(1):564.
14. Frieden TR. Six components necessary for effective public health program implementation. *Am J Public Health*. Jan 2013;104(1):17–22.
15. Oliver K, Innvar S, Lorenc T, Woodman J, Thomas J. A systematic review of barriers to and facilitators of the use of evidence by policymakers. *BMC Health Serv Res*. 2014;14:2.

16. Murphy K, Wolfus B, Lofters A. From complex problems to complex problem-solving: Transdisciplinary practice as knowledge translation. In: Kirst M, Schaefer-McDaniel N, Hwang S, O'Campo P, eds. *Converging Disciplines: A Trans disciplinary Research Approach to Urban Health Problems*. New York, NY: Springer; 2011:111–129.

17. Roussos ST, Fawcett SB. A review of collaborative partnerships as a strategy for improving community health. *Annu Rev Public Health*. 2000;21:369–402.

18. Harper GW, Neubauer LC, Bangi AK, Francisco VT. Transdisciplinary research and evaluation for community health initiatives. *Health Promot Pract*. Oct 2008;9(4):328–337.

19. Stokols D. Toward a science of transdisciplinary action research. *Am J Community Psychol*. Sep 2006;38(1–2):63–77.

20. Kobus K, Mermelstein R. Bridging basic and clinical science with policy studies: The Partners with Transdisciplinary Tobacco Use Research Centers experience. *Nicotine Tob Res*. May 2009;11(5):467–474.

21. Morgan GD, Kobus K, Gerlach KK, et al. Facilitating transdisciplinary research: the experience of the transdisciplinary tobacco use research centers. *Nicotine Tob Res*. Dec 2003;5(Suppl 1):S11–S19.

22. Committee on Accelerating Progress in Obesity Prevention. *Accelerating Progress in Obesity Prevention: Solving the Weight of the Nation*. Washington, DC: Institute of Medicine of The National Academies; 2012.

23. Task Force on Community Preventive Services. Guide to Community Preventive Services. www.thecommunityguide.org. Accessed June 5, 2016.

24. Agency for Healthcare Research and Quality. Guide to Clinical Preventive Services, 2014. http://www.ahrq.gov/professionals/clinicians-providers/guidelines-recommendations/guide/index.html. Accessed October 12, 2016.

25. Cancer Control PLANET. Cancer Control PLANET. Links resources to comprehensive cancer control. http://cancercontrolplanet.cancer.gov/index.html Accessed July 28, 2016.

26. The Cochrane Collaboration. The Cochrane Public Health Group. http://ph.cochrane.org/. Accessed July 28, 2016.

27. SAMHSA. SAMHSA's National Registry of Evidence-based Programs and Practices. http://www.nrepp.samhsa.gov/. Accessed July 28, 2016.

28. Kohatsu ND, Robinson JG, Torner JC. Evidence-based public health: an evolving concept. *Am J Prev Med*. Dec 2004;27(5):417–421.

29. Green LW. Public health asks of systems science: to advance our evidence-based practice, can you help us get more practice-based evidence? *Am J Public Health*. Mar 2006;96(3):406–409.

30. Brownson RC, Allen P, Duggan K, Stamatakis KA, Erwin PC. Fostering more-effective public health by identifying administrative evidence-based practices: a review of the literature. *Am J Prev Med*. Sep 2012;43(3):309–319.

31. Rychetnik L, Bauman A, Laws R, et al. Translating research for evidence-based public health: key concepts and future directions. *J Epidemiol Community Health*. Dec 2012;66(12):1187–1192.

32. Jenicek M. Epidemiology, evidence-based medicine, and evidence-based public health. *J Epidemiol Commun Health*. 1997;7:187–197.

33. Brownson RC, Gurney JG, Land G. Evidence-based decision making in public health. *J Public Health Manag Pract*. 1999;5:86–97.

34. Rychetnik L, Hawe P, Waters E, Barratt A, Frommer M. A glossary for evidence based public health. *J Epidemiol Community Health*. Jul 2004;58(7):538–545.

35. Satterfield JM, Spring B, Brownson RC, et al. Toward a transdisciplinary model of evidence-based practice. *Milbank Q.* Jun 2009;87(2):368–390.
36. Armstrong R, Pettman TL, Waters E. Shifting sands—from descriptions to solutions. *Public Health.* Jun 2014;128(6):525–532.
37. Yost J, Dobbins M, Traynor R, DeCorby K, Workentine S, Greco L. Tools to support evidence-informed public health decision making. *BMC Public Health.* Jul 18 2014;14:728.
38. Viehbeck SM, Petticrew M, Cummins S. Old myths, new myths: challenging myths in public health. *Am J Public Health.* Apr 2015;105(4):665–669.
39. Stevenson A, Lindberg C, eds. *The New Oxford American Dictionary.* 3rd ed. New York, NY: Oxford University Press; 2010.
40. McQueen DV. Strengthening the evidence base for health promotion. *Health Promot Int.* Sep 2001;16(3):261–268.
41. Chambers D, Kerner J. Closing the gap between discovery and delivery. *Dissemination and Implementation Research Workshop: Harnessing Science to Maximize Health.* Rockville, MD; 2007.
42. Rimer BK, Glanz DK, Rasband G. Searching for evidence about health education and health behavior interventions. *Health Educ Behav.* 2001;28(2):231–248.
43. Kerner JF. Integrating research, practice, and policy: what we see depends on where we stand. *J Public Health Manag Pract.* Mar-Apr 2008;14(2):193–198.
44. Mulrow CD, Lohr KN. Proof and policy from medical research evidence. *J Health Polit Policy Law.* Apr 2001;26(2):249–266.
45. Sturm R. Evidence-based health policy versus evidence-based medicine. *Psychiatr Serv.* Dec 2002;53(12):1499.
46. Brownson RC, Royer C, Ewing R, McBride TD. Researchers and policymakers: travelers in parallel universes. *Am J Prev Med.* Feb 2006;30(2):164–172.
47. Li V, Carter SM, Rychetnik L. Evidence valued and used by health promotion practitioners. *Health Educ Res.* Apr 2015;30(2):193–205.
48. Milat AJ, Bauman AE, Redman S, Curac N. Public health research outputs from efficacy to dissemination: a bibliometric analysis. *BMC Public Health.* 2011;11:934.
49. Melbourne School of Population and Global Health. Public Health Insight. http://mspgh.unimelb.edu.au/centres institutes/centre for health-equity/research-group/public-health-insight. Accessed November 24, 2016.
50. Green LW, Glasgow RE. Evaluating the relevance, generalization, and applicability of research: issues in external validation and translation methodology. *Eval Health Prof.* Mar 2006;29(1):126–153.
51. Green LW, Ottoson JM, Garcia C, Hiatt RA. Diffusion theory, and knowledge dissemination, utilization, and integration in public health. *Annu Rev Public Health.* Jan 15 2009;30:151–174.
52. Spencer LM, Schooley MW, Anderson LA, et al. Seeking best practices: a conceptual framework for planning and improving evidence-based practices. *Prev Chronic Dis.* 2013;10:E207.
53. University of Wisconsin Population Health Institute. Using What Works for Health. http://www.countyhealthrankings.org/roadmaps/what-works-for-health/using-what-works-health. Accessed July 28, 2016.
54. Kessler R, Glasgow RE. A proposal to speed translation of healthcare research into practice: dramatic change is needed. *Am J Prev Med.* Jun 2011;40(6):637–644.
55. Nutbeam D. How does evidence influence public health policy? Tackling health inequalities in England. *Health Promot J Aust.* 2003;14:154–158.

56. Ogilvie D, Egan M, Hamilton V, Petticrew M. Systematic reviews of health effects of social interventions: 2. Best available evidence: how low should you go? *J Epidemiol Community Health*. Oct 2005;59(10):886–892.

57. Castro FG, Barrera M, Jr., Martinez CR, Jr. The cultural adaptation of prevention interventions: resolving tensions between fidelity and fit. *Prev Sci*. Mar 2004;5(1):41–45.

58. Kerry R, Eriksen TE, Noer Lie SA, Mumford S, Anjum RL. Causation in evidence-based medicine: in reply to Strand and Parkkinen. *J Eval Clin Pract*. Dec 2014;20(6):985–987.

59. Lorenc T, Tyner EF, Petticrew M, et al. Cultures of evidence across policy sectors: systematic review of qualitative evidence. *Eur J Public Health*. Dec 2014;24(6):1041–1047.

60. Ng E, de Colombani P. Framework for Selecting Best Practices in Public Health: A Systematic Literature Review. *J Public Health Res*. Nov 17 2016;4(3):577.

61. Dobrow MJ, Goel V, Upshur RE. Evidence-based health policy: context and utilisation. *Soc Sci Med*. Jan 2004;58(1):207–217.

62. Marmot M, Allen JJ. Social determinants of health equity. *Am J Public Health*. Sep 2014;104(Suppl 4):S517–S519.

63. Maslov A. A theory of human motivation. *Psychological Review*. 1943;50:370–396.

64. Gibbert WS, Keating SM, Jacobs JA, et al. Training the Workforce in Evidence-Based Public Health: An Evaluation of Impact Among US and International Practitioners. *Prev Chronic Dis*. 2013;10:E148.

65. Lovelace KA, Aronson RE, Rulison KL, Labban JD, Shah GH, Smith M. Laying the groundwork for evidence-based public health: why some local health departments use more evidence-based decision-making practices than others. *Am J Public Health*. Apr 2015;105(Suppl 2):S189–S197.

66. Daar AS, Singer PA, Persad DL, et al. Grand challenges in chronic non-communicable diseases. *Nature*. Nov 22 2007;450(7169):494–496.

67. Braveman PA, Kumanyika S, Fielding J, et al. Health disparities and health equity: the issue is justice. *Am J Public Health*. Dec 2011;101(Suppl 1):S149–S155.

68. Shah SN, Russo ET, Earl TR, Kuo T. Measuring and monitoring progress toward health equity: local challenges for public health. *Prev Chronic Dis*. 2014;11:E159.

69. Pawson R, Greenhalgh T, Harvey G, Walshe K. Realist review: a new method of systematic review designed for complex policy interventions. *J Health Serv Res Policy*. Jul 2005;10(Suppl 1):21–34.

70. Millward L, Kelly M, Nutbeam D. *Public Health Interventions Research: The Evidence*. London: Health Development Agency; 2003.

71. Petticrew M, Roberts H. Systematic reviews: do they "work" in informing decision-making around health inequalities? *Health Econ Policy Law*. Apr 2008;3(Pt 2):197–211.

72. Petticrew M, Cummins S, Ferrell C, et al. Natural experiments: an underused tool for public health? *Public Health*. Sep 2005;119(9):751–757.

73. Tones K. Beyond the randomized controlled trial: a case for "judicial review." *Health Educ Res*. Jun 1997;12(2):i–iv.

74. Steckler A, McLeroy KR, Goodman RM, Bird ST, McCormick L. Toward integrating qualitative and quantitative methods: an introduction. *Health Education Quarterly*. 1992;19(1):1–8.

75. Torrone EA, Thomas JC, Maman S, et al. Risk behavior disclosure during HIV test counseling. *AIDS Patient Care STDS*. Sep 2010;24(9):551–561.

76. Sapkota D, Adhikari SR, Bajracharya T, Sapkota VP. Designing Evidence-Based Family Planning Programs for the Marginalized Community: An Example of Muslim Community in Nepal. *Front Public Health.* 2016;4:122.

77. Griffin TL, Pallan MJ, Clarke JL, et al. Process evaluation design in a cluster randomised controlled childhood obesity prevention trial: the WAVES study. *Int J Behav Nutr Phys Act.* 2014;11:112.

78. Owen L, Youdan B. 22 years on: the impact and relevance of the UK No Smoking Day. *Tob Control.* Feb 2006;15(1):19–25.

79. Brownson RC, Brennan LK, Evenson KR, Leviton LC. Lessons from a mixed-methods approach to evaluating Active Living by Design. *Am J Prev Med.* Nov 2012;43(5 Suppl 4):S271–S280.

80. McQueen DV. The evidence debate. *J Epidemiol Community Health.* Feb 2002;56(2):83–84.

81. Suppe F. *The Structure of Scientific Theories.* 2nd ed. Urbana, IL: University of Illinois Press; 1977.

82. Cavill N, Foster C, Oja P, Martin BW. An evidence-based approach to physical activity promotion and policy development in Europe: contrasting case studies. *Promot Educ.* 2006;13(2):104–111.

83. Shi J, Jiang C, Tan D, et al. Advancing Implementation of Evidence-Based Public Health in China: An Assessment of the Current Situation and Suggestions for Developing Regions. *Biomed Res Int.* 2016;2016:2694030.

84. Bender K, Halverson PK. Quality improvement and accreditation: what might it look like? *J Public Health Manag Pract.* Jan-Feb 2010;16(1):79–82.

85. Public Health Accreditation Board. Public Health Accreditation Board Standards and Measures, version 1.5. 2013. http://www.phaboard.org/wp-content/uploads/SM-Version-1.5-Board-adopted-FINAL-01-24-2014.docx.pdf. Accessed November 20, 2016.

86. Fielding JE. Foreword. In: Brownson RC, Baker EA, Leet TL, Gillespie KN, eds. *Evidence-Based Public Health.* New York, NY: Oxford University Press; 2003:v–vii.

87. Presidential Task Force on Evidence-Based Practice. Evidence-based practice in psychology. *Am Psychol.* May-Jun 2006;61(4):271–285.

88. Gambrill E. Evidence-based practice: Sea change or the emperor's new clothes? *J Social Work Educ.* 2003;39(1):3–23.

89. Mullen E, Bellamy J, Bledsoe S, Francois J. Teaching evidence-based practice. *Research on Social Work Practice.* 2007;17(5):574–582.

90. Melnyk BM, Fineout-Overholt E, Stone P, Ackerman M. Evidence-based practice: the past, the present, and recommendations for the millennium. *Pediatr Nurs.* Jan-Feb 2000;26(1):77–80.

91. Evidence-Based Medicine Working Group. Evidence-based medicine. A new approach to teaching the practice of medicine. *JAMA.* 1992;17:2420–2425.

92. Cochrane A. *Effectiveness and Efficiency: Random Reflections on Health Services.* London: Nuffield Provincial Hospital Trust; 1972.

93. Guyatt G, Rennie D, Meade M, Cook D, eds. *Users' Guides to the Medical Literature. A Manual for Evidence-Based Clinical Practice.* 3rd ed. Chicago, IL: American Medical Association Press; 2015.

94. Canadian Task Force on the Periodic Health Examination. The periodic health examination. Canadian Task Force on the Periodic Health Examination. *Can Med Assoc J.* Nov 3 1979;121(9):1193–1254.

95. Tilson H, Gebbie KM. The public health workforce. *Annu Rev Public Health.* 2004;25:341–356.

96. National Board of Public Health Examiners. Certified in Public Health. http://www.nbphe.org/examinfo.cfm. Accessed November 24, 2014.

97. Thacker SB. Public health surveillance and the prevention of injuries in sports: what gets measured gets done. *J Athl Train.* Apr-Jun 2007;42(2):171–172.

98. Fielding J, Teutsch S, Breslow L. A framework for public health in the United States. *Public Health Reviews.* 2010;32:174–189.

99. Institute of Medicine. *Who Will Keep the Public Healthy? Educating Public Health Professionals for the 21st Century.* Washington, DC: National Academies Press; 2003.

100. Homer JB, Hirsch GB. System dynamics modeling for public health: background and opportunities. *Am J Public Health.* Mar 2006;96(3):452–458.

101. Stokols D. Translating social ecological theory into guidelines for community health promotion. *American Journal of Health Promotion.* 1996;10(4):282–298.

102. Glanz K, Bishop DB. The role of behavioral science theory in development and implementation of public health interventions. *Annu Rev Public Health.* Apr 21 2010;31:399–418.

103. Cargo M, Mercer SL. The value and challenges of participatory research: Strengthening its practice. *Annu Rev Public Health.* Apr 21 2008;29:325–350.

104. Israel BA, Schulz AJ, Parker EA, Becker AB. Review of community-based research: assessing partnership approaches to improve public health. *Annual Review of Public Health.* 1998;19:173–202.

105. Leung MW, Yen IH, Minkler M. Community based participatory research: a promising approach for increasing epidemiology's relevance in the 21st century. *Int J Epidemiol.* Jun 2004;33(3):499–506.

106. Centers for Disease Control and Prevention. *A Practitioner's Guide for Advancing Health Equity: Community Strategies for Preventing Chronic Disease.* Atlanta, GA: CDC; 2013.

107. Slater MD, Kelly KJ, Thackeray R. Segmentation on a shoestring: health audience segmentation in limited-budget and local social marketing interventions. *Health Promot Pract.* Apr 2006;7(2):170–173.

108. Brownson R. Research Translation and Public Health Services & Systems Research. *Keeneland Conference: Public Health Services & Systems Research.* Lexington, KY; 2013.

109. Thacker SB, Berkelman RL. Public health surveillance in the United States. *Epidemiol Rev.* 1988;10:164–190.

110. Thacker SB, Stroup DF. Public health surveillance. In: Brownson RC, Petitti DB, eds. *Applied Epidemiology: Theory to Practice.* 2nd ed. New York, NY: Oxford University Press; 2006:30–67.

111. Oxman AD, Guyatt GH. The science of reviewing research. *Ann N Y Acad Sci.* Dec 31 1993;703:125–133; discussion 133–124.

112. Waters E, Doyle J. Evidence-based public health practice: improving the quality and quantity of the evidence. *J Public Health Med.* Sep 2002;24(3):227–229.

113. Gold MR, Siegel JE, Russell LB, Weinstein MC. *Cost-Effectiveness in Health and Medicine.* New York, NY: Oxford University Press; 1996.

114. Carande-Kulis VG, Maciosek MV, Briss PA, et al. Methods for systematic reviews of economic evaluations for the Guide to Community Preventive Services. Task Force on Community Preventive Services. *Am J Prev Med.* Jan 2000;18(1 Suppl):75–91.

115. Harris P, Harris-Roxas B, Harris E, Kemp L. *Health Impact Assessment: A Practical Guide.* Sydney: Australia: Centre for Health Equity Training, Research and

Evaluation (CHETRE). Part of the UNSW Research Centre for Primary Health Care and Equity, UNSW; August 2007.

116. Cole BL, Wilhelm M, Long PV, Fielding JE, Kominski G, Morgenstern H. Prospects for health impact assessment in the United States: new and improved environmental impact assessment or something different? *J Health Polit Policy Law*. Dec 2004;29(6):1153–1186.

117. Kemm J. Health impact assessment: a tool for healthy public policy. *Health Promot Int*. Mar 2001;16(1):79–85.

118. Mindell J, Sheridan L, Joffe M, Samson-Barry H, Atkinson S. Health impact assessment as an agent of policy change: improving the health impacts of the mayor of London's draft transport strategy. *J Epidemiol Community Health*. Mar 2004;58(3):169–174.

119. De Leeuw E, Peters D. Nine questions to guide development and implementation of Health in All Policies. *Health Promot Int*. Dec 2014;30(4):987–997.

120. Green LW, George MA, Daniel M, et al. *Review and Recommendations for the Development of Participatory Research in Health Promotion in Canada*. Vancouver, British Columbia: The Royal Society of Canada; 1995.

121. Green LW, Mercer SL. Can public health researchers and agencies reconcile the push from funding bodies and the pull from communities? *Am J Public Health*. Dec 2001;91(12):1926–1929.

122. Hallfors D, Cho H, Livert D, Kadushin C. Fighting back against substance abuse: are community coalitions winning? *Am J Prev Med*. Nov 2002;23(4):237–245.

CHAPTER 2

༭ᔑᕮ

Building Capacity for Evidence-Based Public Health

Evidence without capacity is an empty shell.
Mohan Singh

Putting evidence to use in public health settings requires sufficient capacity (i.e., the availability of resources, structures, and workforce to deliver the "preventive dose" of an evidence-based practice or policy).[1,2] *Capacity building* refers to intentional, coordinated, and mission-driven efforts aimed at strengthening the management and governance of public health agencies to improve their performance and impact.[3] Capacity is a determinant of performance; that is, greater capacity is linked with greater public health impact.[4-6] For success in capacity building, public health agencies need to bridge diverse disciplines, build the evidence base across settings, link with the community, and enhance skills in public health sciences among practitioners.[7]

Capacity is needed among both individuals and organizations, which have a reciprocal relationship (Figure 2.1).[8] Success in achieving evidence-based decision making is achieved by building the skills of individuals (e.g., capacity to carry out a program evaluation) and organizations (e.g., achieving a climate and culture that supports innovation). These two facets are interrelated in that individuals shape organizations and organizations support the development of individuals.

This chapter includes three sections. The first describes some barriers to and opportunities for capacity building and implementation of evidence-based approaches. The next section outlines agency-level determinants of public health performance. The third part is an overview of a framework for evidence-based public health (EBPH) practice.

Individuals shape organizations

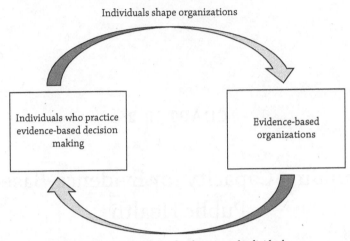

Organizations facilitate the development of individuals

Figure 2.1: The interrelationships between individuals and organizations in supporting evidence-based decision making.[8] This figure was adapted with permission from Figure 0.2 in Muir Gray JA. *Evidence-Based Healthcare: How to Make Decisions About Health Services and Public Health*. 3rd ed. New York and Edinburgh: Churchill Livingstone Elsevier; 2009.

BARRIERS TO BE ADDRESSED THROUGH CAPACITY BUILDING

There are several barriers to EBPH that suggest a variety of capacity-building strategies (Table 2.1).[9-13] Inadequate resources, incentives, vision, time, information, and training in key public health disciplines are chief among these barriers. Possible approaches for overcoming these barriers have been discussed by others.[14,15] For low- and middle-income countries (LMICs), there are particular challenges.[16-18] Among these barriers are (1) the high cost of training programs in Western countries and lack of incentives for LMIC trainees to return home after being educated; (2) the need for more direct field experience; (3) the isolation from ministries of health, local communities, and other scientific disciplines; and (4) the lack of experienced public health practitioners to serve as role models.[19]

The importance of establishing, maintaining, and evaluating training and education for EBPH cannot be overemphasized. Training is not only critical for applying EBPH concepts in a particular content area (e.g., building an effective injury prevention program) but also may serve as an incentive and allow practitioners to make better use of scarce resources.[20,21] Leadership is needed from public health practitioners and policy makers on education about the need for and importance of evidence-based decision making. Such leadership development is evident in training programs, such as the regional leadership network for public health practitioners[22] and the ongoing efforts to develop and

Table 2.1. POTENTIAL EBPH BARRIERS AND SOLUTIONS
FOR BUILDING CAPACITY

Barrier	Potential Solution
Lack of resources	Commitment to increase funding for prevention and reprioritizing existing resources
Lack of leadership and instability in setting a clear and focused agenda for evidence-based approaches	Commitment from all levels of public health leadership to increase the understanding of the value of evidence-based public health (EBPH) approaches
Lack of incentives for using evidence-based approaches	Identification of new ways of shaping organizational culture to support EBPH
Lack of a view of the "long-term horizon" for program implementation and evaluation	Adoption and adherence to causal frameworks and formative evaluation plans
External (including political) pressures drive the process away from an evidence-based approach	Systematic communication and dissemination strategies
Inadequate training in key public health disciplines	Wider dissemination of new and established training programs, including use of distance learning technologies
Lack of time to gather information, analyze data, and review the literature for evidence	Enhanced skills for efficient analysis and review of the literature, computer searching abilities, use of systematic reviews
Lack of evidence on the effectiveness of certain public health interventions for special populations	Increased funding for applied public health research; better dissemination of findings
Lack of information on implementation of interventions	A greater emphasis on building the evidence base for external validity

disseminate evidence-based guidelines for interventions.[23] Finally, establishing or strengthening partnerships across disciplines and agencies will present new opportunities for both shared responsibility and accountability for the public's health, which can be an impetus to increased use and understanding of EBPH.[24] Many of these issues are covered in later chapters.

WHAT TO MEASURE AND ATTEND TO
AT THE AGENCY LEVEL

Capacity building for EBPH is essential at all levels of public health, from national standards to agency-level practices. As noted in chapter 1, the priority of EBPH principles is highlighted in domain 10 of the Public Health Accreditation Board Standards that seeks to "contribute to and apply the evidence base of public health."[25] This standard highlights the importance of using the best available evidence and also the role of health departments in adding to the body of evidence for promising approaches. Accreditation of health departments calls for agencies to meet a set of capacity-related standards and measures that in turn link to enhanced performance in delivering public health services.

At the agency level, a set of administrative and management evidence-based practices have been identified.[4] The underlying premise for administrative evidence-based practices (A-EBPs) is that a high-performing health department requires a combination of applying evidence-based interventions from scientific sources (e.g., the *Community Guide*,[23] the Cochrane Collaboration[26]) and competence in carrying out effective organizational practices in health departments or other agencies. A-EBPs are agency (health department)—and work unit—level structures and activities that are positively associated with performance measures (e.g., achieving core public health functions, carrying out evidence-based interventions).[4] These A-EBPs often fit under the umbrella of public health services and systems research[27,28] and cover five major domains of workforce development: leadership, organizational climate and culture, relationships and partnerships, and financial processes. These practices were delineated in a literature review[4] and are potentially modifiable within a few years, making them useful targets for quality improvement efforts.[29-31] Recent efforts have measured these A-EBPs in research studies,[32,33] developed a tool for practitioners to assess performance,[34] and linked A-EBPs with science-based decision making in state health departments.[35]

INCREASING CAPACITY FOR EVIDENCE-BASED DECISION MAKING

Efforts to strengthen EBPH competencies must consider the diverse education and training backgrounds of the workforce. The emphasis on principles of EBPH is not uniformly taught in all the disciplines represented in the public health workforce. For example, a public health nurse is likely to have had less training than an epidemiologist in how to locate the most current evidence and interpret alternatives. A recently graduated health educator with a Master of Public Health degree is more likely to have gained an understanding of the importance of EBPH than an environmental health specialist holding a bachelor's degree. Currently, it appears that few public health departments have made continuing education about EBPH mandatory.

Although the formal concepts of EBPH are relatively new, the underlying skills are not.[9] For example, reviewing the scientific literature for evidence and evaluating a program intervention are skills often taught in graduate programs in public health or other academic disciplines and are building blocks of public health practice. To support building many of these skills, competencies for more effective public health practice are becoming clearer.[36-38] For example, to carry out the EBPH process, the skills needed to make evidence-based decisions related to programs and policies require a specific set of competencies (Table 2.2).[9,39,40] Many of the competencies on this list illustrate the value of developing partnerships and engaging diverse disciplines in the EBPH process.[41]

To address these and similar competencies, programs have been developed to train university students (at both undergraduate and graduate levels),[42-45] public health professionals,[46-49] and staff of community-based organizations.[50,51] Training programs have been developed across multiple continents and countries.[45,52-55] Some programs show evidence of effectiveness.[47,51] The most common format uses didactic sessions, computer labs, and scenario-based exercises, taught by a faculty team with expertise in EBPH. The reach of these training programs can be increased by employing a train-the-trainer approach.[49] Other formats have been used, including Internet-based self-study,[50,56] CD-ROMs,[57] distance and distributed learning networks, and targeted technical assistance. Training programs may have greater impact when delivered by "change agents" who are perceived as experts, yet share common characteristics and goals with trainees.[58] For example, in data from four states, a train-the-trainer approach was effective in building skills and has some advantages (e.g., contouring to local needs, local ownership).[49] A commitment from leadership and staff to lifelong learning is also an essential ingredient for success in training[59] and is itself an example of evidence-based decision making.[4]

Implementation of training to address EBPH competencies should employ principles of adult learning. These issues were articulated by Bryan and colleagues,[60] who highlighted the need to (1) know why the audience is learning; (2) tap into an underlying motivation to learn by the need to solve problems; (3) respect and build on previous experience; (4) design learning approaches that match the background and diversity of recipients; and (5) actively involve the audience in the learning process.

In this section, a multistage, sequential framework to promote greater use of evidence in day-to-day decision making is briefly described (Figure 2.2).[9,52,61] Each part of the framework is described in detail in later chapters. It is important to note that this process is seldom a strictly prescriptive or linear one, but instead includes numerous feedback loops and processes that are common in many program planning models. This multistage framework

Table 2.2. COMPETENCIES IN EVIDENCE-BASED PUBLIC HEALTH

Title	Domain	Level	Sample competency
1. Community input	C	B	Understand the importance of obtaining community input before planning and implementing evidence-based interventions.
2. Etiologic knowledge	E	B	Understand the relationship between risk factors and diseases.
3. Community assessment	C	B	Understand how to define the health issue according to the needs and assets of the population/community of interest.
4. Partnerships at multilevels	P/C	B	Understand the importance of identifying and developing partnerships in order to address the issue with evidence-based strategies at multiple levels.
5. Developing a concise statement of the issue	EBP	B	Understand the importance of developing a concise statement of the issue in order to build support for it.
6. Grant-writing need	T/T	B	Recognize the importance of grant writing skills including the steps involved in the application process.
7. Literature searching	EBP	B	Understand the process for searching the scientific literature and summarizing search-derived information on the health issue.
8. Literature searching	P	B	Identify evidence-based policy solutions based on quantitative and qualitative data.
9. Leadership and evidence	L	B	Recognize the importance of strong leadership from public health professionals regarding the need and importance of evidence-based public health interventions.
10. Role of behavioral science theory	T/T	B	Understand the role of behavioral science theory in designing, implementing, and evaluating interventions.
11. Leadership at all levels	L	B	Understand the importance of commitment from all levels of public health leadership to increase the use of evidence-based interventions.

Table 2.2. CONTINUED

Title	Domain	Level	Sample competency
12. Evaluation in "plain English"	EV	I	Recognize the importance of translating the impacts of programs or policies in language that can be understood by communities, practice sectors and policy makers.
13. Leadership and change	L	I	Recognize the importance of effective leadership from public health professionals when making decisions in the midst of ever changing environments.
14. Translating evidence-based interventions	EBP	I	Recognize the importance of translating evidence-based interventions to unique "real world" settings.
15. Quantifying the issue	T/T	I	Understand the importance of descriptive epidemiology (concepts of person, place, time) in quantifying the public health issue.
16. Developing an action plan for program or policy	EBP	I	Understand the importance of developing a plan of action which describes how the goals and objectives will be achieved, what resources are required, and how responsibility of achieving objectives will be assigned.
17. Prioritizing health issues	EBP	I	Understand how to choose and implement appropriate criteria and processes for prioritizing program and policy options.
18. Qualitative evaluation	EV	I	Recognize the value of qualitative evaluation approaches including the steps involved in conducting qualitative evaluations.
19. Collaborative partnerships	P/C	I	Understand the importance of collaborative partnerships between researchers and practitioners when designing, implementing, and evaluating evidence-based programs and policies.
20. Nontraditional partnerships	P/C	I	Understand the importance of traditional partnerships as well as those that have been considered non-traditional such as those with planners, department of transportation, and others.

(continued)

Table 2.2. CONTINUED

Title	Domain	Level	Sample competency
21. Systematic reviews	T/T	I	Understand the rationale, uses, and usefulness of systematic reviews that document effective interventions.
22. Quantitative evaluation	EV	I	Recognize the importance of quantitative evaluation approaches including the concepts of measurement validity and reliability.
23. Grant-writing skills	T/T	I	Demonstrate the ability to create a grant including an outline of the steps involved in the application process.
24. Health equity	P/C	A	Demonstrate the ability to address health equity in the development and delivery of public health programs and policies.
25. Role of economic evaluation	T/T	A	Recognize the importance of using economic data and strategies to evaluate costs and outcomes when making public health decisions.
26. Creating policy briefs	P	A	Understand the importance of writing concise policy briefs to address the issue using evidence-based interventions.
27. Evaluation designs	EV	A	Comprehend the various designs useful in program evaluation with a particular focus on quasi-experimental (non-randomized) designs.
28. Communication	P	A	Demonstrate the ability to effectively communicate with a range of policy-related stakeholders using formal (e.g., newsletters) and informal methods (e.g., lunch conversation).
29. Transmitting evidence-based research to policy makers	P	A	Understand the importance of coming up with creative ways of transmitting what we know works (evidence-based interventions) to policy makers in order to gain interest, political support and funding.

A = advanced; B = beginner; C = community-level planning; E = etiology; EBP = evidence-based process; EV = evaluation; I = intermediate; L = leadership; P = policy; P/C = partnerships & collaboration; "T/T = theory & analytic tools.
Adapted from Brownson et al.[9,39] and Luck et al.[40]

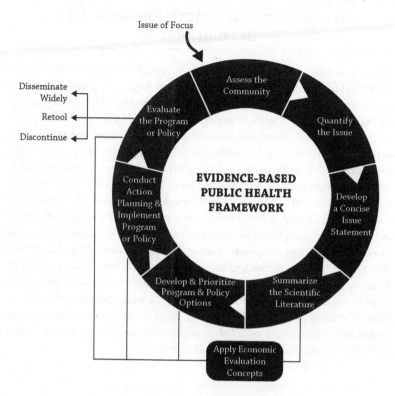

Figure 2.2: Training approach to evidence-based public health.[9,52,61]

can be applied in a number of ways. It can be used as a basis for training future public health practitioners (Box 2.1).[45] The approach can also help in focusing attention and resources on key public health issues such as obesity (Box 2.2).[62,63] And with some modification, the framework can be applied to emerging issues such as climate change.[64]

Assess the Community

Community assessment typically occurs before the development of a program or policy and seeks to understand the public health issues and priorities in a given community by exploring the strengths and challenges faced by community members and the agencies that serve them. Data are sometimes available through surveillance systems and national and local data sets. Other information that is useful at this stage is documentation of the social, economic, and physical environment contextual factors that influence health. Finally, it is essential to identify stakeholders and capture data on community perceptions and preferences. Community assessment data can be collected through

Box 2.1

TRAINING FUTURE PRACTITIONERS IN EBPH IN SAUDI ARABIA

There is a need to increase capacity in evidence-based public health (EBPH) skills in the Eastern Mediterranean Region.[45] There are several important barriers to EBPH in the region, including the lack of systems for incorporating evidence into decision making, lack of relevant publications from the Arab region, and the need for stronger communication between practitioners and researchers. In a graduate program at King Saud University, College of Medicine, Riyadh, students were trained to better integrate the best available evidence in public health decision making. Courses in EBPH were designed based on the sequential framework in Figure 2.2. A postcourse survey was conducted in which 45 students were invited to complete a validated self-administered questionnaire that assessed knowledge, opinions, and attitudes toward EBPH. More than 80% had sound knowledge and could appreciate the importance of EBPH. A strong majority of students (80% to 90%) reported understanding the steps in the EBPH process; however, only 64% were confident about their skills of critical appraisal. The findings from development, delivery, and evaluation of the course establish a solid foundation for capacity building in EBPH in Saudi Arabia and the Arab world.

Box 2.2

APPLYING AN EVIDENCE-BASED PLANNING FRAMEWORK IN COLORADO

The Colorado Department of Public Health and Environment embarked on a systematic planning process to more effectively address obesity, the top prevention priority for the state.[62] Using a well-established framework for evidence-based public health,[63] the team sought to stimulate comprehensive and effective action. A total of 45 department staff members were trained to review the literature on physical activity and nutrition interventions. Using group facilitation and Web-based surveys, the group worked with an extensive set of external stakeholders to prioritize strategies. In the literature review phase, three sources were used: systematic reviews, journal articles, and gray literature. Using a typology to classify each strategy across one of five levels (proven, likely effective, promising, emerging, not recommended), 58 interventions were categorized. To prioritize the strategies, five criteria were invoked: likelihood of population impact, capacity to implement, impact on health disparities, political and community support, and ability to measure. The initial list of 58 strategies was narrowed to a high-priority list of 12 strategies. This groundwork led to a more efficient action planning and evaluation to address one of the leading public health issues. Additional benefits included capacity building among staff, enhanced partnerships, and better alignment of public health priorities.

quantitative (questionnaires) or qualitative (individual or group interviews) methods.

Quantify the Issue

After developing a working description of the public health issue of interest, it is necessary to objectively quantify it to answer the question, "How big is the issue?" An initial approach to quantification is to identify sources of existing data. Such descriptive data may be available from ongoing vital statistics data (birth and death records), surveillance systems, special surveys, or national studies.

Descriptive studies can take several forms. In public health, the most common type of descriptive study involves a survey of a scientifically valid sample (a representative cross section) of the population of interest. These cross-sectional studies are not intended to change health status (as an intervention would), but rather to quantify the prevalence of behaviors, characteristics, exposures, and diseases at some point (or period) of time in a defined population. This information can be valuable for understanding the scope of the public health problem at hand. Descriptive studies commonly provide information on patterns of occurrence according to such attributes as person (e.g., age, gender, ethnicity), place (e.g., county of residence), and time (e.g., seasonal variation in disease patterns). Additionally, under certain circumstances, cross-sectional data can provide information for use in the design of analytic studies (e.g., baseline data to evaluate the effectiveness of a public health intervention).

Develop a Concise Issue Statement

The practitioner should next develop a concise statement of the issue or problem being considered, answering the question, "How important is the issue?" To build support for any issue (with an organization, policy makers, or a funding agency), the issue must be clearly articulated. This problem definition stage has some similarities to the beginning steps in a strategic planning process, which often involve describing the mission, internal strengths and weaknesses, external opportunities and threats, and the vision for the future. It is often helpful to describe gaps between the current status of a program or organization and the desired goals. The key components of an issue statement include the health condition or risk factor being considered, the populations affected, the size and scope of the problem, prevention opportunities, and potential stakeholders.

Summarize the Scientific Literature

After the issue to be considered has been clearly defined, the practitioner needs to become knowledgeable about previous or ongoing efforts to address the issue in order to determine the cause of the problem and *what should be done about it*. This step includes a systematic approach to identify, retrieve, and evaluate relevant reports on scientific studies, panels, and conferences related to the topic of interest. The most common method for initiating this investigation is a formal literature review. There are many databases available to facilitate such a review. Common among them for public health purposes are PubMed, PsycINFO, and Google Scholar (see chapter 8). Some databases can be accessed by the public through institutions (such as the National Library of Medicine [http://www.nlm.nih.gov], universities, and public libraries); others can be subscribed to by an organization or selectively found on the Internet. There also are many organizations that maintain Internet sites that can be useful for identifying relevant information, including many state health departments, the Centers for Disease Control and Prevention (e.g., https://chronicdata.cdc.gov/), and the National Institutes of Health. It is important to remember that not all intervention (Type 2) studies will be found in the published literature.

Develop and Prioritize Program and Policy Options

Based largely on the first three steps, a variety of health program or policy options are examined, answering the question, "What are we going to do about the issue?" The list of options can be developed from a variety of sources. The initial review of the scientific literature may highlight various intervention options. More often, expert panels provide program or policy recommendations on a variety of issues. Summaries of available evidence-base program and policy options are often available in systematic reviews and practice guidelines. There are several assumptions or contexts underlying any development of options. These fall into five main categories: political/regulatory, economic, social values, demographic, and technological.[65]

In particular, it is important to assess and monitor the political process when developing health policy options. To do so, stakeholder input may be useful. The stakeholder for a policy might be the health policy maker. Supportive policy makers can frequently provide advice regarding timing of policy initiatives, methods for framing the issues, strategies for identifying sponsors, and ways to develop support among the general public. In contrast, the stakeholder for a coalition-based community intervention might be a community member. In this case, additional planning data may be garnered from community members through key informant interviews, focus groups, or coalition member surveys.[66]

Develop an Action Plan and Implement the Program or Policy

This aspect of the process again deals largely with strategic planning issues that answer the question, "How are we going to address the issue, when, and what are our expected results?" After an option has been selected, a set of goals and objectives is developed. A goal is a long-term desired change in the status of a priority health need, and an objective is a short-term, measurable, specific activity that leads toward achievement of a goal. The plan of action describes how the goals and objectives will be achieved, what resources are required, and how responsibility for achieving objectives will be assigned.

Evaluate the Program or Policy

In simple terms, evaluation is the determination of the degree to which program or policy goals and objectives are met, answering the question, "How will we know if we have made a difference?" If they follow any research design, most public health programs and policies are evaluated through "quasi-experimental" designs—that is, designs lacking random assignment to intervention and comparison groups. In general, the strongest evaluation designs acknowledge the roles of both quantitative and qualitative evaluation. Furthermore, evaluation designs need to be flexible and sensitive enough to assess intermediate changes, even those that fall short of changes in behavior. Genuine change takes place incrementally over time, in ways that are often not visible to those too close to the intervention.

Apply Economic Evaluation Concepts

Key concepts from economic evaluation can inform numerous steps in an evidence-based decision-making process. It is useful for practitioners to be familiar with common terms and types of economic evaluations. For most practitioners, the goal is not to teach them how to do an economic evaluation, but rather to understand core perspectives of economic evaluation and how to use the concepts to further program and policy development, and to be able to identify and document relevant costs.

The multistage framework of evidence-based public health summarized in this chapter is similar to an eight-step approach first described by Jenicek.[67] Frameworks such as the one shown in Figure 2.2 can be used to mobilize action and identify analytic tools in public health departments (e.g., economic evaluation).[62] An additional logical step focuses on teaching others how to practice EBPH.[67]

SUMMARY

Capacity building (e.g., moving training toward prevention, increasing the skills of professionals) has been noted as a "grand challenge" for public health.[68] Despite the critical importance of capacity building for public health performance, relatively little is known about how best to structure and carry out capacity-building approaches.[69,70] It is important that workforce training on EBPH concepts be available at local, national, and international levels. Future work will require expanding and improving the access of training initiatives as well as building research capacity to guide evidence-based action on the social determinants of health (including health equity). This chapter has focused primarily on capacity building within public health agencies, but similar capacity is needed for public health partners and stakeholders.[71]

KEY CHAPTER POINTS

- To build capacity for EBPH in practice settings (e.g., health departments), several important contextual factors should be considered: organizational culture, the role of leadership, political challenges, funding challenges, and workforce training needs.
- A set of administrative and management evidence-based practices have been identified; these A-EBPs can predict performance and can be measured reliably.
- A multistage, sequential framework can be useful in promoting greater use of evidence in day-to-day decision making in public health practice.
- Future work will require expanding and improving the access of training initiatives as well as building research capacity to guide evidence-based action on the social determinants of health (including health equity).

SUGGESTED READINGS AND SELECTED WEBSITES

Suggested Readings

Brownson RC, Allen P, Duggan K, Stamatakis KA, Erwin PC. Fostering more-effective public health by identifying administrative evidence-based practices: a review of the literature. *Am J Prev Med.* Sep 2012;43(3):309–319.

Gibbert WS, Keating SM, Jacobs JA, Dodson E, Baker E, Diem G, Giles W, Gillespie KN, Grabauskas V, Shatchkute A, Brownson RC. Training the workforce in evidence-based public health: an evaluation of impact among US and international practitioners. *Prev Chronic Dis.* 2013;10:E148.

Jacob RR, Baker EA, Allen P, Dodson EA, Duggan K, Fields R, Sequeira S, Brownson RC. Training needs and supports for evidence-based decision making among the public health workforce in the United States. *BMC Health Serv Res.* 2014;14:564.

Leeman J, Calancie L, Hartman MA, et al. What strategies are used to build practitioners' capacity to implement community-based interventions and are they effective? A systematic review. *Implement Sci*. May 29 2015;10:80.

Meyer AM, Davis M, Mays GP. Defining organizational capacity for public health services and systems research. *J Public Health Manag Pract*. Nov 2012;18(6):535–544.

Pettman TL, Armstrong R, Jones K, Waters E, Doyle J. Cochrane update: building capacity in evidence-informed decision-making to improve public health. *J Public Health (Oxf)*. Dec 2013;35(4):624–627.

Yarber L, Brownson CA, Jacob RR, Baker EA, Jones E, Baumann C, Deshpande AD, Gillespie KN, Scharff DP, Brownson RC. Evaluating a train-the-trainer approach for improving capacity for evidence-based decision making in public health. *BMC Health Serv Res*. 2015;15:547.

Yost J, Ciliska D, Dobbins M. Evaluating the impact of an intensive education workshop on evidence-informed decision making knowledge, skills, and behaviours: a mixed methods study. *BMC Med Educ*. 2014;14:13.

Selected Websites

Centers for Disease Control and Prevention (CDC) Community Health Resources <http://www.cdc.gov/nccdphp/dch/online-resource/index.htm>. This searchable site provides access to CDC's best resources for planning, implementing, and evaluating community health interventions and programs to address chronic disease and health disparities issues. The site links to hundreds of useful planning guides, evaluation frameworks, communication materials, behavioral and risk factor data, fact sheets, scientific articles, key reports, and state and local program contacts.

Evidence-based behavioral practice (EBB)) <http://www.ebbp.org/>. The EBBP.org project creates training resources to bridge the gap between behavioral health research and practice. An interactive website offers modules covering topics such as the EBBP process, systematic reviews, searching for evidence, critical appraisal, and randomized controlled trials. This site is ideal for practitioners, researchers, and educators.

Evidence-Based Public Health (Association of State and Territorial Health Officials [ASTHO])<http://www.astho.org/programs/evidence-based-public-health/>.For more than 10 years, ASTHO has collaborated with the Centers for Disease Control and Prevention to promote evidence-based public health, particularly through adoption of the Task Force recommendations in the *Guide to Community Preventive Services*. The site includes state success stories and a set of tools for using the Community Guide and other related resources.

Evidence-Based Public Health (Washington University in St. Louis) < http://www.evidencebasedpublichealth.org/> The purpose of this site is to provide public health professionals and decision makers with resources and tools to make evidence-based public health practice accessible and realistic. The portal includes a primer on EBPH, resources, and a training program for practitioners.

PH Partners: From Evidence-Based Medicine to Evidence-Based Public Health <https://phpartners.org/tutorial/04-ebph/2-keyConcepts/4.2.1.html>. The PH Partners portal is designed to support the public health workforce on issues related to information access and management. The site seeks to allow users to find reliable and authoritative consumer-oriented materials to support health education; retrieve statistical information and access data sets relevant to public health; and retrieve and evaluate information in support of evidence-based practice.

Public Health Services and Systems Research and the Public Health Practice-Based Research Networks: Administrative Evidence-Based Practices Assessment Tool. http://tools.publichealthsystems.org/tools/tool?view=about&id=134. This tool helps managers and practitioners at local and state public health departments assess the extent to which their departments utilize administrative evidence-based practices (A-EBPs), leading to improved efficiency and public health outcomes and building competency for accreditation. This tool provides an assessment of the extent to which a health department currently supports the adoption of A-EBPs across five key domains: workforce development, leadership, organizational climate and culture, relationships and partnerships, and financial processes. The tool also allows comparison to a national, stratified sample of local health departments.

REFERENCES

1. Hanusaik N, Sabiston CM, Kishchuk N, Maximova K, O'Loughlin J. Association between organizational capacity and involvement in chronic disease prevention programming among Canadian public health organizations. *Health Educ Res*. Apr 2014;30(2):206–222.
2. World Health Organization Regional Office for Europe. Report on the 23rd Annual Meeting of Countrywide Integrated Noncommunicable Diseases Intervention (CINDI) Programme Directors. Paper presented at: CINDI Meeting; October 16-17, 2006, 2009; Banff, Canada.
3. Create the Future. Capacity Building Overview. http://www.createthefuture.com/capacity_building.htm. Accessed November 20, 2016.
4. Brownson RC, Allen P, Duggan K, Stamatakis KA, Erwin PC. Fostering more-effective public health by identifying administrative evidence-based practices: a review of the literature. *Am J Prev Med*. Sep 2012;43(3):309–319.
5. Meyer AM, Davis M, Mays GP. Defining organizational capacity for public health services and systems research. *J Public Health Manag Pract*. Nov 2012;18(6):535–544.
6. Schenck AP, Meyer AM, Kuo TM, Cilenti D. Building the evidence for decision-making: the relationship between local public health capacity and community mortality. *Am J Public Health*. Apr 2015;105(Suppl 2):S211–S216.
7. Turnock BJ. *Public Health: What It Is and How It Works*. 6th ed. Sudbury, MA: Jones and Bartlett Publishers; 2016.
8. Muir Gray JA. *Evidence-Based Healthcare: How to Make Decisions About Health Services and Public Health*. 3rd ed. New York and Edinburgh: Churchill Livingstone Elsevier; 2009.
9. Brownson RC, Baker EA, Leet TL, Gillespie KN, True WR. *Evidence-Based Public Health*. 2nd ed. New York, NY: Oxford University Press; 2011.
10. Hausman AJ. Implications of evidence-based practice for community health. *Am J Community Psychol*. Jun 2002;30(3):453–467.
11. Jacobs JA, Dodson EA, Baker EA, Deshpande AD, Brownson RC. Barriers to evidence-based decision making in public health: a national survey of chronic disease practitioners. *Public Health Rep*. Sep-Oct 2010;125(5):736–742.
12. Ramanadhan S, Crisostomo J, Alexander-Molloy J, et al. Perceptions of evidence-based programs among community-based organizations tackling health disparities: a qualitative study. *Health Educ Res*. Aug 2011;27(4):717–728.

13. Van Lerberghe W, Conceicao C, Van Damme W, Ferrinho P. When staff is underpaid: dealing with the individual coping strategies of health personnel. *Bull World Health Organ.* 2002;80(7):581–584.

14. Baker EA, Brownson RC, Dreisinger M, McIntosh LD, Karamehic-Muratovic A. Examining the role of training in evidence-based public health: a qualitative study. *Health Promot Pract.* Jul 2009;10(3):342–348.

15. Oliver K, Innvar S, Lorenc T, Woodman J, Thomas J. A systematic review of barriers to and facilitators of the use of evidence by policymakers. *BMC Health Serv Res.* 2014;14:2.

16. McMichael C, Waters E, Volmink J. Evidence-based public health: what does it offer developing countries? *J Public Health (Oxf).* Jun 2005;27(2):215–221.

17. Puchalski Ritchie LM, Khan S, Moore JE, et al. Low- and middle-income countries face many common barriers to implementation of maternal health evidence products. *J Clin Epidemiol.* Aug 2016;76:229–237.

18. Singh KK. Evidence-based public health: barriers and facilitators to the transfer of knowledge into practice. *Indian J Public Health.* Apr-Jun 2015;59(2):131–135.

19. Beaglehole R, Dal Poz MR. Public health workforce: challenges and policy issues. *Hum Resour Health.* Jul 17 2003;1(1):4.

20. Simoes EJ, Land G, Metzger R, Mokdad A. Prioritization MICA: a Web-based application to prioritize public health resources. *J Public Health Manag Pract.* Mar-Apr 2006;12(2):161–169.

21. Simoes EJ, Mariotti S, Rossi A, et al. The Italian health surveillance (SiVeAS) prioritization approach to reduce chronic disease risk factors. *Int J Public Health.* Aug 2012;57(4):719–733.

22. Wright K, Rowitz L, Merkle A, et al. Competency development in public health leadership. *Am J Public Health.* Aug 2000;90(8):1202–1207.

23. Task Force on Community Preventive Services. Guide to Community Preventive Services. www.thecommunityguide.org. Accessed June 5, 2016.

24. Institute of Medicine. Committee on Public Health. *Healthy Communities: New Partnerships for the Future of Public Health.* Washington, DC: National Academy Press; 1996.

25. Public Health Accreditation Board. Public Health Accreditation Board Standards and Measures, version 1.5. 2013. http://www.phaboard.org/wp-content/uploads/SM-Version-1.5-Board-adopted-FINAL-01-24-2014.docx.pdf. Accessed November 20, 2016.

26. The Cochrane Collaboration. The Cochrane Public Health Group. http://ph.cochrane.org/. Accessed July 28, 2016.

27. Mays GP, Scutchfield FD. Advancing the science of delivery: public health services and systems research. *J Public Health Manag Pract.* Nov 2012;18(6):481–484.

28. Scutchfield FD, Patrick K. Public health systems research: the new kid on the block. *Am J Prev Med.* Feb 2007;32(2):173–174.

29. Beitsch LM, Leep C, Shah G, Brooks RG, Pestronk RM. Quality improvement in local health departments: results of the NACCHO 2008 survey. *J Public Health Manag Pract.* Jan-Feb 2010;16(1):49–54.

30. Drabczyk A, Epstein P, Marshall M. A quality improvement initiative to enhance public health workforce capabilities. *J Public Health Manag Pract.* Jan-Feb 2012;18(1):95–99.

31. Erwin PC. The performance of local health departments: a review of the literature. *J Public Health Manag Pract.* Mar-Apr 2008;14(2):E9–E18.

32. Brownson RC, Reis RS, Allen P, et al. Understanding administrative evidence-based practices: findings from a survey of local health department leaders. *Am J Prev Med*. Jan 2013;46(1):49–57.

33. Erwin PC, Harris JK, Smith C, Leep CJ, Duggan K, Brownson RC. Evidence-based public health practice among program managers in local public health departments. *J Public Health Manag Pract*. Sep-Oct 2014;20(5):472–480.

34. Public Health Services and Systems Research and the Public Health Practice-Based Research Networks. Administrative Evidence-Based Practices Assessment Tool. http://tools.publichealthsystems.org/tools/tool?view=about&id=134. Accessed November 20, 2016.

35. Jacob R, Allen P, Ahrendt L, Brownson R. Learning about and using research evidence among public health practitioners. *Am J Prev Med*. 2017;52(3S3):S304–S308.

36. Birkhead GS, Davies J, Miner K, Lemmings J, Koo D. Developing competencies for applied epidemiology: from process to product. *Public Health Rep*. 2008;123(Suppl 1):67–118.

37. Birkhead GS, Koo D. Professional competencies for applied epidemiologists: a roadmap to a more effective epidemiologic workforce. *J Public Health Manag Pract*. Nov-Dec 2006;12(6):501–504.

38. Gebbie K, Merrill J, Hwang I, Gupta M, Btoush R, Wagner M. Identifying individual competency in emerging areas of practice: an applied approach. *Qual Health Res*. Sep 2002;12(7):990–999.

39. Brownson RC, Ballew P, Kittur ND, et al. Developing competencies for training practitioners in evidence-based cancer control. *J Cancer Educ*. 2009;24(3):186–193.

40. Luck J, Yoon J, Bernell S, et al. The Oregon Public Health Policy Institute: Building Competencies for Public Health Practice. *Am J Public Health*. Aug 2015;105(8):1537–1543.

41. Haire-Joshu D, McBride T, eds. *Transdisciplinary Public Health: Research, Education, and Practice*. San Francisco, CA: Jossey-Bass Publishers; 2013.

42. Carter BJ. Evidence-based decision-making: practical issues in the appraisal of evidence to inform policy and practice. *Aust Health Rev*. Nov 2010;34(4):435–440.

43. Fitzpatrick VE, Mayer C, Sherman BR. Undergraduate public health capstone course: teaching evidence-based public health. *Front Public Health*. 2016;4:70.

44. O'Neall MA, Brownson RC. Teaching evidence-based public health to public health practitioners. *Ann Epidemiol*. Aug 2005;15(7):540–544.

45. Wahabi HA, Siddiqui AR, Mohamed AG, Al-Hazmi AM, Zakaria N, Al-Ansary LA. Evidence-based decision making in public health: capacity building for public health students at King Saud University in Riyadh. *Biomed Res Int*. 2016;2015:576953.

46. Jansen MW, Hoeijmakers M. A masterclass to teach public health professionals to conduct practice-based research to promote evidence-based practice: a case study from The Netherlands. *J Public Health Manag Pract*. Jan-Feb 2012;19(1):83–92.

47. Gibbert WS, Keating SM, Jacobs JA, et al. Training the workforce in evidence-based public health: an evaluation of impact among US and international practitioners. *Prev Chronic Dis*. 2013;10:E148.

48. Yost J, Ciliska D, Dobbins M. Evaluating the impact of an intensive education workshop on evidence-informed decision making knowledge, skills, and behaviours: a mixed methods study. *BMC Med Educ*. 2014;14:13.

49. Yarber L, Brownson CA, Jacob RR, et al. Evaluating a train-the-trainer approach for improving capacity for evidence-based decision making in public health. *BMC Health Serv Res*. 2015;15(1):547.

50. Maxwell ML, Adily A, Ward JE. Promoting evidence-based practice in population health at the local level: a case study in workforce capacity development. *Aust Health Rev.* Aug 2007;31(3):422–429.

51. Maylahn C, Bohn C, Hammer M, Waltz E. Strengthening epidemiologic competencies among local health professionals in New York: teaching evidence-based public health. *Public Health Rep.* 2008;123(Suppl 1):35–43.

52. Brownson RC, Diem G, Grabauskas V, et al. Training practitioners in evidence-based chronic disease prevention for global health. *Promot Educ.* 2007;14(3):159–163.

53. Oliver KB, Dalrymple P, Lehmann HP, McClellan DA, Robinson KA, Twose C. Bringing evidence to practice: a team approach to teaching skills required for an informationist role in evidence-based clinical and public health practice. *J Med Libr Assoc.* Jan 2008;96(1):50–57.

54. Diem G, Brownson RC, Grabauskas V, Shatchkute A, Stachenko S. Prevention and control of noncommunicable diseases through evidence-based public health: implementing the NCD 2020 action plan. *Glob Health Promot.* Sep 2016;23(3):5–13.

55. Pettman TL, Armstrong R, Jones K, Waters E, Doyle J. Cochrane update: building capacity in evidence-informed decision-making to improve public health. *J Public Health (Oxf).* Dec 2013;35(4):624–627.

56. Linkov F, LaPorte R, Lovalekar M, Dodani S. Web quality control for lectures: Supercourse and Amazon.com. *Croat Med J.* Dec 2005;46(6):875–878.

57. Brownson RC, Ballew P, Brown KL, et al. The effect of disseminating evidence-based interventions that promote physical activity to health departments. *Am J Public Health.* Oct 2007;97(10):1900–1907.

58. Proctor EK. Leverage points for the implementation of evidence-based practice. *Brief Treatment and Crisis Intervention.* Sep 2004;4(3):227–242.

59. Chambers LW. The new public health: do local public health agencies need a booster (or organizational "fix") to combat the diseases of disarray? *Can J Public Health.* Sep-Oct 1992;83(5):326–328.

60. Bryan RL, Kreuter MW, Brownson RC. Integrating adult learning principles into training for public health practice. *Health Promot Pract.* 2009 Oct;10(4):557–563.

61. Brownson RC, Gurney JG, Land G. Evidence-based decision making in public health. *J Public Health Manag Pract.* 1999;5:86–97.

62. Kaplan GE, Juhl AL, Gujral IB, Hoaglin-Wagner AL, Gabella BA, McDermott KM. Tools for identifying and prioritizing evidence-based obesity prevention strategies, Colorado. *Prev Chronic Dis.* 2013;10:E106.

63. Brownson RC, Fielding JE, Maylahn CM. Evidence-based public health: a fundamental concept for public health practice. *Annu Rev Public Health.* Apr 21 2009;30:175–201.

64. Hess JJ, Eidson M, Tlumak JE, Raab KK, Luber G. An evidence-based public health approach to climate change adaptation. *Environ Health Perspect.* Nov 2014;122(11):1177–1186.

65. Ginter PM, Duncan WJ, Capper SA. Keeping strategic thinking in strategic planning: macro-environmental analysis in a state health department of public health. *Public Health.* 1992;106:253–269.

66. Florin P, Stevenson J. Identifying training and technical assistance needs in community coalitions: a developmental approach. *Health Education Research.* 1993;8:417–432.

67. Jenicek M. Epidemiology, evidence-based medicine, and evidence-based public health. *J Epidemiol Commun Health*. 1997;7:187–197.
68. Daar AS, Singer PA, Persad DL, et al. Grand challenges in chronic non-communicable diseases. *Nature*. Nov 22 2007;450(7169):494–496.
69. Leeman J, Calancie L, Hartman MA, et al. What strategies are used to build practitioners' capacity to implement community-based interventions and are they effective? A systematic review. *Implement Sci*. May 29 2015;10:80.
70. Mitton C, Adair CE, McKenzie E, Patten SB, Waye Perry B. Knowledge transfer and exchange: review and synthesis of the literature. *Milbank Q*. Dec 2007;85(4):729–768.
71. Mays GP, Scutchfield FD. Improving public health system performance through multiorganizational partnerships. *Prev Chronic Dis*. Nov 2010;7(6):A116.

CHAPTER 3

ᴄᴧᴐ

Assessing Scientific Evidence
for Public Health Action

It is often necessary to make a decision on the basis of information sufficient for action
but insufficient to satisfy the intellect.
Immanuel Kant

In most areas of public health and clinical practice, decisions on when to intervene and which program or policy to implement are not simple and straightforward. These decisions are often based on three fundamental questions: (1) Should public health action be taken to address a particular public health issue (Type 1, etiologic evidence)? (2) What action should be taken (Type 2, intervention evidence)? and (3) How can a particular program or policy most effectively be implemented in a local setting (Type 3, contextual or translational evidence)? This chapter primarily explores the first and second questions. That is, it focuses on several key considerations in evaluating scientific evidence and determining when a scientific basis exists for some type of public health action. It deals largely with the interpretation of epidemiologic studies that seek to identify health risks and intervention programs and policies that seek to improve population health. The third question is explored in more detail in later chapters (especially chapters 9 and 10).

Public health information for decision making is founded on science, and science is based on the collection, analysis, and interpretation of data.[1,2] Data in public health are generally derived from two overlapping sources: research studies and public health surveillance systems. Here, we focus on information from research studies; an emphasis on public health surveillance is provided in chapter 7. Research studies are primarily conducted in five broad areas[3]: (1) to understand the (etiologic) links between behaviors and health (e.g., Does fruit and vegetable intake influence the risk for coronary heart disease?); (2) to develop methods for measuring the behavior (e.g., What are the most valid and reliable methods by which to measure fruit and vegetable consumption?); (3) to identify the factors that influence the behavior (e.g., Which populations are at highest risk for low consumption of fruits and vegetables?; (4) to determine whether public health interventions are successful in meeting their stated objectives for risk reduction (e.g., Is a media campaign to increase fruit and vegetable intake effective?); and (5) to translate (or disseminate) research to practice (e.g., How does one "scale-up" an effective intervention promoting fruit and vegetable consumption so that it will widely improve population health?). In general, too much emphasis has been placed on the discovery of etiologic knowledge compared with the development, adaptation, implementation, and dissemination of effective interventions.[4-6]

BACKGROUND

In this era when public and media interest in health issues is intense, the reasons for not taking action based on an individual research study, even if it was carefully designed, successfully conducted, and properly analyzed and interpreted, need to be emphasized. Public health research is incremental, with a body of scientific evidence building up over years or decades. Therefore, although individual studies may contribute substantially to public health decision making, a single study rarely constitutes a strong basis for action. The example in Box 3.1 regarding the contamination of drinking water in Flint, Michigan is unusual because action was warranted based on a small but convincing body of scientific evidence.[7, 8]

When considering the science, strong evidence from epidemiologic (and other) studies may suggest that prevention and control measures should be taken. Conversely, evidence may be equivocal, so that taking action would be premature. Often the strength of evidence is suggestive, but not conclusive; yet one has to make a decision about the desirability of taking action. Here, other questions come to mind:

- Is the public health problem large and growing?
- Are there effective interventions for addressing the problem?
- Is a particular program or policy worth doing (i.e., is it better than alternatives?), and will it provide a satisfactory return on investment, measured in monetary terms or in health impacts?
- What information about the local context related to this particular intervention is helpful in deciding its potential use in the situation at hand?

Box 3.1

CONTAMINATION OF DRINKING WATER IN FLINT, MICHIGAN

In 2014, the city of Flint, Michigan temporarily changed its drinking water supply from Lake Huron to the Flint River in an effort to save money. After this change, residents expressed concerns about water color, taste, and odor, along with a range of health complaints (e.g., skin rashes).[8] Bacteria were detected in excess of Safe Drinking Water standards. The switch in water source increased the likelihood for corrosion and leaching of lead into drinking water, in part due to the aging distribution system in Flint. Because lead in drinking water is neurotoxic and affects numerous developments processes (e.g., intelligence, behavior), an investigative team analyzed blood lead levels in children younger than 5 years before and after Flint introduced a more corrosive water supply. The incidence of elevated blood lead levels increased from 2.4% to 4.9% ($p < 0.05$) after the source change, and neighborhoods with the highest water lead levels experienced a 6.6% increase.[8] The most socioeconomically disadvantaged neighborhoods showed the highest blood lead level increases. Based on a single epidemiologic study, investigators uncovered one of the most vivid examples of health inequalities in the United States. In the Flint example, Flint citizens, mostly blacks, already had a disparity in lead exposure that was widened by the change in water source and lack of government action.[7] The Flint situation is a vivid example of the public health need to maintain a modern water infrastructure along with the need to address health inequalities framed by a history of racial discrimination, "white flight," declining tax revenues, and a city government's inability to provide basic services.[8]

If the answer to the first three questions is "yes," then the decision to take action is relatively straightforward. In practice, unfortunately, decisions are seldom so simple.

EXAMINING A BODY OF SCIENTIFIC EVIDENCE

As practitioners, researchers, and policy makers committed to improving population health, we have a natural tendency to scrutinize the scientific literature for new findings that would serve as the basis for prevention or intervention programs. In fact, the main motivation for conducting research should be to stimulate appropriate public health action. Adding to this inclination to intervene may be claims from investigators regarding the critical importance of their findings, media interpretation of the findings as the basis for immediate action, political pressure for action, and community support for responding to the striking new research findings with new or modified programs. The importance of community action in motivating public health efforts was shown in the Long Island Breast Cancer Study Project (LIBCSP). Community advocates in Long Island raised concerns about the high incidence of breast cancer and possible linkages with environmental chemicals and radiation. More than 10 research project have been conducted by the New York State Health Department, along with scientists from universities and the National Institutes of Health. In each Long Island–area county, breast cancer incidence increased over a 10-year period, while mortality from breast cancer decreased.[9] At the conclusion of the study, the LIBCSP could not identify a set of specific environmental agents that could be responsible for the high rates of breast cancer incidence. The exceptions may be breast cancer risk associated with exposure to polyaromatic hydrocarbon and living in proximity to organochlorine-containing hazardous waste sites.[10] The LIBCSP is an important example of participatory research in which patient advocates play important roles in shaping the research (participatory approaches are discussed in more detail in chapters 5 and 10).

Finding Scientific Evidence

Chapter 8 describes systematic methods for seeking out credible, peer-reviewed scientific evidence. Modern information technologies have made searching the scientific literature quick and accessible. There are also numerous websites that summarize research and provide ready access to surveillance data. The ready access to information may also present a paradox, in that more access is better to the extent one can synthesize contrary findings and recognize good science and advice from bad. Often, various tools are helpful in examining and synthesizing an entire body of evidence, rather than reviewing the literature study-by-study. These summary approaches, described in chapters 4 and 8, include systematic reviews of the literature, evidence-based guidelines, summaries of best practices, health impact assessments, and economic evaluations.

The Roles of Peer Review and Publication Bias

In assessing evidence, it is important to understand the role of peer review. Peer review is the process of reviewing research proposals, manuscripts submitted for publication by journals, and abstracts submitted for presentation at scientific meetings. These materials are judged for scientific and technical merit by other scientists in the same field.[11] Reviewers are commonly asked to comment on such issues as the scientific soundness of the methods used, innovation, generalizability, and appropriateness of a scientific article to the audience. Although peer review has numerous limitations, including a large time commitment, complexity, and expense, it remains the closest approximation to a gold standard when determining the merits of scientific endeavor.

Through the process of peer review and dissemination of science, it is important to guard against publication bias—that is, the higher likelihood for journal editors to publish positive or "new" findings in contrast to negative studies or those that do not yield statistically significant results. Studies have shown that positive findings tend to get published more often and more quickly.[12] Recent work provides direct empirical evidence for the existence of publication bias.[13] There are numerous possible reasons for publication bias, including researchers' tendency to submit positive rather than negative studies, peer reviewers who are more likely to recommend publication of positive studies, and journal editors who favor publication of positive studies.[14] The net effect of publication bias may be an overrepresentation of false-positive findings in the literature.

It is also important to be aware of potential publication bias when reading or conducting a systematic review relying rely solely on the published literature and not seeking out unpublished studies. When a sufficient number of studies is available, funnel plots may be an effective method by which to determine whether publication bias is present in a particular body of evidence.[14,15] Figure 3.1 presents hypothetical data showing the effects of publication bias. In the plot on the right-hand side, smaller studies are represented in the literature only when they tend to show a positive effect. Thus, the left side of the inverted funnel is missing, and publication bias may be present. Steps to

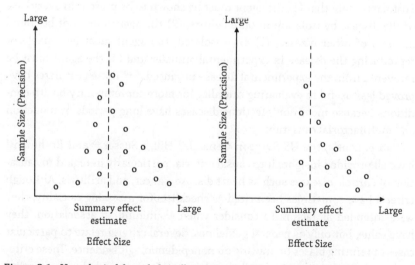

Figure 3.1: Hypothetical funnel plots illustrating the effect of publication bias.

address publication bias include making strenuous efforts to find all published and unpublished work when conducting systematic reviews[16] and the establishment of reporting guidelines that specifically address publication bias (also see chapter 8).[17]

ASSESSING CAUSALITY IN ETIOLOGIC RESEARCH

A cause of a disease is an event, condition, characteristic, or combination of factors that plays an important role in the development of the disease or health condition.[18] An epidemiologic study assesses the extent to which there is an association between these factors and the disease or health condition. An intervention (program, policy, or other public health action) is based on the presumption that the associations found in these epidemiologic studies are causal rather than arising through bias or for some other spurious reason.[19] Unfortunately, in most instances in observational research, there is no opportunity to prove absolutely that an association is causal. Nonetheless, numerous frameworks have been developed that are useful in determining whether a cause-and-effect relationship exists between a particular risk factor and a given health outcome. This is one of the reasons for assembling experts to reach scientific consensus on various issues.

Criteria for Assessing Causality

The earliest guidelines for assessing causality for infectious diseases were developed in the 1800s by Jacob Henle and Robert Koch. The Henle-Koch Postulates state that (1) the agent must be shown to be present in every case of the disease by isolation in pure culture; (2) the agent must not be found in cases of other disease; (3) once isolated, the agent must be capable of reproducing the disease in experimental animals; and (4) the agent must be recovered from the experimental disease produced.[11,20] These postulates have proved less useful in evaluating causality for more contemporary health conditions because most noninfectious diseases have long periods of induction and multifactorial causation.

Subsequently, the US Surgeon General,[21] Hill,[22] Susser,[23] and Rothman[24] have all provided insights into causal criteria, particularly in regard to causation of chronic diseases such as heart disease, cancer, and arthritis. Although criteria have sometimes been cited as checklists for assessing causality, they were intended as factors to consider when examining an association: they have value, but only as general guidelines. Several criteria relate to particular cases of refuting biases or drawing on nonepidemiologic evidence. These criteria have been discussed in detail elsewhere.[19,25] In the end, belief in causality is based on an individual's judgment, and different individuals may in good faith reach different conclusions from the same available information. The six key issues below have been adapted from Hill[22] and Weed.[26] Each is described by a definition and a rule of evidence. These are also illustrated in Table 3.1 by examining two risk factor–disease relationships.

1. *Consistency*
   Definition: The association is observed in studies in different settings and populations, using various methods.
   Rule of evidence: The likelihood of a causal association increases as the proportion of studies with similar (positive) results increases.

2. *Strength*
   Definition: This is defined by the size of the relative risk estimate. In some situations, meta-analytic techniques are used to provide an overall, summary risk estimate.
   Rule of evidence: The likelihood of a causal association increases as the summary relative risk estimate increases. Larger effect estimates are generally less likely to be explained by unmeasured bias or confounding.

3. *Temporality*
   Definition: This is perhaps the most important criterion for causality—some consider it an absolute condition. Temporality refers to the temporal relationship between the occurrence of the risk factor and the occurrence of the disease or health condition.
   Rule of evidence: The exposure (risk factor) must precede the disease.

4. *Dose-response relationship*
   Definition: The observed relationship between the dose of the exposure and the magnitude of the relative risk estimate.
   Rule of evidence: An increasing level of exposure (in intensity or time) increases the risk when hypothesized to do so.

5. *Biological plausibility*
   Definition: The available knowledge on the biological mechanism of action for the studied risk factor and disease outcome.
   Rule of evidence: There is not a standard rule of thumb except that the more likely the agent is biologically capable of influencing the disease, the more probable that a causal relationship exists.

6. *Experimental evidence*
   Definition: The presence of findings from a prevention trial in which the factor of interest is removed from randomly assigned individuals.

Table 3.1. DEGREE TO WHICH CAUSAL CRITERIA ARE MET FOR TWO
CONTEMPORARY PUBLIC HEALTH ISSUES

Issue	Physical Activity and Coronary Heart Disease (CHD)	Extremely Low Frequency Electromagnetic Fields (EMFs) and Childhood Cancer[a]
Consistency	More than 50 studies since 1953; most studies show positive association	Based on a relatively small number of studies, the preponderance of the evidence favors a judgment of no association
Strength	Median relative risk of 1.9 for a sedentary lifestyle across studies, after controlling for other risk factors	Early studies showed relative risks in the range of 1.5 to 2.5. Most subsequent studies with larger sample sizes and more comprehensive exposure methods have not shown positive associations
Temporality	Satisfied, based on prospective cohort study design	Not satisfied; very difficult to assess because of ubiquitous exposure and the rarity of the disease
Dose-response relationship	Most studies show an inverse relationship between physical activity and risk for CHD	Because there is little biological guidance into what components of EMF exposure may be problematic, exposure assessment is subject to a high degree of misclassification. True dose gradients are therefore very hard to classify reliably
Biological plausibility	Biological mechanisms are demonstrated, including atherosclerosis, plasma and lipid changes, blood pressure, ischemia, and thrombosis	No direct cancer mechanism is yet known because EMFs produce energy levels far too low to cause DNA damage or chemical reactions
Experimental evidence	Trials have not been conducted related to CHD but have been carried out for CHD intermediate factors such as blood pressure, lipoprotein profile, insulin sensitivity, and body fat	Numerous experimental studies of EMF exposure have been conducted to assess indirect mechanisms for carcinogenesis in animals and via in vitro cell models. The few positive findings to date have not been successfully reproduced in other laboratories

[a]Predominantly childhood leukemia and brain cancer.

Rule of evidence: A positive result (i.e., reduction in a health condition) after removal of the risk factor provides evidence of a causal association.

In practice, evidence for causality is often established through the elimination of noncausal explanations for an observed association. For example, some studies have suggested that alcohol use might increase the risk for breast cancer. Other studies have not found such an association. Further studies would need to be conducted to determine whether there might be confounding or other biases that account for the findings. By whittling away alternative explanations, the hypothesis asserting that alcohol use causes breast cancer becomes increasingly credible. It is the job of researchers to propose and test noncausal explanations so that when the association has withstood a series of such challenges, the case for causality is strengthened.

Because most associations involve unknown confounders, a key issue becomes the extent to which causal conclusions or public health recommendations should be delayed until all or nearly all potential confounders are discovered or better measured.[27] As noted earlier, those who argue that causality must be established with absolute certainty before interventions are attempted may fail to appreciate that their two alternatives—action and inaction—each have risks and benefits. When searching for causal relationships, researchers generally seek those that are modifiable and potentially amenable to some type of public health intervention. For example, if researchers studied youth and discovered that age of initiation of smoking was strongly related to the ethnicity of the teen and exposure to advertising, the latter variable would be a likely target of intervention efforts.

INTERVENTION STUDY DESIGN AND EXECUTION: ASSESSING INTERNAL VALIDITY

As described in chapter 1, public health practitioners are often interested in finding Types 2 and 3 evidence (e.g., Which interventions are effective? How do I implement the intervention?). A body of intervention research is often judged on the basis of internal validity, which is the degree to which the treatment or intervention effects changed the dependent variable. For a study or program evaluation to be internally valid, the study and comparison groups should be selected and compared in a way that the observed differences in dependent variables are attributed to the hypothesized effects under study (apart from sampling error).[11] In other words, can the observed results be attributed to the risk factor being studied or intervention being implemented, or are there plausible alternate explanations? These concepts are illustrated in Figure 3.2.

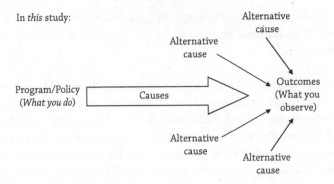

Figure 3.2: Illustration of internal validity in establishing a cause-and-effect relationship.
Source: <http://www.socialresearchmethods.net/kb/>.

Although it is beyond the scope of this chapter to discuss these issues in detail, an overview of key issues (so-called threats to validity) is provided, along with entry points into a larger body of literature. The internal validity of a given study can be assessed based on the study design and study execution.

In public health research, a variety of study designs are used to assess health risks and to measure intervention effectiveness. Commonly, these are not "true" experiments in which study participants are randomized to an intervention or control condition. These generally quasi-experimental or observational designs are described in chapter 7. A hierarchy of designs shows that a randomized trial tends to be the strongest type of study, yet such a study is often not feasible in community settings (Table 3.2).[28,29] Interestingly, when summary results from the same topic were based on observational studies and on randomized controlled trials, the findings across study designs were remarkably similar.[30]

The quality of a study's execution can be determined by many different standards. In general, internal validity is threatened by all types of systematic error, and error rates are influenced by both study design and study execution. Systematic error occurs when there is a tendency within a particular study to produce results that vary in a systematic way from the true values.[18] Dozens of specific types of bias have been identified. Among the most important are the following[11]:

1. *Selection bias:* error due to systematic differences in characteristics between those who take part in the study and those who do not.
2. *Information bias:* a flaw in measuring exposure or outcomes that results in different quality (accuracy) of information between study groups.
3. *Confounding bias:* distortion of the estimated effect of an exposure on an outcome, caused by the presence of an extraneous factor associated with both the exposure and the outcome.

Table 3.2. HIERARCHY OF STUDY DESIGNS

Suitability	Examples	Attributes
Greatest	Randomized group or individual trial; prospective cohort study; time series study with comparison group	Concurrent comparison groups and prospective measurement of exposure and outcome
Moderate	Case-control study; time-series study without comparison group	All retrospective designs or multiple premeasurements or postmeasurements but no concurrent comparison group
Least	Cross-sectional study; case series; ecological study	Before-after studies with no comparison group or exposure and outcome measured in a single group at the same point in time

Source: Adapted from Briss et al., 2000[28] and Briss et al., 2004.[29]

In ongoing work of the US Public Health Service,[31] study execution is assessed according to six categories, each of which may threaten internal validity: (1) study population and intervention descriptions; (2) sampling; (3) exposure and outcome measurement; (4) data analysis; (5) interpretation of results (including follow-up, bias, and confounding); and (6) other related factors.

THE NEED FOR A STRONGER FOCUS ON EXTERNAL VALIDITY

Most research in public health to date has tended to emphasize internal validity (e.g., well-controlled efficacy trials), while giving limited attention to external validity (i.e., the degree to which findings from a study or set of studies can be generalizable to and relevant for populations, settings, and times other than those in which the original studies were conducted).[5] Green succinctly summarized a key challenge related to external validity in 2001[32]:

> Where did the field get the idea that evidence of an intervention's efficacy from carefully controlled trials could be generalized as THE best practice for widely varied populations and settings? (p. 167)

Much of the information needed to assess external validity relates to so-called Type 3 (or contextual) evidence,[33] as described in chapter 1. Too often, this evidence is incomplete or missing completely in the peer-reviewed literature. For example, Klesges and colleagues reviewed 77 childhood obesity studies to assess the extent to which dimensions of external validity were reported.[34] Importantly, the work of Klesges shows that some key contextual variables (e.g., representativeness of settings, program sustainability) are missing entirely in the peer-reviewed literature on obesity treatment. This finding is likely to apply across most other areas of public health.

To develop a stronger literature base for external validity, there is a need for guidelines and better reporting of key variables.[35,36] The essential questions are outlined in Table 3.3 and follow the SPOT guidelines (Settings and populations; Program/policy implementation and adaptation; Outcomes for decision making; Time for maintenance and institutionalization).[37] By answering these questions, public health practitioners can better determine whether a program or study is relevant to their particular setting. This often includes consideration of the target audience, available resources, staff capacity, and availability of appropriate measures.

For public health practitioners, these data on external validity are likely to be as important as information on the internal validity of a particular program or policy. Yet detailed information on external validity is often missing in journal articles. Similarly, systematic reviews have difficulty in examining whether factors that may affect external validity (e.g., training and involvement of staff, organizational characteristics) function as important effect modifiers.[38] For certain public health issues, documentation is available on how to implement programs that have been shown to be internally valid. Such guidance is sometimes called an "implementation guide," which might assist a practitioner in adapting a scientifically proven intervention to local contextual conditions. Implementation guides have been developed for many areas of public health.

In other cases, it is worth the effort to seek additional data on external validity. This gathering of information relates to the concept of "pooling"— that is, a step in the intervention process in which one reviews and pools the best experience from prior attempts at behavioral, environmental, or policy change.[39] Key informant interviews are one useful tool to collect these data.[40] Persons to interview may include stakeholders at the local level (e.g., program delivery agents, target populations) who have indigenous wisdom about the context for a particular intervention,[37] or the lead investigator or project manager in a research study. Less intensive (yet more superficial) ways to gather this information may involve emailing colleagues or posting specific questions on LISTSERVs.

Table 3.3. QUALITY RATING CRITERIA FOR EXTERNAL VALIDITY

1. Settings and populations
   A. Participation: Are there analyses of the participation rate among potential settings, delivery staff, and patients (consumers)?
   B. Target audience: Is the intended target audience stated for adoption (at the intended settings such as worksites, medical offices, etc.) and application (at the individual level)?
   C. Representativeness—settings: Are comparisons made of the similarity of settings in study to the intended target audience of program settings—or to those settings that decline to participate?
   D. Representativeness—individuals: Are analyses conducted of the similarity and differences between patients, consumers, or other subjects who participate versus either those who decline or the intended target audience?

2. Program or policy implementation and adaptation
   A. Consistent implementation: Are data presented on the level and quality of implementation of different program components?
   B. Staff expertise: Are data presented on the level of training or experience required to deliver the program or quality of implementation by different types of staff?
   C. Program adaptation: Is information reported on the extent to which different settings modified or adapted the program to fit their setting?
   D. Mechanisms: Are data reported on the processes or mediating variables through which the program or policy achieved its effects?

3. Outcomes for decision making
   A. Significance: Are outcomes reported in a way that can be compared to either clinical guidelines or public health goals?
   B. Adverse consequences: Do the outcomes reported include quality of life or potential negative outcomes?
   C. Moderators: Are there any analyses of moderator effects—including of different subgroups of participants and types of intervention staff—to assess robustness versus specificity of effects?
   D. Sensitivity: Are there any sensitivity analyses to assess dose-response effects, threshold level, or point of diminishing returns on the resources expended?
   E. Costs: Are data on the costs presented? If so, are standard economic or accounting methods used to fully account for costs?

4. Time: Maintenance and institutionalization
   A. Long-term effects: Are data reported on longer term effects, at least 12 months after treatment?
   B. Institutionalization: Are data reported on the sustainability (or reinvention or evolution) of program implementation at least 12 months after the formal evaluation?
   C. Attrition: Are data on attrition by condition reported, and are analyses conducted of the representativeness of those who drop out?

Adapted from Green and Glasgow, 2006.[37]

OTHER IMPORTANT ISSUES WHEN CONSIDERING PUBLIC HEALTH ACTION

In addition to understanding scientific causality and validity (both internal and external), several related issues are important to consider when weighing public health action.

Overarching Factors Influencing Decision Making in Public Health

There are many factors that influence decision making in public health (Table 3.4).[19,41-43] Some of these factors are under the control of the public health practitioner, whereas others are nearly impossible to modify. A group of experts may systematically assemble and present a persuasive body of

Table 3.4. FACTORS INFLUENCING DECISION MAKING AMONG PUBLIC HEALTH ADMINISTRATORS, POLICY MAKERS, AND THE GENERAL PUBLIC

Category	Influential Factor
Information	• Sound scientific basis, including knowledge of causality • Source (e.g., professional organization, government, mass media, friends)
Clarity of contents	• Formatting and framing • Perceived validity • Perceived relevance • Cost of intervention • Strength of the message (i.e., vividness)
Perceived values, preferences, beliefs	• Role of the decision maker • Economic background • Previous education • Personal experience or involvement • Political affiliation • Willingness to adopt innovations • Willingness to accept uncertainty • Willingness to accept risk • Ethical aspect of the decision
Context	• Culture • Politics • Timing • Media attention • Financial or political constraints

Adapted from Bero et al.[41] and Anderson et al.[64]

scientific evidence such as recommendations for clinical or community-based interventions, but even when they convene in a rational and evidence-based manner, the process is imperfect, participants may disagree, and events may become politically charged, as noted in Box 3.2.[44-50] In addition, one may have little control over the timing of some major public health event (e.g., prostate cancer diagnosis in an elected leader) that may have a large impact on the awareness and behaviors of the general public and policy makers.[51] Therefore, for success in the policy process, one often needs to proactively analyze and assemble data so that evidence is ready when a policy window or opportunity emerges.[52] Generally, evidence for public policy decisions should be viewed

---

Box 3.2

THE EVOLUTION OF BREAST CANCER SCREENING GUIDELINES

Breast cancer screening guidance for women aged 40 to 49 years has been the subject of considerable debate and controversy. Breast cancer is the most common cancer type among US women, accounting for 246,660 new cases and 40,450 deaths in 2016.[45] It is suggested that appropriate use of screening mammography may lower death rates due to breast cancer by as much as 30%. Official expert guidance from the US government was first issued in 1977 when the National Cancer Institute (NCI) recommended annual mammography screening for women aged 50 years and older but discouraged screening for younger women.[46] In 1980, the American Cancer Society dissented from this guidance and recommended a baseline mammogram for women at age 35 years and annual or biannual mammograms for women in their 40s.[65] The NCI and other professional organizations differed on recommendations for women in their 40s throughout the late 1980s and 1990s. To resolve disagreement, the director of the National Institutes of Health called for a Consensus Development Conference in January 1997. Based on evidence from randomized controlled trials, the consensus group concluded that the available data did not support a blanket mammography recommendation for women in their 40s. The panel issued a draft statement that largely left the decision regarding screening up to the woman.[47] This guidance led to widespread media attention and controversy. Within 1 week, the US Senate passed a 98-to-0 vote resolution calling on the NCI to express unequivocal support for screening women in their 40s, and within 60 days, the NCI had issued a new recommendation.

The controversy regarding breast cancer screening resurfaced in 2009. The US Preventive Services Task Force (USPSTF) was first convened by the Public Health Service in 1984. Since its inception, it has been recognized as an authoritative source for determining the effectiveness of clinical preventive services, and its methods have been adapted by guidelines groups worldwide. In December 2009, the Task Force revised its guideline on mammography screening, which in part recommended against routine screening mammography in women aged 40 to 49 years.[48] The change from the earlier guideline was based on benefit-risk calculations including the likelihood of false-positive tests that result in additional x-rays, unnecessary biopsies, and significant anxiety. This recommendation was met with unprecedented media attention and charges by some groups (like the American College of Radiology) that the guidelines were changed in response to the Obama administration's wish to save health care dollars.[50] The US Department of Health and Human Services, which appoints and vets the Task Force, also distanced itself from the updated recommendation. In 2015, the USPSTF updated its recommendation again, encouraging women between 40 and 49 years old, at average risk, to make the decision individually on whether they should start biennial screening mammography. This example points to the interplay of science, politics, timing, and health communication when assessing the evidence for public health interventions.

across a continuum of certainty (i.e., a range of rational policy options) rather than as a dichotomy.[19]

Estimating Population Burden and the Prevented Fraction

As noted earlier, many factors enter into decisions about public health interventions, including certainty of causality, validity, relevance, economics, and political climate (Table 3.4). Measures of burden may also contribute substantially to science-based decision making. The burden of infectious diseases, such as measles, has been primarily assessed through incidence, measured in case numbers or rates. For chronic or noninfectious diseases like cancer, burden can be measured in terms of morbidity, mortality, and disability. The choice of measure should depend on the characteristics of the condition being examined. For example, mortality rates are useful in reporting data on a fatal condition such as lung cancer. For a common, yet generally nonfatal condition such as arthritis, a measure of disability would be more useful (e.g., limitations in activities of daily living). When available, measures of the population burden of health conditions are extremely useful (e.g., quality-adjusted life-years).

When assessing the scientific basis for a public health program or policy, quantitative considerations of preventable disease can help us make a rational choice. This can be thought of as "preventable burden." When presented with an array of potential causal factors for disease, we need to evaluate how much might be gained by reducing or eliminating each of the hazards. For example, can we predict in numerical terms the benefits that one or more interventions might yield in the community?

Epidemiologic measures, such as relative risk estimates, indicate how strongly exposure and disease are associated, but they do not indicate directly the benefits that could be gained through modifying the exposure. Of still greater potential value is the incorporation of information on how common the exposure is. Although some exposures exert a powerful influence on individuals (i.e., a large relative risk), they are so rare that their public health impact is minimal. Conversely, some exposures have a modest impact but are so widespread that their elimination could have great benefit. To answer the question, "What proportion of disease in the total population is a result of the exposure?" the *population-attributable risk* (PAR) is used. The PAR is calculated as follows:

$$\frac{P_e(\text{relative risk} - 1)}{1 + P_e(\text{relative risk} - 1)},$$

where P_e represents the proportion of the population that is exposed. Assuming that the relative risk for lung cancer due to cigarette smoking is 15 (i.e., smokers have 15 times the risk for lung cancer compared with nonsmokers) and that 30% of the population are smokers, the PAR is 0.81, or 81%. This would suggest that 81% of the lung cancer burden in the population is caused by cigarette smoking and could be eliminated if the exposure were eliminated. Table 3.5 describes a variety of risk factors for coronary heart disease.[53] This list demonstrates that the greatest population burden (PAR) would be affected by eliminating elevated cholesterol and physical inactivity, even though the relative risk values for these risk factors are in the moderate or weak range.[53]

A related metric is the prevented fraction (PF). In an intervention in which "exposure" to a program or policy may protect against disease, the PF is the proportion of disease occurrence in a population averted because of a protective risk factor or public health intervention.[54] The PF is calculated as follows:

$$P_e(1 - \text{relative risk}),$$

where P_e represents the prevalence of exposure to the protective factor and relative risk is a protective effect estimate (i.e., exposure to the preventive measure protects against acquiring a specific health problem). This formula for the PF is the same one used to calculate vaccine efficacy and has also been used to estimate the benefits of disease screening programs.[55] Thacker and colleagues examined 702 population-based interventions and found PF

Table 3.5. MODIFIABLE RISK FACTORS FOR CORONARY HEART DISEASE, UNITED STATES

Magnitude	Risk Factor	Best Estimate (%) of Population-Attributable Risk (Range)
Strong (relative risk >4)	None	
Moderate (relative risk 2–4)	High blood pressure (>140/90 mm Hg)	25 (20–29)
	Cigarette smoking	22 (17–25)
	Elevated cholesterol (>200 mg/dL)	43 (39–47)
	Diabetes (fasting glucose S140 mg/dL)	8 (1–15)
Weak (relative risk <2)	Obesity[a]	17 (7–32)
	Physical inactivity	35 (23–46)
	Environmental tobacco smoke exposure	18 (8–23)
	Elevated plasma C-reactive protein (>3.mg/L)	19 (11–25)
	Elevated fibrinogen (>3.74 g/L)	21 (17–25)
	Elevated plasma homocysteine (>15 μmol/L)	5 (2–9)
Possible	Psychological factors	
	Alcohol use[b]	
	Infectious agents	

[a]Based on body mass index >30 kg/m^2.
[b]Moderate to heavy alcohol use may increase risk, whereas light use may reduce risk.
From Liu et al.[52]

data on only 31 (4.4%), suggesting the need to expand the evidence base on prevention.[56]

Assessing Time Trends

Numerous other factors may be considered when weighing the need for public health action. One important factor to consider involves temporal trends. Public health surveillance systems can provide information on changes over time in a risk factor or disease of interest. Through use of these data, one may determine whether the condition of interest is increasing, decreasing, or remaining constant. One may also examine the incidence or prevalence of a condition in relation to other conditions of interest. For example, if a public health practitioner were working with a statewide coalition to control cancer, it would be useful to plot both the incidence and mortality rates for various cancer sites (Figure 3.3).[57] The researcher might reach

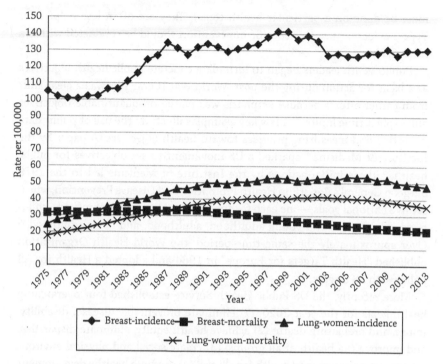

Figure 3.3: Trends in incidence and mortality for lung and breast cancer in women, United States, 1975–2013.
Source: Howlander et al., 2016.[56]

different conclusions on the impact and changing magnitude of various cancers when examining incidence versus mortality rates across the state. When working at a local level, however, it would be important to note that sample sizes might be too small for many health conditions, making rates unstable and subject to considerable fluctuations over time. In addition, a formal time-series analysis requires numerous data points (approximately 50 for the most sophisticated statistical methods). A simple and often useful time-series analysis can often be conducted with ordinary least-squares regression techniques, which are amenable to fewer data points than formal time-series analyses.

Priority Setting Through National Health Goals

Determining public health and health care priorities in a climate of limited resources is a demanding task. In some cases, priority setting from experts and governmental bodies can help to focus areas for public health action. These efforts are particularly useful in evaluating Type 1 evidence (i.e., something must be done on a particular health topic). They are often less helpful for Type 2 evidence (i.e., this specific intervention should be conducted within a local area).

Public health leaders began to formulate concrete public health objectives as a basis for action during the post–World War II era. This was a clear shift from earlier efforts because emphasis was placed on quantifiable objectives and explicit time limits.[58] A few key examples illustrate the use of public data in setting and measuring progress toward health objectives. A paper by the Institute of Medicine[59] sparked a US movement to set objectives for public health.[58] These initial actions by the Institute of Medicine led to the 1979 Surgeon General's Report on Health Promotion and Disease Prevention, which set five national goals—one each for the principal life stages of infancy, childhood, adolescence and young adulthood, adulthood, and older adulthood.[60] Over approximately the same time period, the World Health Organization published "Health Targets for Europe" in 1984 and adopted a Health for All policy with 38 targets.[61]

More recently, the US Public Health Service established four overarching health goals for the year 2020: (1) eliminate preventable disease, disability, injury, and premature death; (2) achieve health equity, eliminate disparities, and improve the health of all groups; (3) create social and physical environments that promote good health for all; and (4) promote healthy development and healthy behaviors across every stage of life.[62] As discussed in the final chapter in this book, addressing social and physical determinants of health raises important questions about the types of evidence that is appropriate and how we track progress.

SUMMARY

The issues covered in this chapter highlight one of the continuing challenges for public health practitioners and policy makers—determining when scientific evidence is sufficient for public health action. In nearly all instances, scientific studies cannot demonstrate causality with absolute certainty. The demarcation between action and inaction is seldom distinct and requires careful consideration of scientific evidence as well as assessment of values, preferences, costs, and benefits of various options. The difficulty in determining scientific certainty was eloquently summarized by A. B. Hill[22]:

> All scientific work is incomplete—whether it be observational or experimental. All scientific work is liable to be upset or modified by advancing knowledge. That does not confer upon us a freedom to ignore the knowledge we already have, or to postpone the action that it appears to demand at a given time.

Because policy cannot wait for perfect information, one must consider actions wherein the benefit outweighs the risk. This was summarized by Szklo as, "How much do we stand to gain if we are right?" and "How much do we stand to lose if we are wrong?"[63]

In many instances, waiting for absolute scientific certainty would mean delaying crucial public health action. For example, the first cases of acquired immunodeficiency syndrome (AIDS) were described in 1981, yet the causative agent (a retrovirus) was not identified until 1983.[64] Studies in epidemiology and prevention research, therefore, began well before gaining a full understanding of the molecular biology of AIDS transmission.

KEY CHAPTER POINTS

- When considering public health measures, it is helpful to consider the consequences of taking action or no action.
- The demarcation between action and inaction is seldom distinct and requires careful consideration of scientific evidence as well as assessment of values, preferences, costs, and benefits of various options.
- Advances in public health research are generally incremental, suggesting the need for intervention as a body of literature accumulates.
- When evaluating literature and determining a course of action, both internal and external validity should be considered.
- A set of standardized criteria can be useful in assessing the causality of an association.
- Many factors beyond science, such as resource constraints, sources of information, timing, and politics, influence decision making in public health.

SUGGESTED READINGS AND SELECTED WEBSITES

Suggested Readings

Green LW, Glasgow RE. Evaluating the relevance, generalization, and applicability of research: issues in external validation and translation methodology. *Eval Health Prof.* Mar 2006;29(1):126–153.

Rothman KJ. Causes. *Am J Epidemiol.* 1976;104:587–592.

Redwood R, Remington PL, Brownson RC. Methods in chronic disease epidemiology. In: Remington PL, Brownson RC, Wegner M, eds. *Chronic Disease Epidemiology and Control.* 4th ed. Washington, DC: American Public Health Association; 2016.

Weed DL. On the use of causal criteria. *Int J Epidemiol.* 1997;26(6):1137–1141.

Zaza S, Briss PA, Harris KW, eds. *The Guide to Community Preventive Services: What Works to Promote Health?* New York, NY: Oxford University Press; 2005.

Selected Websites

Disease Control Priorities Project (DCPP) <http://www.dcp2.org>. The DCPP is an ongoing effort to assess disease control priorities and produce evidence-based analysis and resource materials to inform health policymaking in developing countries. DCPP has produced three volumes providing technical resources that can assist developing countries in improving their health systems and, ultimately, the health of their people.

Health Evidence Network (HEN), World Health Organization Regional Office for Europe <http://www.euro.who.int/HEN>. The HEN is an information service primarily for public health and health care policy makers in the European Region. HEN synthesizes the huge quantity of information and evidence available in the fields of public health and health care·that is dispersed among numerous databases and other sources. HEN provides summarized information from a wide range of existing sources, including websites, databases, documents, national and international organizations, and institutions. It also produces its own reports on topical issues.

Healthy People <http://www.healthypeople.gov/>. Healthy People provides science-based, 10-year national objectives for promoting health and preventing disease in the United States. Since 1979, Healthy People has set and monitored national health objectives to meet a broad range of health needs, encourage collaborations across sectors, guide individuals toward making informed health decisions, and measure the impact of prevention activity.

Office of the Surgeon General <http://www.surgeongeneral.gov/>. The Surgeon General serves as America's chief health educator by providing Americans with the best scientific information available on how to improve their health and reduce the risk for illness and injury. The Surgeon General's public health priorities, reports, and publications are available on this site.

Partners in Information Access for the Public Health Workforce <http://phpartners.org/>. Partners in Information Access for the Public Health Workforce is a collaboration of US government agencies, public health organizations, and health sciences libraries that provides timely, convenient access to selected public health resources on the Internet.

Research Methods Knowledge Base <http://www.socialresearchmethods.net/kb/>. The Research Methods Knowledge Base is a comprehensive Web-based textbook that covers the entire research process, including formulating research questions, sampling, measurement (surveys, scaling, qualitative, unobtrusive), research design (experimental and quasi-experimental), data analysis, and writing the research paper. It uses an informal, conversational style to engage both the newcomer and the more experienced student of research.

University of California, San Francisco (UCSF) School of Medicine: Virtual Library in Epidemiology <http://www.epibiostat.ucsf.edu/epidem/epidem.html>. UCSF maintains an extensive listing of websites in epidemiology and related fields. Among the categories are government agencies and international organizations, data sources, and university sites.

World Health Organization (WHO) <http://www.who.int/en/>. The WHO is the directing and coordinating authority for health within the United Nations system. It is responsible for providing leadership on global health matters, shaping the health research agenda, setting norms and standards, articulating evidence-based policy options, providing technical support to countries, and monitoring and assessing health trends. From this site, one can access *The World Health Report*, WHO's leading publication that provides an expert assessment on global health with a focus on a specific subject each year.

REFERENCES

1. Brownson RC, Baker EA, Leet TL, Gillespie KN, True WR. *Evidence-Based Public Health.* 2nd ed. New York, NY: Oxford University Press; 2011.
2. Fielding JE, Briss PA. Promoting evidence-based public health policy: can we have better evidence and more action? *Health Aff (Millwood).* Jul-Aug 2006;25(4):969–978.
3. Sallis JF, Owen N, Fotheringham MJ. Behavioral epidemiology: a systematic framework to classify phases of research on health promotion and disease prevention. *Ann Behav Med.* 2000;22(4):294–298.
4. Brunner JW, Sankare IC, Kahn KL. Interdisciplinary priorities for dissemination, implementation, and improvement science: frameworks, mechanics, and measures. *Clin Transl Sci.* Dec 2015;8(6):820–823.
5. Green LW, Ottoson JM, Garcia C, Hiatt RA. Diffusion theory, and knowledge dissemination, utilization, and integration in public health. *Annu Rev Public Health.* Jan 2009;30:151–174.
6. Brownson R, Colditz G, Proctor E, eds. *Dissemination and Implementation Research in Health: Translating Science to Practice.* New York, NY: Oxford University Press; 2012.
7. Gostin LO. Politics and public health: the Flint drinking water crisis. *Hastings Cent Rep.* Jul 2016;46(4):5–6.
8. Hanna-Attisha M, LaChance J, Sadler RC, Champney Schnepp A. elevated blood lead levels in children associated with the Flint drinking water crisis: a spatial analysis of risk and public health response. *Am J Public Health.* Feb 2015;106(2):283–290.
9. US Department of Health and Human Services. *Report to the U.S. Congress: The Long Island Breast Cancer Study Project.* Bethesda, MD: National Institutes of Health; 2004.
10. Winn DM. Science and society: the Long Island Breast Cancer Study Project. *Nat Rev Cancer.* Dec 2005;5(12):986–994.
11. Porta M, ed. *A Dictionary of Epidemiology.* 6th ed. New York, NY: Oxford University Press; 2014.
12. Olson CM, Rennie D, Cook D, et al. Publication bias in editorial decision making. *JAMA.* Jun 5 2002;287(21):2825–2828.
13. Dwan K, Gamble C, Williamson PR, Kirkham JJ. Systematic review of the empirical evidence of study publication bias and outcome reporting bias: an updated review. *PLoS One.* 2013;8(7):e66844.
14. Guyatt G, Rennie D, Meade M, Cook D, eds. *Users' Guides to the Medical Literature. A Manual for Evidence-Based Clinical Practice.* 3rd ed. Chicago, IL: American Medical Association Press; 2015.
15. Petitti DB. *Meta-analysis, Decision Analysis, and Cost-Effectiveness Analysis: Methods for Quantitative Synthesis in Medicine.* 2nd ed. New York, NY: Oxford University Press; 2000.
16. Delgado-Rodriguez M. Systematic reviews of meta-analyses: applications and limitations. *J Epidemiol Community Health.* Feb 2006;60(2):90–92.
17. Liberati A, Altman DG, Tetzlaff J, et al. The PRISMA statement for reporting systematic reviews and meta-analyses of studies that evaluate healthcare interventions: explanation and elaboration. *BMJ.* 2009;339:b2700.

18. Bonita R, Beaglehole R, Kjellstrom T. *Basic Epidemiology*. 2nd ed. Geneva, Switzerland: World Health Organization; 2006.
19. Savitz DA. *Interpreting Epidemiologic Evidence. Strategies for Study Design and Analysis*. New York, NY: Oxford University Press; 2003.
20. Rivers TM. Viruses and Koch's postulates. *Journal of Bacteriology*. 1937;33:1–12.
21. US Department of Health, Education, and Welfare. *Smoking and Health. Report of the Advisory Committee to the Surgeon General of the Public Health Service*. Vol. Publication (PHS) 1103. Washington, DC: Centers for Disease Control; 1964.
22. Hill AB. The environment and disease: association or causation? *Proc R Soc Med*. 1965;58:295–300.
23. Susser M. *Causal Thinking in the Health Sciences: Concepts and Strategies in Epidemiology*. New York, NY: Oxford University Press; 1973.
24. Rothman KJ. Causes. *Am J Epidemiol*. 1976;104:587–592.
25. Rothman K, Greenland S, Lash T. *Modern Epidemiology*. 3rd ed. Philadelphia, PA: Lippincott Williams & Wilkins; 2012.
26. Weed DL. Epidemiologic evidence and causal inference. *Hematol Oncol Clin North Am*. 2000;14(4):797–807.
27. Ward AC. The role of causal criteria in causal inferences: Bradford Hill's "aspects of association." *Epidemiol Perspect Innov*. 2009;6:2.
28. Briss PA, Zaza S, Pappaioanou M, et al. Developing an evidence-based Guide to Community Preventive Services: methods. The Task Force on Community Preventive Services. *Am J Prev Med*. 2000;18(1 Suppl):35–43.
29. Briss PA, Brownson RC, Fielding JE, Zaza S. Developing and using the Guide to Community Preventive Services: lessons learned about evidence-based public health. *Annu Rev Public Health*. Jan 2004;25:281–302.
30. Concato J, Shah N, Horwitz RI. Randomized, controlled trials, observational studies, and the hierarchy of research designs. *N Engl J Med*. 2000;342:1887–1892.
31. Zaza S, Briss PA, Harris KW, eds. *The Guide to Community Preventive Services: What Works to Promote Health?* New York, NY: Oxford University Press; 2005.
32. Green LW. From research to "best practices" in other settings and populations. *Am J Health Behav*. 2001;25(3):165–178.
33. Rychetnik L, Hawe P, Waters E, Barratt A, Frommer M. A glossary for evidence based public health. *J Epidemiol Community Health*. Jul 2004;58(7):538–545.
34. Klesges LM, Williams NA, Davis KS, Buscemi J, Kitzmann KM. External validity reporting in behavioral treatment of childhood obesity: a systematic review. *Am J Prev Med*. Feb 2012;42(2):185–192.
35. Glasgow RE. What types of evidence are most needed to advance behavioral medicine? *Ann Behav Med*. Jan-Feb 2008;35(1):19–25.
36. Glasgow RE, Green LW, Klesges LM, et al. External validity: we need to do more. *Ann Behav Med*. Apr 2006;31(2):105–108.
37. Green LW, Glasgow RE. Evaluating the relevance, generalization, and applicability of research: issues in external validation and translation methodology. *Eval Health Prof*. Mar 2006;29(1):126–153.
38. Green LW, Glasgow RE, Atkins D, Stange K. Making evidence from research more relevant, useful, and actionable in policy, program planning, and practice slips "twixt cup and lip". *Am J Prev Med*. Dec 2009;37(6 Suppl 1):S187–S191.
39. Green LW, Kreuter MW. *Health Promotion Planning: An Educational and Ecological Approach*. 4th ed. New York, NY: McGraw-Hill; 2005.
40. Yin RK. *Case Study Research: Design and Methods*. 5th ed. Thousand Oaks, CA: Sage Publications; 2014.

41. Anderson LM, Brownson RC, Fullilove MT, et al. Evidence-based public health policy and practice: promises and limits. *Am J Prev Med.* Jun 2005;28(5 Suppl):226–230.

42. Bero LA, Jadad AR. How consumers and policy makers can use systematic reviews for decision making. In: Mulrow C, Cook D, eds. *Systematic Reviews. Synthesis of Best Evidence for Health Care Decisions.* Philadelphia, PA: American College of Physicians; 1998:45–54.

43. Mays GP, Scutchfield FD. Improving population health by learning from systems and services. *Am J Public Health.* Apr 2015;105(Suppl 2):S145–S147.

44. Ernster VL. Mammography screening for women aged 40 through 49: a guidelines saga and a clarion call for informed decision making. *Am J Public Health.* 1997;87(7):1103–1106.

45. American Cancer Society. *Cancer Facts and Figures 2016.* Atlanta, GA: American Cancer Society; 2016.

46. Breslow L, Agran L, Breslow DM, Morganstern M, Ellwein L. Final Report of NCI Ad Hoc Working Groups on Mammography in Screening for Breast Cancer. *J Natl Cancer Inst.* 1977;59(2):469–541.

47. National Institutes of Health Consensus Development Panel. National Institutes of Health Consensus Development Conference Statement: Breast Cancer Screening for Women Ages 40-49, January 21-23, 1997. *J Natl Cancer Inst.* 1997;89:1015–1026.

48. Screening for breast cancer: U.S. Preventive Services Task Force recommendation statement. *Ann Intern Med.* Nov 17 2009;151(10):716–726, W-236.

49. U.S. Preventive Services Task Force. Final Recommendation Statement: Breast Cancer: Screening. 3rd, http://www.uspreventiveservicestaskforce.org/Page/Document/RecommendationStatementFinal/breast-cancer-screening1. Accessed September 2, 2016.

50. Kolata G. Mammogram debate took group by surprise. *The New York Times.* November 20, 2009.

51. Oliver TR. The politics of public health policy. *Annu Rev Public Health.* 2006;27:195–233.

52. Brownson RC, Chriqui JF, Stamatakis KA. Understanding evidence-based public health policy. *Am J Public Health.* Sep 2009;99(9):1576–1583.

53. Liu L, Nelson J, Newschaffer C. Cardiovascular disease. In: Remington PL, Brownson RC, Wegner M, eds. *Chronic Disease Epidemiology and Control.* 3rd ed. Washington, DC: American Public Health Association; 2016.

54. Gargiullo PM, Rothenberg RB, Wilson HG. Confidence intervals, hypothesis tests, and sample sizes for the prevented fraction in cross-sectional studies. *Stat Med.* 1995;14(1):51–72.

55. Straatman H, Verbeek AL, Peeters PH. Etiologic and prevented fraction in case-control studies of screening. *J Clin Epidemiol.* 1988;41(8):807–811.

56. Thacker SB, Ikeda RM, Gieseker KE, et al. The evidence base for public health informing policy at the Centers for Disease Control and Prevention. *Am J Prev Med.* Oct 2005;29(3):227–233.

57. Howlader N, Noone A, Krapcho M, et al. *SEER Cancer Statistics Review, 1975-2013.* Bethesda, MD: National Cancer Institute; 2016.

58. Breslow L. The future of public health: prospects in the United States for the 1990s. *Annu Rev Public Health.* 1990;11:1–28.

59. Nightingale EO, Cureton M, Kamar V, Trudeau MB. *Perspectives on Health Promotion and Disease Prevention in the United States. [staff paper].* Washington, DC: Institute of Medicine, National Academy of Sciences; 1978.

60. U.S. Department of Health, Education, and Welfare. *Healthy People. The Surgeon General's Report on Health Promotion and Disease Prevention.* Washington, DC: U.S. Department of Health, Education, and Welfare; 1979. Publication no. 79-55071.

61. Irvine L, Elliott L, Wallace H, Crombie IK. A review of major influences on current public health policy in developed countries in the second half of the 20th century. *J R Soc Promot Health.* Mar 2006;126(2):73–78.

62. Fielding J, Kumanyika S. Recommendations for the concepts and form of Healthy People 2020. *Am J Prev Med.* Sep 2009;37(3):255–257.

63. Szklo M. Translating epi data into public policy is subject of Hopkins symposium. Focus is on lessons learned from experience. *The Epidemiology Monitor.* 1998(August/September).

64. Wainberg MA, Jeang KT. 25 years of HIV-1 research: progress and perspectives. *BMC Med.* 2008;6:31.

65. American Cancer Society. Report on the cancer-related health checkup. *CA: Cancer J Clin.* 1980;30:193–196.

CHAPTER 4

cҳɔ

Understanding and Applying Economic Evaluation and Other Analytic Tools

There are in fact two things: science and opinion. One begets knowledge, the latter ignorance.

Hippocrates

The preceding chapters have underlined the desirability of using evidence to inform decision making in public health. The first chapter gave an overview and definitions of evidence-based practice. The second chapter made the case for expanding capacity for evidence-based public health. The third chapter described the scientific factors to consider when determining whether some type of public health action is warranted. This chapter describes several useful tools for evidence-based public health practice that help practitioners answer the question, "Is this program or policy worth doing?" The primary focus is on economic evaluation, which compares the costs and benefits of a program or policy as one way to address this question. Six other analytic tools are also presented. Epidemiology, which is its own area of analytics, is presented in the seventh chapter.

Chapter 4 has five main parts. First, we describe some context for these methods. Then we describe economic evaluation, a set of methods for comparing benefits and costs. One particular type of economic evaluation, cost-effectiveness analysis (CEA), is described in greater detail. The third part discusses several analytic tools for measuring intervention impact and effectiveness. In the fourth section, several challenges and opportunities in using these analytic tools are discussed. A major goal of this chapter is to help readers develop an understanding of these evidence-based methods and an appreciation of their usefulness. The number of publications using these methods, particularly economic evaluation, has grown exponentially over the years.

We seek to assist practitioners in becoming informed consumers of these publications.

BACKGROUND

Economic evaluation aims at improving the allocation of scarce resources. Given that we cannot afford to do everything, how do we choose among projects? Economic evaluation identifies and weighs the relative costs and benefits of competing alternatives so that the project with the least costs for a given benefit, or the greatest benefits for a given cost, can be identified and chosen. Economic evaluations can be conducted before implementation of an intervention to assess feasibility, alongside interventions,[1-5] or after the intervention has concluded. Economic evaluations can use prospective data to determine the cost-effectiveness of a new project, use the existing literature to forecast the impact of a proposed program or policy, or use a combination of both prospective data and the existing literature. The number of economic evaluations has grown over the years, and public health decision makers can now search the literature for economic evaluations of a potential intervention to help them decide whether to undertake that intervention.

Several quantitative techniques help support economic evaluations. For example, a key component in economic evaluation is the cost of the illness or disease that the intervention is designed to address. Resources will be saved by preventing the condition or treating it more effectively. Cost of illness studies measure the direct and indirect costs of diseases and conditions, giving an estimate of the anticipated number of individuals experiencing the condition and the potential costs saved by preventing the illness or disease and its sequelae.

Another useful quantitative method for economic evaluation is decision analysis. A necessary step in all economic evaluations is the specification of all alternatives and their costs and benefits. For example, some participants in a smoking cessation program may quit smoking, some may quit smoking and relapse, and some may continue to smoke. These groups may then differ in their probability of having lung cancer later in life. This part of the analysis can be complex, with multiple alternatives, each with their own probability of occurrence. Decision analysis is an analytic tool designed to assist with complex decision making.

Finally, only effective interventions should be assessed with economic evaluation, so knowing the effectiveness of interventions is key. Several quantitative methods are relevant to determining the effectiveness of an intervention. Meta-analysis and pooled analysis are two methods to quantitatively combine the results of multiple studies. Risk assessment is a method to determine the risks to people due to an adverse exposure. Health impact assessments are a related method that determines the risk and benefits to health posed by interventions commonly thought to be non–health related, such as subsidized housing or public transportation.

ECONOMIC EVALUATION: A TOOL FOR COMPARING OPTIONS AND WEIGHING BENEFITS VERSUS COSTS

Economic evaluation is the comparison of costs and benefits to determine the most efficient allocation of scarce resources. We undertake economic evaluations all the time in everyday life, though we seldom think of the process explicitly. For example, ordering lunch at a fast-food restaurant requires weighing the costs (monetary and caloric) versus the benefits (nutrition and flavor) of all of the options. Then, we choose a meal that is the "best" use of our resources—the best value for the money. This implicit weighing of costs and benefits is almost automatic, though we've probably all faced a menu that seemed to offer too many options at one time or another. In most public health applications, however, weighing the costs and benefits does not happen so automatically.

What are the distinguishing features of public health that require a formal economic evaluation? Consider three features of the restaurant example. First, the costs and benefits are all borne by one person, the diner, who has an incentive to compare costs and benefits and make a wise choice. Second, the information needed for the choice is fairly easy to obtain. In many fast-food restaurants, the food choices are described and listed along with the prices and calories. The diner knows his or her own palate and preferences. Finally, the stakes are fairly low. A bad decision can be remedied by ordering another item (though this has costs) or by avoiding the food choice or restaurant the next time the diner eats out.

All three of these characteristics are absent from most public health decisions. First, by their nature, public health programs are aimed at improving the health of a community, so benefits will be spread over a large number of people. Costs are also typically spread over a large group, often through taxation. Second, the information about costs and benefits may not be easy to obtain. Benefits and costs must be measured over many people. Often, the benefits include hard-to-measure items like improved health status. Third, the stakes are often relatively high. Programs may be expensive and resources scarce, so only a few of a large range of interventions may be funded. A bad choice cannot easily be remedied.

Types of Economic Evaluation

There are four interrelated types of economic evaluation: cost-benefit analysis (CBA), cost-effectiveness analysis (CEA), cost-utility analysis (CUA), and cost-minimization analysis (CMA). This chapter explains these methods, focusing primarily on CEA and CUA. These are the recommended methods of the US Public Health Service Panel on Cost-Effectiveness in Health and Medicine[6] and the most commonly used methods today.

The four methods differ primarily in the way that they measure benefits. CBA measures benefits in monetary units (e.g., dollars, Euros), whereas CEA measures benefits in a naturally occurring health unit (e.g., lives saved, years of life saved). CUA is a type of CEA in which benefits are adjusted for quality of life and quantified with a health utility measure (usually quality-adjusted life-years, or QALYs). CMA is only used when the benefits of the two interventions are identical, so the unit of measurement of benefits is not an issue. Because CBA uses the most "generic" outcome measure (many things can be measured in currency, including the value of transportation projects and educational interventions), it allows for the comparison of the most programs. As we move to CEA, then to CUA, and finally to CMA, the range of programs that can be compared narrows.

Economic evaluation is closely related to return-on-investment (ROI) analysis, business plans, and capital investment decision tools. All of these business tools are undertaken within businesses to compare the costs and benefits of a proposed project or investment to the business entity. As in the fast-food restaurant example, these methods assume that all of the costs are borne by the business and all of the benefits accrue to the business. Economic evaluations use many of the same analytic methods but differ by including costs and benefits that accrue to multiple parties, such as the individual, his or her social network, and society.

All economic evaluations compare one intervention or program to another. Figure 4.1 provides a diagram of an economic evaluation. As shown in the figure, the alternative program can be "standard care" or "no program," but the analysis is always framed as, "What are the extra, or incremental, costs and the extra, or incremental, benefits of this program compared with another program?" This requirement is helpful to the analyst because it is often easier to determine the incremental costs and benefits than the total costs and benefits. The primary outcome of an economic evaluation is the incremental cost-effectiveness ratio (ICER):

$$ICER = \frac{Incremental\,costs}{Incremental\,benefits}$$

The particular items included in the numerator and denominator will depend on the intervention and the type of economic evaluation.

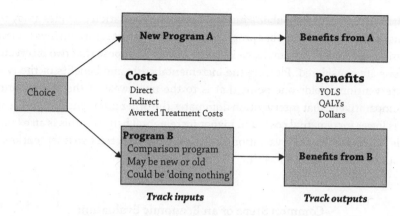

Figure 4.1: Diagram of an economic evaluation. QALYs = quality-adjusted life-years; YOLS = years of life saved.

Outcomes of an Economic Evaluation

Figure 4.2 shows the potential outcomes of an economic evaluation.[7] Consider the four quadrants of the graph. Programs that improve health and save money (quadrant IV) are obviously worthwhile and should be undertaken. Similarly, programs that worsen health and add to costs (quadrant II) are undesirable and should not be initiated or continued. The remaining two quadrants (I and III) are where the dilemmas lie and where economic evaluation can be informative.

Historically, as public health systems develop, interventions and programs begin in quadrant IV, with those programs that are both cost saving and improve health. Many early public health interventions, such as sanitation systems, fall in quadrant IV. As more of these interventions are implemented, attention turns to quadrant I, programs that improve health at some cost. In times of budgetary pressures, quadrant III programs are considered: programs that reduce costs, but at some loss of health status. For both of these quadrants, the question is, "What is the return on the investment (or

	Aggregate Health Benefits	
Quadrant IV		*Quadrant I*
Saves money, Improves health		Costs money, Improves health
		Aggregate Costs
Saves money, Worsens health		Costs money, Worsens health
Quadrant III		*Quadrant II*

Figure 4.2: Possible outcomes of an economic evaluation.
Source: Adapted from Drummond et al.[7]

disinvestment) of the public's funds?" Economic evaluation provides a way to answer this question so that programs with the greatest return on investment can be selected. For example, consider quadrant I. Suppose that two interventions are considered. Plotting the incremental costs and benefits of the two interventions yields one point that is to the northwest of the other point. Comparatively, that intervention dominates the other intervention because it has lower incremental costs and higher incremental benefits. This is an example in which economic evaluation can help choose between two interventions, both of which improve health.

Common Steps of an Economic Evaluation

Whether one wants to conduct an economic evaluation or use the results of an existing evaluation, it is helpful to understand the mechanics of these analyses. Every economic evaluation includes nine steps:

1. Identify an effective intervention for the problem and people at risk
2. Select the perspective of the analysis
3. Select the type of economic evaluation to perform
4. Measure costs
5. Measure outcomes
6. Discount costs and benefits as needed
7. Construct the ICER
8. Conduct a sensitivity analysis
9. Compare the ICER to external standards or use internally

In this section, the first three steps are considered. The remaining steps are considered separately.

The first step is to identify the intervention and the group. Unless the economic evaluation is to be conducted alongside a new intervention, the intervention should have already been demonstrated to be effective. There is nothing to be gained from an economic evaluation of an ineffective intervention. The intervention and the group it applies to should be specified as completely as possible, including identifying the expected benefits of the program.

The second element is the selection of the perspective of the economic evaluation. Any intervention can be considered from several points of view, often characterized as moving from narrow to broad. The narrowest perspective is that of the agency or organization directly involved in delivering the proposed intervention. A next level might be the perspective of insurers, or payers, especially in health, where consumers and payers are often two separate groups. The broadest perspective is that of society as a whole. The Panel on Cost-Effectiveness in Health and Medicine recommends this broad perspective for all economic evaluations,[6] and it is required in several countries with national health systems. The societal perspective is the most appropriate in public health because interventions are designed to benefit the public and taxpayers who fund the costs.

However, an analyst may wish to conduct an economic evaluation from two perspectives, or highlight some aspects of an analysis for particular stakeholders. For example, a workplace injury prevention program can be analyzed from a societal perspective, counting the avoided pain and suffering of workers as a major benefit. Another benefit to the employer is the avoided lost productivity and avoided medical claims. Highlighting these benefits for the employer may encourage employer participation and may even justify some payment for the program by the employer.

The perspective of the analysis will determine which costs and benefits are included in the analysis. In general, the broader the perspective, the more costs and benefits that are included. This chapter focuses on the societal perspective and thus lists all of the possible costs and benefits that can be included. If a narrower perspective is taken, some of the costs or benefits in the text and tables may not be counted. The perspective can be thought of as a fishing net—the broader the perspective, the larger the net that is cast, and the more that is "caught," or included.

The third step is the selection of the appropriate type of economic evaluation. Table 4.1 shows the different types of economic evaluation and their defining characteristics.[8-10]

Selection of the type of economic evaluation primarily depends on the benefits of the program. If they can be easily measured in monetary units, then CBA is appropriate. If there is a primary benefit that can be measured as a naturally occurring health unit, then CEA can be used. If there are multiple health benefits, such as mortality and morbidity reductions, then CUA is appropriate. Finally, if the benefits of the programs being compared are identical, then a CMA can be used.

Measure Costs

The fourth step is the identification and measurement of all incremental costs of a program, option, or intervention. Incremental costs are the additional costs related to the program. The scope of the costs is determined by the perspective of the analysis. If such costs are concentrated among a small group of people, this step will be relatively easy. As costs are more dispersed, it may become more difficult to identify all potential costs. Measurement of the identified costs may similarly be complicated by issues of units of measurement (e.g., monetary wages vs. donated labor time) and timing (e.g., costs incurred over a 5-year interval).

Table 4.1. TYPES OF ECONOMIC EVALUATIONS AND MEASUREMENT OF BENEFITS

Type of Analysis	Benefit (Outcome) and Example	Measurement of Benefits
Cost-minimization analysis (CMA)	Identical, but costs are different *Can we do it for less?*	None (identical measure and amount of benefit)
	CMA compares the costs of different programs that produce the same health-related outcomes. **Example:** Program A. Participants walk 4 days per week. • Lowers cardiovascular disease (CVD) risk by 10% • Costs $3000 per participant per year Program B. Participants reduce fat from 40% to 30% of calories • Lowers CVD risk by 10% • Costs $2500 per participant per year Both programs are equally effective in lowering CVD risk, so compare data on costs only. Decision: Choose the reduced fat intake intervention	
Cost-benefit analysis (CBA)	Single or multiple benefits (outcomes) standardized into a single monetary value (in present dollars) *Is there a reasonable return on investment?*	Monetary units (e.g., dollars, Euros)
	CBA compares the costs and benefits of 2 or more programs using monetary outcomes. It is the gold standard for economic evaluation (EE) and is the most common form of EE in business (also called return-on-investment [ROI] analysis). Lower cost-benefit ratios and higher net benefits are desirable. Ratios <1 indicate that the program is cost saving. **Example:**[8] Intervention: Neighborhood-based program to prevent teen pregnancy Program costs: $9,386 per participant per year Effects: reduced teen pregnancy from 94/1000 to 40/1000 When combined with effects, the cost per birth averted is $26,142 The savings per birth averted (or benefits) are $81,256 The incremental cost-effectiveness ratio (ICER) for the program is $26,142/$81,256, or 0.32. The net benefits are $55,114 (=$81,256 – $26,142) per birth averted	

Table 4.1. CONTINUED

Type of Analysis	Benefit (Outcome) and Example	Measurement of Benefits
Cost-effectiveness analysis (CEA)	Single common benefit (or outcome) *Are the (natural) outcomes worth the cost?* CEA compares the costs and benefits of different programs using the same outcome measure. Outcome measures are naturally occurring health outcomes, such as cases found, years of life saved, or injuries prevented. CEA is easy to understand in the health field and avoids converting health outcomes to dollars. It is limited in its ability to compare interventions because those compared must have the same outcome. The result of a CEA (its ICER) is the cost per unit of health outcome (e.g., cost per year of life saved). Lower ratios are preferred. **Example:**[9] Intervention: Smoking cessation program in the workplace Costs measured: All costs of the cessation program for all 100 participants—$8940 Effect measured: Number of people who quit smoking (quitters)—15 quitters The incremental cost-effectiveness ratio (ICER) = $596 per additional quitter	Natural units, e.g. life years gained, lower A1C levels, improved physical activity
Cost-utility analysis (CUA)	1 or more benefits (outcomes) standardized into a single value *Are standardized outcomes worth the cost?* CUA compares the costs and benefits of a program, with benefits measured in health-related quality of life-years (QALYs). CUA allows for comparison of many projects with health-related outcomes and is useful when both morbidity and mortality are affected or the programs have a wide range of outcomes but all have an effect on healthy years of life. Translating health outcomes, particularly morbidity, to years of healthy life is controversial. The result of a CUA (its ICER) is the cost per QALY ($/QALY). Lower values are preferred. **Example**[10]: Intervention: Diabetes self-management programs in primary care settings Program costs: $866 per participant per year, total lifetime costs of program $11,760 Several effects: 87.5% benefited, A1c -0.5%, total cholesterol. -10% Using QALYs to add up all effects results in lifetime gain of 0.2972 QALYs ICER: $39,563/QALY saved	QALYs

After all costs are identified and counted, they will be summed to form the numerator of the ICER. Table 4.2 shows the types of costs and their usual measures. The labels and definitions for the types of costs vary across disciplines and across textbooks. The important objective of the cost portion of the analysis is the identification and determination of *all* costs, regardless of their labels.

The first category of costs is direct, or program, costs. One caution in stating these costs is that the true economic cost of providing the program should be identified. This is the resource cost of the program, also referred to as the opportunity cost. If this program is undertaken, what other program will we forego? What opportunity must be passed up in order to fund this program? In health, there is often a distinction between *charges* and *costs*. For example, a screening test for diabetes may be billed at $200; however, the cost of providing the test may be $150. From a societal standpoint, the $150 figure should be used. But from the replication standpoint, the charge of $200 is relevant because this is what it would cost to replicate the program.

Direct costs include labor costs, often measured by the number of full-time equivalent employees (FTEs) and their wages and fringe benefits. If volunteers will be used, the value of their time should be imputed using either their own wage rates or the average wage rate for similarly skilled work within the community. Other direct costs are supplies and overhead. (Table 4.3 provides a detailed worksheet for determining direct costs.)

Indirect costs are the other main component of costs. By indirect, we mean that they are not directly paid by the sponsoring agency or organization or directly received by the program participants. In other words, these are costs that "spill over," and they are often referred to as spillover costs. These can be subdivided into five categories. Three of these (time and travel costs, the cost of treating side effects, and the cost of treatment during gained life expectancy) are positive costs and are added to the numerator. The other two (averted treatment costs and averted productivity losses) are negative costs (i.e., benefits) that are subtracted from the numerator. They are included in the numerator because they directly affect the public health budget. This is especially true in a nation with a global health budget but is also recommended for the United States.

The first category of indirect costs is time and travel costs to the participants. From a societal standpoint, these costs should be attributed to the program. Often, to obtain these costs, a survey of program participants must be conducted. In addition, if other family members or friends are involved as caregivers to the program participants, their time and travel costs should be included. An example of this category of indirect costs would occur with a diabetes case management program that featured extra provider visits, group meetings, and recommended exercise. The time spent in all of these aspects of the program should be valued and counted, as well as any related

Table 4.2 TYPES OF COSTS INCLUDED IN
ECONOMIC EVALUATIONS

Category of Cost	Usual Measures and Examples
	Direct or Program Costs
Labor	Wages and fringe benefits
Supplies	Supplies for the intervention, including office supplies, materials
Overhead	Allocation for office space, rent, utilities
	Indirect or Spillover Costs

Positive indirect costs; to be added to costs

Time and travel costs	Time costs to participants, including lost wages
	Travel costs to participants, including transportation and child care
	Caregiver costs, including both time and travel
	Any costs of the program incurred by other budgetary groups
	The value of volunteer labor, measured using the cost to replace it
Cost of treating side effects	Cost of treatment; using actual cost or charge data or imputed, using local, regional, or national averages
Cost of treatment during gained life expectancy	National data on average cost of treatment per year, multiplied by extended life expectancy

Negative indirect costs (benefits); to be subtracted from costs

Averted treatment costs	Future health care treatment costs that will be saved as a result of a program or policy. Measured as the weighted sum of the cost of treatment, including alternative options and complications. Weights reflect the proportion of people projected to have each alternative treatment or complication. Data can be from administrative databases, such as claims data, or imputed, using local, regional, or national average costs or charges
Averted productivity losses	The present value of future wages earned because of disease or injury prevention. Includes costs to employers of replacing absent workers (recruitment, training, etc.). Wages and fringe benefits of participants; for persons not in the labor force, average wages of similarly aged persons or local, regional, or national average wages

Table 4.3. WORSHEET FOR COLLECTING ECONOMIC INFORMATION

Line Item	Internal Resources (new budget allocation)	Internal In-Kind (reallocation of existing resources)	External Resources (grants, contracts, other public or private sources)	External In-Kind (donated services or nonfinancial resources)
Personnel (staff or contractors)				
Examples:				
Coordinator				
Data manager				
Health educator				
Evaluator				
Administrative support staff				
Technical support/ consultants				
Subject matter experts				
Meeting facilitators				
Graphic designer				
Marketing/public relations specialist				
Copy writer/editor				
Website designer				
Fringe benefits				
Equipment and Materials				
Examples:				
Office supplies				
Meeting supplies				
Computer supplies				
Graphic design software				
Data software				
Audio equipment				
Presentation equipment				
Other equipment purchase				
Computer/copier				
Maintenance				
Facilities				
Examples:				
Clinical space				
Space for group meetings				
Conference and meeting rooms				

Table 4.3. CONTINUED

Line Item	Internal Resources (new budget allocation)	Internal In-Kind (reallocation of existing resources)	External Resources (grants, contracts, other public or private sources)	External In-Kind (donated services or nonfinancial resources)
Travel				
Examples:				
Staff meeting travel, lodging, and per diem				
Steering group travel and lodging				
Mileage associated with program implementation				
Other Nonpersonnel Service Costs				
Examples:				
Conference call services				
Long-distance services				
Website service				
Transcription costs for focus group tapes				
Indirect/overhead costs				
Total costs				

transportation expenses. How is the time to be valued? This is explained in the averted productivity losses section below.

The second category of indirect costs is the cost of treating side effects. If the intervention causes any side effects, the cost of treating them should be charged to the intervention. Most public health interventions do not cause substantial side effects, but some may have potential adverse effects. For example, there may be injuries among participants in an exercise program that promotes running.

The third component of indirect costs is the cost of treatment during gained life expectancy. If a person's life is extended because of an intervention, he or she will consume additional health care resources in those additional years. Should these costs be added to the numerator of the cost-utility ratio? Proponents of their inclusion argue that these costs are part of the health budget and will affect its future size. Thus, these costs are included in many studies conducted in countries with global health budgets, such as the United Kingdom. Those opposed point out that these persons will also be paying taxes, thus helping to support their additional consumption of health care. Why single out one aspect of their future spending? Most US-based studies do not include these costs. The Panel on Cost-Effectiveness in Health and Medicine did not make a recommendation with respect to this issue.[6]

The fourth group of indirect costs is averted treatment costs. These are future treatment costs that will be saved as a result of the intervention. For example, screening for diabetes might identify cases earlier and thus limit or prevent some complications and early mortality. These are complications that will not need to be treated (if prevented) or that will not need to be treated as expensively (if delayed). The onset of diabetes and the incidence of complications with and without the program must be estimated and then multiplied by the costs of treatment to obtain the averted treatment costs. Information on the natural course of a disease and the costs of its treatment are often available from the published literature or publicly available data sources. Cost of illness studies, described below, provide estimates of disease burden.

The fifth category is averted productivity losses. These represent the savings to society from avoiding reduced productivity and lost work time. This will be appropriate for workplace injury prevention programs, but many interventions lead to reduced absenteeism and increased productivity. For example, an asthma management program may lead to fewer sick days. In addition, as noted previously, the donated labor of caregivers or volunteers needs to be valued because it is a real cost, even if unbilled and unpaid. If others wish to replicate the intervention and do not have volunteers, they have an estimate of the labor expense.

Ideally, productivity losses are measured directly using the wages and fringe benefits of participants. Often this information is not available—either it was not collected, or it does not exist because the participants are not in the labor force. In this case, the average wages and fringe benefits of similar persons, or of the average person, can be used to estimate this negative cost. In the United States, average wages by profession can be found at the Bureau of Labor Statistics website, and similar sites exist for many other countries. Sources such as these are useful for valuing volunteer labor, as well.

There are several tools and instruments available for estimating productivity costs, including absenteeism and the value of unpaid time.[11,12] These surveys ask about occupation, other activities (differentiating caregiving tasks from other activities), and time usually spent at paid work or engaged in unpaid productive activities. They then provide a methodology to map the answers to an estimate of productivity costs.

Averted productivity losses are used in CBA and CEA but not in CUA. Benefits in a CUA are measured in terms of health utility, which in turn depends on a person's ability to work and earn an income. Thus, the negative costs of averted productivity losses are incorporated in the benefit measure in CUA. However, even in this method, it is often useful to calculate the averted productivity losses so that they can be highlighted for some stakeholders.

Measure Outcomes

The fifth step is the identification and measurement of all outcomes, or benefits. Again, the incremental benefits are of interest: what additional benefits will this program provide, compared with some specified alternative? This step is often more complicated than the identification and measurement of costs. In public health, benefits can include improved health status (cases prevented) and improved mortality outcomes (deaths averted). Clearly, these benefits will be difficult to measure and will be partially subjective.

Another complicating factor for public health is the selection of the relevant time period. The aim of a program or intervention is the improvement of health, so the output to be measured is improved health status. This is a final outcome that may take many years to achieve. Often, a program can only track participants for a brief period of time, and any evaluation will, of necessity, measure intermediate outcomes, such as the number of persons exercising. In such cases, the literature can often be used to extrapolate the effect of the intermediate outcome on health. For example, suppose that one were evaluating a program designed to increase physical activity levels. Other studies have demonstrated that increased physical activity reduces the risk for cardiac events. These studies can be used to estimate the anticipated final outcomes of the intervention.

The benefits of the program or intervention are the improvement in health and are thus conceptually identical, regardless of the type of economic evaluation. However, the unit of measurement and the specific elements included differ by type of evaluation. In a CMA, when the benefits of the intervention and its alternative are demonstrated to be identical, no further measurement of benefits is needed. CBA measures the benefits in money. Thus, improvements to health must be converted to currency amounts. If years of life are saved, then these years must be valued in monetary units. There are several suggested methods to make this conversion. All of them are subject to heated debate.[6]

In response to dissatisfaction with the measurement of health benefits in monetary units, particularly the wide range of values found using different methods, some analysts argued for measuring benefits in a naturally occurring health unit, such as years of life saved. This led to the development of CEA, which uses a single health measure (years of life saved, cases averted) as the measure of benefits. This has the advantage of not requiring reductions of different outcomes to a single scale, but a single health measure cannot capture all the benefits of most interventions. Most programs yield morbidity and mortality improvements. By being forced to select one health measure, only morbidity or mortality can be used to determine the cost-effectiveness of the project. This underestimates the cost-effectiveness of projects because the total costs are divided by only a portion of the benefits. In addition, only programs with outcomes measured in the same unit (e.g., lives saved) can be compared.

Partly in response to the shortcomings of CEA, some analysts argued for the development of a health utility measure of benefits. Such a measure combines morbidity and mortality effects into a single metric and is based on the utility, or satisfaction, that health status gives to a person. Individuals' self-reports of their valuation of health form the basis of the health utility measure.

Several measures that meet these criteria have been developed. They include the quality-adjusted life-year (QALY), the disability-adjusted life-year (DALY), and the healthy year equivalent. The most widely used of these is the QALY, defined as the amount of time in perfect health that would be valued the same as a year with a disease or disability. For example, consider a year with end-stage renal disease, requiring dialysis. Conceptually, the QALY for this condition is the fraction of a year in perfect health that one would value the same as a full year with the condition. Thus, QALYs range from 0 to 1, with 0 defined as dead and 1 as a year in perfect health. The QALY assigned to this condition will vary across persons, with some considering the condition worse than others. If many individuals are surveyed, however, the average QALY assigned to this condition can be obtained.

There are several ways to elicit QALY weights from individuals. These include the visual rating scale, time trade-off method, and standard gamble. There is debate about the theoretically appropriate method and the consistency of results obtained from the different methods.[13] With the visual rating scale, survey participants are presented with a list of health conditions. Beside each description of a condition, there is a visual scale, or line, that ranges from 0 to 1. Participants are asked to indicate on the lines their QALY valuation of each health condition by making a mark. A participant might mark "0.6," for example, for the year with end-stage renal disease.

To measure the benefits in CUA, the analyst must identify all the morbidity and mortality effects of the intervention. These are then weighted by the appropriate QALY value. In practice, there are three ways to assign QALY weights to different conditions. The first is to directly elicit QALY weights from participants, as described earlier. The second is to use a multi-attribute utility function, such as the Euroqol 5 Dimension (EQ-5D) or the Health Utilities Index (HUI).[14,15] These are brief survey instruments that ask one to rate various attributes of health. For example, the EQ-5D rates five aspects of health (mobility, self-care, usual activities, pain/discomfort, and anxiety/depression) from 1 to 3. The responses are then scored to give a QALY value. The weights used for the scoring were obtained from surveys of the general population. The third way to obtain QALY values is by searching the literature or using the Internet. QALY values for many diseases and conditions can be found. Some studies report QALY weights for only one or a few diseases or conditions (e.g., end-stage renal disease), whereas others include tables of QALY values for numerous health states.[16-19]

For example, suppose that an intervention among 1,000 persons yields 50 years of life saved. However, these years saved will be lived with some disability. Review of the literature indicates that this disability has a QALY weight of 0.7. The benefits of the 50 years of life saved would be valued at 50 • 0.7, or 35 QALYs. Similarly, suppose that the intervention also prevents morbidity among 500 of the participants for one year. If the QALY weight of the averted condition is 0.9, then (1 − 0.9), or 0.1 QALYs, is saved for each of the 500 persons, yielding a benefit of 50 QALYs. The total benefits for this program would be 35 + 50, or 85 QALYs. This summary measure thus combines both the morbidity and the mortality effects of the intervention. An illustration of the use of QALYs in measuring the impact of screening for diabetes is shown in Box 4.1.[20-24]

Discount Costs and Benefits as Needed

Discounting refers to the conversion of amounts (usually currency) received over different periods to a common value in the current period. For example, suppose that one were to receive $100 on today's date of each year for 5 years. Though the amount of money is the same, most people prefer, and value, the nearer payments more than the distant payments. The payment received today will be the most valuable because it can be spent today. One might be willing to trade a slightly smaller payment received today for the payment to be received 1 year from today, an even slightly smaller payment today for the payment due in 2 years, and so forth. Discounting is a formal way to determine the current payments that would be equal in value to distant payments.

In economic evaluation, costs occurring in the future should be discounted to current values. This puts outlays, or expenditures, to be paid in the future on an equal footing with current expenditures. The interest rate should reflect either the real rate of growth of the economy or the social rate of discount.[25] The social discount rate reflects a society's time preference. In practice, a discount rate of 2% to 3% is suggested by both methods. The Panel on Cost-Effectiveness in Health and Medicine recommends an interest rate between 0% and 8%,[6] and many studies use rates from 0% to 10%.

Box 4.1

COSTS OF SCREENING FOR TYPE 2 DIABETES

Type 2 diabetes is a chronic disease that usually develops during adulthood and can have multiple complications, including blindness, lower leg amputations, kidney failure, and cardiac problems. These complications can be delayed, minimized, or avoided entirely if the disease is well managed, with good control of blood sugar levels and screening for the onset of complications. Because the disease develops slowly, over a period of years, it is often called the "silent killer": people can live with undetected diabetes for several years, and then the disease is more advanced and the complication rate is higher when they are finally diagnosed. Screening for type 2 diabetes is thus an important prevention issue.

In the 1990s the Centers for Disease Control formed the Diabetes Cost-Effectiveness Study Group. As one part of their work, the Study Group considered opportunistic screening for type 2 diabetes and estimated its cost-effectiveness.[20] The costs and benefits of screening all adults, 25 years and older, at a regular physician visit were estimated.

Costs were estimated using national average charges for physician visits, screening tests, and treatments for the various complications. The occurrence of these costs was estimated, using a computer model that followed a hypothetical cohort of 10,000 adults from the age of screening to death. First, the cohort was assumed to have no routine screening. Second, the cohort was assumed to have screening at the next regular physician visit. The two cohorts were then compared with respect to morbidity and mortality. Because of the earlier detection and treatment of diabetes in the second cohort, those persons had slightly lower diabetes-related mortality, a lower incidence of complications, and delayed onset of complications.

The benefits of screening come at a cost, though. Screening of the entire adult US population would cost $236,449 per additional year of life saved, or $56,649 per quality-adjusted life-year (QALY). These ratios were relatively high compared with other screening programs and other reimbursed interventions. The Task Force also considered subgroups of adults as candidates for screening and found that it was much more cost-effective to screen black people and younger cohorts. Screening 25- to 34-year-olds was estimated to cost $35,768 per additional life-year saved and $13,376 per QALY. For blacks aged 25 to 34 years, the ratios were $2219 per life-year and $822 per QALY.

Because the American Diabetes Association recommends triannual screening of those 45 years and older, based on the presence of risk factors,[21] and the economic evaluation was somewhat sensitive to some key assumptions, the Task Force did not definitively recommend changing screening guidelines. However, it did note that the subgroup analyses strongly suggest that younger cohorts, who have a longer life span over which to accrue benefits, and minority cohorts, who have a higher incidence of diabetes, could benefit the most from screening.

In 2004, with concern about the increasing prevalence of diabetes rising, a new cost-effectiveness analysis of screening for diabetes was published.[23] This analysis followed the methods of the 1998 study, using computer modeling to estimate the costs and benefits of screening the US adult population. However, the authors incorporated new evidence that hypertension is a strong risk factor for diabetes. Subgroup analyses were run for adults with hypertension in 10-year age cohorts. For all ages, the cost-utility ratios were more favorable for persons with hypertension than for the entire population. For example, the cost per QALY for screening 55-year-olds with hypertension was $34,375, whereas the cost per QALY for screening all persons aged 55 years was $360,966. Screening 55- to 75-year-olds with hypertension was cost-effective, with cost-utility ratios below $50,000 per QALY.

In June 2008 the Task Force released updated guidelines, recommending with a grade of B that asymptomatic adults with sustained elevated blood pressure (>135/80 mm Hg, treated or untreated) be screened.[22] In its recommendation the Task Force noted that there is evidence that early detection and treatment of diabetes can delay or prevent the onset of macro- and micro-vascular complications, especially in persons with hypertension.

Revised guidelines were released by the Task Force in 2015.[24] A review of studies published from 2008 to 2105 found good evidence that progression to diabetes among people with impaired fasting glucose can be delayed by modifying diet and exercising. This was especially true for overweight and obese persons as well as those with hypertension. Accordingly, the Task Force broadened their recommendations, stating that all overweight or obese adults aged 40 to 70 years should be tested for abnormal blood sugar as part of a cardiovascular risk assessment.

Should benefits also be discounted? The Panel on Cost-Effectiveness in Health and Medicine recommends that they should be, arguing that, like money, nearer health states are preferred to farther ones. In other words, saving the life of a person today is more immediate, and hence more valuable, than saving the life of a person 30 years hence. On the other hand, money is liquid—that is, it can be stored in banks or financial instruments and withdrawn at later dates. Health cannot be "banked" in this way. In practice, many studies do not discount health benefits.

Construct the Incremental Cost-Effectiveness Ratio

The seventh step is the comparison of costs and benefits. This is found by forming the ICER, with costs in the numerator and benefits in the denominator. Table 4.4 shows the ICER for CBA, CEA, and CUA. These formulas reflect analyses conducted in the United States from a societal perspective. Note that the costs of treatment during gained life expectancy have not been included. This is true for analyses conducted in the United States. These costs may be included in studies conducted in other countries, such as the United Kingdom and Canada.

The numerator of the ICER is the same for CBA and CEA. Averted productivity losses are not included in cost-utility analysis because they enter into the determination of the QALY weights for the condition of interest.

In CBA, all the costs and benefits are measured in dollars, so the ratio becomes a single number reflecting the ratio of costs to benefits. For example, a ratio of 1.6 means that it will cost $1.60 for each $1.00 saved. Ratios below 1 indicate cost-saving interventions. Because both the numerator and the denominator are in currency units, the difference between benefits and costs, or net benefits, is often reported instead of a ratio. Net benefits greater than zero indicate a cost-saving intervention. In a CEA, benefits are measured in a naturally occurring health unit, so the ratio will be expressed in terms of that unit. For example, a project might cost $25,000 per life saved. The product of a CUA is stated in terms of QALYs—it costs $x for each QALY gained.

Conduct a Sensitivity Analysis

A final issue to consider is sensitivity analysis. Numerous assumptions are made in constructing the ICER. For example, the average effectiveness of an intervention as reported in a review article or meta-analysis may have been used in a CUA. The costs and benefits of the intervention depend on its effectiveness and will vary if the effectiveness is higher or lower than anticipated. Sensitivity analysis provides a way to estimate the effect of changing key assumptions used in the economic evaluation.

There are several ways to conduct a sensitivity analysis. All start by identifying the key assumptions and parameters that have been used in the economic evaluation. One method is to construct best-case and worst-case scenarios for the intervention, systematically varying all of the assumptions to favor and then to bias against the intervention. The ICER is recalculated for the best-case and worst-case scenarios and then reported along with the original ratio. Another method is to vary the key assumptions one at a time, recalculating the ICER each time. A table or figure is usually provided to report the ICERs for the different assumptions.

Table 4.4. INCREMENTAL COST EFFECTIVENESS RATIOS

CBA	CEA	CUA
$ICER = \dfrac{\text{Direct} + \text{indirect costs} - \text{Averted treatment costs} - \text{Averted productivity losses}}{\text{Monetary value of improved health}}$	$ICER = \dfrac{\text{Direct} + \text{indirect costs} - \text{Averted treatment costs} - \text{Averted productivity losses}}{\text{Naturally occurring health outcome}}$	$ICER = \dfrac{\text{Direct} + \text{indirect costs} - \text{Averted treatment costs}}{\text{QALYs}}$

The most common method is to use probabilistic sensitivity analysis techniques, specifying the distributions of key parameters and then randomly sampling from those distributions in multiple simulations.[26] The analyst then reports the original, or base case, ICER and the range of the ICER in 95% of the simulations. This is similar to a confidence interval but is based on the simulation results rather than statistical calculation. The sensitivity analysis can also indicate how sensitive the ICER is to various parameters used in the modeling.

Sensitivity analysis often identifies several parameters that influence the ICER. Consideration of these parameters can then lead to the identification of subgroups for which the intervention is more or less cost-effective. For example, perhaps the ICER is found to be sensitive to the age of the participants. The analyst may then calculate and report the ICER for different age groups. This may help to redefine the appropriate target audience for the intervention. Regardless of the method used, a sensitivity analysis is a vital component of an economic evaluation. The less variation there is in the ICER as key assumptions are varied, the more confident one can be in the results.

Compare the Incremental Cost-Effectiveness Ratio to External Standards or Use Internally

The final step is the interpretation of the results. If one finds, for example, that a program costs $27,000 per life saved, is the program worthwhile? There are numerous ways to approach this question, involving ethics, practical considerations, political realities, and economics. One could argue that, clearly, a life is worth $27,000, and the program is worthwhile. If, however, there is another program that costs $15,000 per life saved and the budget allows only one to be funded, an argument can be made that the latter program is more worthwhile than the former. There are two principal ways to interpret and use the ICER. The first compares the cost-utility ratio internally to other competing programs; the other uses external references, comparing the ratio to an established threshold value. Interventions below the threshold are considered worthwhile.

If several economic evaluations of competing programs have been conducted within an organization, or if information on the cost-effectiveness of several interventions can be obtained, then an internal comparison is warranted. The programs can be ranked from the lowest ICER to the highest. Programs with the lowest ratios should generally be funded first, after other considerations are taken into account. For example, a program manager and policy maker also need to consider the amount of resources required to establish and maintain a program, the ethics of various approaches, and the socio-political environment.

Comparison with similar programs helps the practitioner decide whether the proposed program is relatively efficient. If existing screening programs for diabetes cost $25,000 per QALY and the proposed screening program is estimated to cost $15,000 per QALY, then it represents a more efficient screening method.

The alternative way to decide whether a given ICER justifies a program is to compare that ratio with an external threshold value for the ratio. In the United States, a threshold of $50,000 per QALY (approximately $100,000 in current dollars) has often been referenced, with periodic calls for higher values or the use of multiple, or tiered, thresholds.[27] How is the threshold value determined? There are two main approaches. One looks at programs that have already been funded, reasoning that society must value such programs. Comparison with programs that are already funded helps the practitioner argue for funding by insurers or public agencies. For example, the Medicare program provides mammography for women aged 65 years and older. This coverage is partially based on economic evaluations of breast cancer screening that estimated cost-utility ratios of between $12,000 and $20,000 per QALY.[28] In 2015 dollars, these ratios are $25,037 to $41,728 per QALY. A recent extension of this approach in the United States considered all health care spending, whether federally financed or not, and compared it to improvements in health status to determine a threshold range of $184,000 to $264,000 per QALY.[29]

The alternative approach looks at the average wages of workers and their implied preferences about health and well-being. In the United States, Garber and Phelps[30] used this approach to determine a $50,000 per QALY threshold, based on the average wages of American workers and the context of other publicly funded programs. At the time of the study, $50,000 was roughly twice the average annual wage of an American worker. At current dollar values, the $50,000 per QALY threshold would be approximately $100,000 per QALY. Others have argued for two to three times the average wage as a QALY threshold in developing countries.[31,32] The National Institute for Health and Clinical Excellence (NICE) in Great Britain uses a threshold range of £20,000 to £30,000.[33] Regardless of the method used, there is considerable debate about the appropriate threshold value, particularly in the United States.[27, 34-36]

An important final step in an economic evaluation is the reporting of the results, particularly the ICER, in the literature. There are now several catalogs of ICERs available in the literature and on the Internet, many of which are listed in the websites section at the end of this chapter. Often, the public health practitioner can refer to these sources to determine what is already known about the cost-effectiveness of a public health intervention.

CHALLENGES AND OPPORTUNITIES IN USING ECONOMIC EVALUATIONS

Analytic tools such as economic evaluation can be extremely valuable for assessing the cost-effectiveness of an intervention. However, when undertaking or reading an economic evaluation, several considerations should be kept in mind.

Ensuring Consistency in Quality

Reviews of the economic evaluation literature have found that studies that are labeled economic evaluations are often only cost studies, only descriptive, or use the methods inappropriately.[37-39] However, there have been guidelines and checklists developed to assist those conducting and reviewing economic evaluations.[40] More recent reviews find evidence of increased consistency in economic evaluations.[41]

Addressing Methodological Issues

There are areas of debate about the appropriate ways to conduct economic evaluations. Analysts can use established methods inappropriately or employ methods still being debated and developed. Four particular areas of concern are as follows: choosing the type of economic evaluation, estimating costs, standardization of reporting, and measuring benefits using QALYs.

Although CUA is the preferred method in the United Kingdom and elsewhere, there has been controversy over its use in the United States. This methodology was initially recommended by the Panel on Cost-Effectiveness in Health and Medicine.[6] However, CBA is preferred by many federal agencies, including the US Environmental Protection Agency (EPA). The broader term of cost-effectiveness is used in many US guidelines and publications to refer to both CEA and CUA. Currently, there is no clear preference between these two types of analysis in US federal policy.

It is difficult to measure or estimate costs accurately in many public health settings.[38] Sometimes costs are estimated from national or regional data sets, and their local applicability may be questionable. In addition, some programs have high fixed costs, such as equipment or personnel, making it difficult to achieve cost-effectiveness. In studies of a new intervention there may be research costs that would not be included in a replication of the intervention. Including these in the economic evaluation is warranted, but the researchers should note that replication would have lower costs and thus a lower ICER.

Averted productivity losses, an indirect cost, are often difficult to measure. There is debate about the appropriate method—human capital or friction costs—to use to measure these costs, and the estimates obtained from the two methods are quite different.[11] Valuing unpaid caregiver time, such as a parent caring for a sick child at home, is difficult. But the unpaid time can be critical in determining the cost-effectiveness of the intervention.[42]

There have been frequent calls for standardization of methods and reporting of economic evaluations. However, there is not always consensus. For example, whether the reference case should discount future health benefits is a matter of debate. Another area of concern is the conduct and reporting of sensitivity analysis. Some have suggested the reporting of ICERs based on both average and median values.[43] Others have focused on the choice of sensitivity analysis methods and the appropriate reporting of sensitivity analysis results to accurately reflect the degree of uncertainty in the ICER.[44]

The most frequently used outcome measure in CUA, the QALY, has been criticized for a number of reasons. First, there are issues related to the precision and consistency of measurement. Any indicator is imperfect and includes some level of error. When ranking interventions, the QALY score used for a particular condition helps determine the cost-utility ratio. Different QALY values may change an intervention's relative cost-effectiveness. There are several QALY score instruments, such as the EQ-5D, and a growing set of catalogs of QALY weights available. Unfortunately, these do not always report the same values for the same conditions and interventions. Further, the existing instruments and catalogs are sometimes not sensitive enough to detect small changes in QALYs.[45, 46]

A related issue is whether to use QALYs only for direct participants in an intervention or for other persons, particularly caregivers,[47] as well. In addition, for interventions aimed at a family or community level, it may be difficult to assess the QALYs of all participants.

There are many critiques of QALYs related to ethical issues, including concerns that they may favor the young over the old,[48,49] men over women,[50] the able-bodied over the disabled,[51,52] and the rich over the poor.[53] By design, QALYs reflect societal preferences and are inherently subjective. However, systematic biases and measurement errors should be minimized as much as possible. The use of QALYs has also been criticized because they rely on utilitarianism as their underlying ethical framework.[54] With utilitarianism, the assumed goal of society is the greatest good for the greatest number, regardless of the distribution of good. Weighting schemes have been proposed to incorporate other allocation frameworks and goals, such as a preference for saving lives over avoiding morbidity.[55-57] Regardless of these critiques, the use of QALYs has become widely accepted and provides a useful starting point for discussions of the appropriate allocation of scarce health resources.

TOOLS FOR ASSESSING INTERVENTION IMPACT AND EFFECTIVENESS

A number of analytic tools are available to describe complex interventions or to synthesize the results of multiple studies to measure the effectiveness of a particular public health intervention. Other tools have an etiologic focus and assess risk for exposure to a particular factor (e.g., cigarette smoking, lack of mammography screening) or assess the health impacts of a nonhealth intervention. Here, we describe cost of illness studies, decision analysis, meta-analysis, pooled analysis, risk assessment, and health impact assessment.

Cost of Illness Studies

Cost of illness studies, also called burden of illness studies, measure the direct and indirect costs of an illness or condition. When combined with data on the number of people with a particular condition, they estimate the economic costs to society of that condition. Thus they can be used to give an estimate of the economic benefits of prevention or more efficient treatment.

The direct expenses of a condition are the health system resources expended on that condition for treatment. This includes all expenditures, whether incurred by the health system directly or paid by a combination of insurance reimbursements and out-of-pocket expenditures by the consumer. In most countries direct costs can be obtained from diagnostic codes and national survey data or national health accounts data.

Indirect costs are productivity losses due to the condition. These include days missed from work, school, or usual activities and their associated costs. If employed, individuals lose income or potential income, and their employers incur costs to replace them while they are absent. As noted elsewhere in the chapter, productivity losses can be estimated with two basic methods: the human capital and the friction cost approaches. Survey-based tools are available to estimate these losses.

Cost of illness studies often rely on national surveys that include diagnostic, medical expenditure, and productivity information. Persons with the condition are identified using the diagnostic information. Their medical expenditures and their productivity losses are calculated and summed. The medical expenditures and productivity losses of the remaining survey respondents are also calculated and summed. The difference between the two totals is the estimate of the cost of illness for this condition. Another approach uses multiple data sources, rather than a single survey, and combines the information from these sources into a model that is used to estimate total cost. For example, data from 27 surveys and databases were linked and used in a spreadsheet-based model to estimate the costs of asthma in the United Kingdom and its member nations at more than £1.1 billion annually.[58] Similarly, a cost of diabetes model developed by the American Diabetes Association estimates the annual US cost of diabetes at $245 billion, with $176 billion in direct medical expenditures and the remainder due to productivity losses.[59]

Decision Analysis

Decision analysis is a derivative of operations research and game theory that involves the identification of all available choices and potential outcomes of each in a visual series of decisions.[60] Along with each choice in the "decision tree," probabilities of outcomes are estimated that arise at decision nodes. An example of a decision tree is shown in Figure 4.3.[7] This tree is based on a study of Oseltamivir treatment for influenza among patients at high risk for complications.[61] The study estimated what would happen in the Netherlands if persons with a high risk for complications from influenza were treated with Oseltamivir or not. To estimate the effects of Oseltamivir treatment, the authors had to identify all of the outcomes relevant to influenza (the branches of the tree) and use the literature to find the prevalence of these events within a year (the probabilities below the branches of the tree). This study could help inform pandemic preparedness.

Decision analysis has historically been used to help inform complex decisions under conditions of uncertainty. It has been widely used by clinicians to make decisions about individual patients. Increasingly, decision analysis has been used to develop policies about the management of groups of patients by looking for the "best" outcome for the most value and is often a fundamental component of an economic evaluation.[7] In the latter case, the tree is modified to include the costs and benefits of each branch as well as the probabilities.

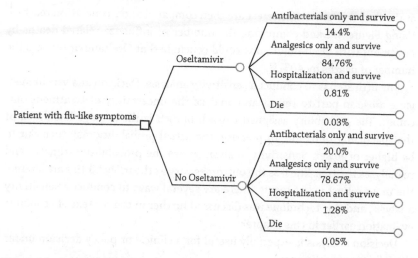

Figure 4.3: Sample decision tree for Oseltamivir treatment of influenza among persons at high risk for complications.
Source: Based on data from Postma et al.[61]

There are five steps in a decision analysis[62]:

1. Identifying and bounding the problem
2. Structuring the problem
3. Gathering information to fill the decision tree
4. Analyzing the decision tree
5. Harnessing uncertainty by conducting a sensitivity analysis

The first two steps help one to draw the decision tree. Step 3, "gathering information," can be done by using new data or by surveying the literature. For a standard decision tree, the probability of reaching each branch and the number of persons who will enter the tree are the two essential pieces of information. For an economic evaluation, the tree must also include the costs and benefits of each branch.

The decision tree is analyzed by starting a number of persons at the base of the tree. The number of persons could be derived from population data or a hypothetical cohort. Based on the probabilities found at each branching point, a certain number of persons go to different branches. The process stops when all of the persons have reached one of the far right-hand branches, which represent the final outcomes. For example, suppose that 10,000 persons in the Netherlands are at high risk for complications from influenza. If Oseltamivir is prescribed to all of these persons, 3 will die from influenza (10,000 × 0.0003). If, alternatively, these persons do not receive Oseltamivir, 5 of them will die from influenza (10,000 × 0.0005). The numbers of people at the final outcomes of interest are then compared and a conclusion reached. Using Figure 4.1 and comparing the number of influenza-related deaths by treatment with Oseltamivir, one could conclude that Oseltamivir reduces the number of deaths by 40%.[61]

The fifth step is to conduct a sensitivity analysis. Decision analysis in medicine arose in part to reflect and analyze the uncertainty of treatment outcomes. The probability assigned to each branch is the average likelihood of that particular outcome. In practice, the actual probability may turn out to be higher or lower. Sensitivity analysis varies the probability estimates and reanalyzes the tree. The less the outcomes vary as the probabilities are altered, the more robust is the result. There are several ways to conduct a sensitivity analysis, and this technique was discussed further in the context of economic evaluation earlier in this chapter.

Decision analysis is especially useful for a clinical or policy decision under the following conditions:

- The decision is complex and information is uncertain.
- Viable choices exist that are legal, ethical, and not cost-prohibitive.
- The decision is a close call, and consequences are important.

Decision analysis can be informative because it forces the analyst to explicitly list all the potential outcomes and pathways and the likelihood of each. Often, the process itself is illuminating, especially if there are complex pathways involved.

Meta-Analysis

Meta-analysis is a specific subtype of a systematic review in which original studies are combined to produce a summary estimate and an estimate of variability.[63] This quantitative synthesis can be particularly valuable in making use of multiple studies when there is a consistent treatment effect. Meta-analysis has the potential to combine studies, thus enhancing statistical power and precision. When there are adequate data, and studies are similar enough, meta-analysis may be useful for summarizing an intervention effect.

Meta-analysis also allows researchers to test subgroup effects (e.g., by gender or age group) that are sometimes difficult to assess in a single, smaller study. For example, a recent meta-analysis of the effectiveness of community engagement in public health interventions for disadvantaged groups identified 131 studies for inclusion.[64] These studies measured several different outcomes. In 105 of the studies, health behavior change was measured, with each reporting the average change in health behavior, the standard deviation of that change, and the number of study participants. These average changes were then pooled using a random effects statistical model to obtain an average effect size for health behavior. The effect was positive, indicating that community engagement is effective in public health interventions for disadvantaged groups. The authors then investigated different types of community engagement and to see if certain types of interventions were more effective. Meta-analysis is covered in more detail in chapter 8.

Pooled Analysis

Pooled analysis refers to the analysis of data from multiple studies at the level of the individual participant. Meta-analysis uses aggregate data from multiple studies. The goals of a pooled analysis are the same as a meta-analysis, that is, obtaining a quantitative estimate of effect. This type of analysis is less common than meta-analysis and has received less formal treatment in the literature. Nonetheless, it has proved informative in characterizing dose-response relationships for certain environmental risks that may be etiologically related to a variety of chronic diseases. For example, pooled analyses have been published on radiation risks for nuclear workers[65]; the relationship between alcohol, smoking, and head and neck cancer[66]; and whether vitamin D can prevent fractures.[67]

Recent efforts by journals and granting agencies encouraging and requiring the posting of study data have made pooled studies more feasible.[68,69] Methodological and software advances have also spurred an increase in these types of studies. Pooled studies using shared data can be particularly useful for studying emerging infections, such as the Zika virus.[70] Although pooled analyses can simply pool the individual data and estimate effect size, they usually either weight the data or include variables indicating study characteristics and use a fixed or random effects modeling strategy. The increased availability of individual data due to journal reporting requirements and electronic medical records means that pooled analysis will be used more in public health analysis.[71]

Risk Assessment

Quantitative risk assessment is a widely used term for a systematic approach to characterizing the risks posed to individuals and populations by environmental pollutants and other potentially adverse exposures.[72] In the United States, its use is either explicitly or implicitly required by a number of federal statutes, and its application worldwide is increasing. Risk assessment has become an established process through which expert scientific input is provided to agencies that regulate environmental or occupational exposures.[73] Four key steps in risk assessment are hazard identification, risk characterization, exposure assessment, and risk estimation. An important aspect of risk assessment is that it frequently results in classification schemes that take into account uncertainties about exposure-disease relationships. For example, the EPA developed a five-tier scheme for classifying potential and proven cancer-causing agents that includes the following: (1) Carcinogenic to Humans, (2) Likely to Be Carcinogenic to Humans; (3) Suggestive Evidence of Carcinogenic Potential; (4) Inadequate Information to Assess Carcinogenic Potential; and (5) Not Likely to Be Carcinogenic to Humans.[74]

Health Impact Assessment

Another assessment tool is the HIA, which measures the impact of a nonhealth sector intervention on the health of a community.[75-77] For example, zoning changes to require sidewalks can increase physical activity, thus improving the health of the community. The number of existing HIAs has been growing rapidly throughout the world, and there have been calls for more use of this methodology.[78,79] For example, numerous HIAs have investigated the impact of transportation policies designed to encourage more active transportation, such as cycling.[80] In the United States this method can be viewed as an extension of the environmental impact statement, an assessment of the intended and unintended consequences of new development on the environment required for some projects.

Dannenberg and colleagues[78] reviewed 27 HIAs completed in the United States from 1999 to 2007. Topics studied ranged from policies about living wages and after-school programs to projects about power plants and public transit. Within this group of 27 HIAs, an excellent illustration is the assessment of a Los Angeles living wage ordinance.[81] Researchers used estimates of the effects of health insurance and income on mortality to project and compare potential mortality reductions attributable to wage increases and changes in health insurance status among workers covered by the Los Angeles City living wage ordinance.[81] Estimates demonstrated that the health insurance provisions of the ordinance would have a much larger health benefit than the wage increases, thus providing valuable information for policy makers who may consider adopting living wage ordinances in other jurisdictions or modifying existing ordinances.

There are five steps to an HIA: screening, scoping, appraisal, reporting, and monitoring.[77] The screening step is used to determine whether the proposed program or intervention will have significant impacts on health, necessitating an HIA. In the scoping step, the relevant community and the health impacts associated with the proposed program are identified. Next, the health impacts on the community are projected and measured. This appraisal step can be done in a relatively quick manner or can be accomplished with a more detailed comprehensive approach such as computer modeling or systematic review. Multiple simulation models have been developed focusing on different geographic areas, public health areas, or economic sectors (e.g., transportation). For example, the DYNAMO-HIA model was developed for use in European countries and has been applied to estimate the health impacts of lifestyle-related health risk factors in 11 European countries.[82,83] In the fourth step, reporting, the positive and negative health impacts of the proposed program are reported, along with suggestions on how best to mitigate negative outcomes and enhance positive ones. Finally, if the proposed program is implemented, its actual impact on health should be monitored and reported to add to the existing evidence base. As a recent US review of 23 HIAs and interviews with 144 HIA practitioners found, HIAs can be useful tools for documenting the impact of policies on health and influencing policy.[79]

FINDING AND TRANSLATING ECONOMIC EVALUATION EVIDENCE INTO RECOMMENDATIONS AND PUBLIC HEALTH ACTION

The economic evaluation literature has grown exponentially over the years. A recent review found 2,844 economic evaluations in health published over a 28-month period.[4] Using a search of PubMed, there have been 3,771 economic evaluations of public health topics in the past 5 years, compared with 1,761 public health economic evaluations in the prior 5 years. This increase in publication can be a boon to public health practitioners because it is more likely that interventions being considered for adoption have already been assessed for cost-effectiveness. The increase in publication has also been accompanied by the development of more guidelines for economic evaluations and several specialized databases focusing on economic evaluation that follow standardized abstracting guidelines.

There are challenges in using economic evaluations in policy. Economic evaluations, though used extensively in other countries, particularly those with national health plans, have a checkered history within the United States.[37,84,85] A review of economic evaluations in public health areas in the United States, such as tobacco control, injury prevention, and immunizations, found inconsistency in the conduct of economic evaluations both across and within topical areas. Further, the results of the economic evaluations were influential in decision making in some public health topic areas but not others. Clearly, there is room for improvement.[86]

Another issue is adapting national or state standards for local needs. Economic evaluations usually take a societal perspective, defined as at least at the state, province, or regional level but more often at the national level. To apply the results of these studies, the practitioner has to consider whether national costs should be adjusted to local costs and whether there are specific state or local characteristics that would influence implementation of results from national data. For example, suppose that a policy maker has found an economic evaluation that supports the use of mass media campaigns to increase physical activity levels. If the city or county in which the policy maker works bans billboard advertising, then the economic evaluation results would have to be adjusted for this restriction.

Finally, there is the matter of training and accessibility. For many in public health, the key question may be, "How does a practitioner learn about or make appropriate use of these tools?" To make better use of economic evaluations and related methods, enhanced training is needed both during graduate education and through continuing education of public health professionals working in community settings.

Despite its limitations, economic evaluation can be a useful tool for managers and policy makers. When doing an economic evaluation, one must specify the intervention and its intended audience; identify the perspective, or scope, of the investigation; list and identify all the costs; and list and identify all the benefits. Then, after discounting to account for differential timing, the costs and benefits are brought together in an ICER. Finally, the stability of the ICER is assessed by varying the assumptions of the analysis in a sensitivity analysis. All of these steps may not provide a definitive answer. Economic evaluation is ultimately a decision aid, not a decision rule. But the clarification provided by the analysis and the insight into the trade-offs that must be made between costs and health are critical aids to managers, planners, and decision makers.[87]

In general, prevention programs are a good value for the money invested.[88] A few interventions are cost-saving, such as the routine childhood immunization schedule in the United States.[89] Most prevention programs will not be cost-saving, but they will provide a good return on investment. Of course, not all prevention programs are cost-effective, but there are many prevention programs that provide increased health outcomes at a lower cost than medical interventions. In the United States, hundreds of thousands of lives could be saved if smokers were advised to quit, those at risk for heart disease took a low-dose aspirin, people received flu shots, and people were screened for colorectal, breast, and cervical cancer.[90] Most of these lives would be saved at a lower cost per life saved than the comparable medical intervention required to treat the associated diseases.

SUMMARY

This chapter has presented economic evaluation, a useful tool for developing and practicing evidence-based public health. Economic evaluation quantifies the costs and benefits of an intervention and provides an assessment of its effectiveness (i.e., "Are the costs reasonable to obtain the likely benefits?"). Cost of illness studies, decision analysis, meta-analysis, pooled analysis, risk assessment, and health impact assessment are all tools to help organize and assess complex topics.

All of these techniques are relatively sophisticated and are generally carried out by persons with specialized training (e.g., an economist would conduct a CUA). The aim of this chapter has been to explain these techniques to public health practitioners so that they can be educated consumers of these methods.

KEY CHAPTER POINTS

- Economic evaluations and related techniques can provide reliable tools for decision making among public health professionals and policy makers.
- These techniques are relatively sophisticated, but their underlying logic and structure can be understood.
- Economic evaluation is the comparison of costs and benefits to determine the most efficient allocation of scarce resources.
- Several challenges (inconsistent quality, methodologic issues, difficulties in implementation) should be kept in mind when considering the use of economic evaluations.
- Cost of illness studies document the direct and indirect burden of disease on society.
- Decision analysis provides a visual tool, the tree diagram, to display complex interventions with multiple outcomes and different probabilities of occurrence. The tree can be calculated to give a score for each of the main outcomes.
- Meta-analysis and pooled analysis are both methods to synthesize the results of several quantitative studies to give a summary measure of effectiveness.
- Risk assessment is a tool to assess complicated pathways of exposure and risk, such as in environmental exposures.

- Health impact assessment is a technique to estimate the health impact of nonhealth interventions, such as minimum wage laws or transportation policies.
- These methods will be increasingly used, especially in times of limited public health resources, and practitioners must be able to understand them so that they can argue for setting appropriate public health priorities.

SUGGESTED READINGS AND SELECTED WEBSITES
Suggested Readings

Birley M. *Health Impact Assessment: Principles and Practice.* New York, NY: Routledge, 2011.

Briss PA, Brownson RC, Fielding JE, Zaza S. Developing and using the Guide to Community Preventive Services: lessons learned about evidence-based public health. *Annu Rev Public Health.* Jan 2004;25:281–302.

Drummond MF, Sculpher MJ, Claxton K, Stoddart GL, Torrance GW. *Methods for the Economic Evaluation of Health Care Programmes.* 4th ed. New York, NY: Oxford University Press; 2015.

Gold MR, Siegel JE, Russell LB, Weinstein MC. *Cost-Effectiveness in Health and Medicine.* New York, NY: Oxford University Press, 1996.

Haddix AC, Teutsch SM, Corso PS. *Prevention Effectiveness. A Guide to Decision Analysis and Economic Evaluation.* 2nd ed. New York, NY: Oxford University Press; 2002.

Kemm J, Parry J, Palmer S, eds. *Health Impact Assessment: Concepts, Theory, Techniques and Applications.* New York, NY: Oxford University Press; 2004.

Muennig P, Bounthavong M. *Cost-Effectiveness Analysis in Health: A Practical Approach.* 3rd ed. San Francisco, CA: Jossey-Bass Publishers, 2016.

Petitti DB. *Meta-analysis, Decision Analysis, and Cost-Effectiveness Analysis: Methods for Quantitative Synthesis in Medicine.* 2nd ed. New York, NY: Oxford University Press, 2000.

Selected Websites

Association of Public Health Observatories, The HIA Gateway <http://www.apho.org.uk/default.aspx?QN=P_HIA>. This UK-based website provides resources for health impact assessments, including sample causal diagrams and a searchable catalog of HIAs.

Cochrane Collaboration <http://www.cochrane.org>. The Cochrane Collaboration is an international organization that aims to help people make well-informed decisions about health care by preparing, maintaining, and promoting the accessibility of systematic reviews of the effects of health care interventions. The Collaboration conducts its own systematic reviews, abstracts the systematic reviews of others, and provides links to complementary databases.

Chronic Disease Cost Calculator Version 2, Centers for Disease Control and Prevention <http://www.cdc.gov/chronicdisease/calculator/index.html>. This tool provides state-level estimates of the cost of several chronic diseases in the United States. Cost is measured as medical expenditures and absenteeism costs. Diseases covered are arthritis, asthma, cancer, cardiovascular diseases, depression, and diabetes.

Cost-Effectiveness Analysis Registry, Center for the Evaluation of Value and Risk in Health, Institute for Clinical Research and Health Policy Studies, Tufts Medical Center <http://healtheconomics.tuftsmedicalcenter.org/cear4/Home.aspx>. Originally based on the articles by Tengs et al.,[19,91] this website includes a detailed database of cost-effectiveness analyses, cost-effectiveness ratios, and QALY weights.

Evaluation, National Association of Chronic Disease Directors <http://www.chronicdisease.org/?page=Evaluation>. The evaluation page of this US website includes resources on return-on-investment analysis. The accompanying guide presents the different forms of economic evaluation under the umbrella of return on investment.

Guide to Clinical Preventive Services, Third Edition <http://www.ahrq.gov/clinic/uspstfix.htm>. The US Preventive Services Task Force developed and updates this guide, intended for primary care clinicians, other allied health professionals, and students. It provides recommendations for clinical preventive interventions—screening tests, counseling interventions, immunizations, and chemoprophylactic regimens—for more than 80 target conditions. Systematic reviews form the basis for the recommendations. The Guide is provided through the website of the Agency for Healthcare Research and Quality.

Guide to Community Preventive Services <http://www.thecommunityguide.org>. Under the auspices of the US Public Health Service, the Task Force on Community Preventive Services developed the Guide to Community Preventive Services. The Guide uses systematic reviews to summarize what is known about the effectiveness of population-based interventions for prevention and control in 18 topical areas. Interventions that are rated effective are then evaluated for cost-effectiveness.

Health Impact Assessment, Centers for Disease Control Health Places <http://www.cdc.gov/healthyplaces/hia.htm>. This website provides definitions, examples, and links to other catalogs and archives of HIAs.

Health Impact Assessment, National Association of County & City Health Officials <http://www.naccho.org/programs/community-health/healthy-community-design/health-impact-assessment/>. Includes resources for local health departments to assist them in the use of HIA.

Health Impact Project, The Pew Charitable Trusts <http://www.pewtrusts.org/en/projects/health-impact-project/health-impact-assessment>. Includes an overview, a description of the HIA process, links to toolkits and other resources, and multiple case studies.

World Health Organization Health Impact Assessment <http://www.who.int/hia/en/>. The World Health Organization provides resources, examples, toolkits, and a catalog of worldwide HIAs.

REFERENCES

1. Marshall DA, Hux M. Design and analysis issues for economic analysis alongside clinical trials. *Med Care.* Jul 2009;47(7 Suppl 1):S14–S20.
2. Ramsey S, Willke R, Briggs A, et al. Good research practices for cost-effectiveness analysis alongside clinical trials: the ISPOR RCT-CEA Task Force report. *Value Health.* Sep-Oct 2005;8(5):521–533.

3. Petrou S, Gray A. Economic evaluation alongside randomised controlled trials: design, conduct, analysis, and reporting. *BMJ*. 2011;342:d1548.
4. Pitt C, Goodman C, Hanson K. Economic evaluation in global perspective: a bibliometric analysis of the recent literature. *Health Econ*. Feb 2016;25(Suppl 1):9–28.
5. Ramsey S, Willke R, Glick H, et al. Cost-effectiveness analysis alongside clinical trials. II: An ISPOR Good Research Practices Task Force report. *Value Health*. 2015;18(2):161–172.
6. Gold MR, Siegel JE, Russell LB, Weinstein MC. *Cost-Effectiveness in Health and Medicine*. New York, NY: Oxford University Press; 1996.
7. Drummond M, Sculpher M, Torrance G, O'Brien B, Stoddart G. *Methods for the Economic Evaluation of Health Care Programmes*. 3rd ed. New York, NY: Oxford University Press; 2005.
8. Rosenthal MS, Ross JS, Bilodeau R, Richter RS, Palley JE, Bradley EH. Economic evaluation of a comprehensive teenage pregnancy prevention program: pilot program. *Am J Prev Med*. Dec 2009;37(6 Suppl 1):S280–S287.
9. Tanaka H, Yamato H, Tanaka T, et al. Effectiveness of a low-intensity intraworksite intervention on smoking cessation in Japanese employees: a three-year intervention trial. *J Occup Health*. May 2006;48(3):175–182.
10. Brownson CA, Hoerger TJ, Fisher EB, Kilpatrick KE. Cost-effectiveness of diabetes self-management programs in community primary care settings. *Diabetes Educ*. Sep-Oct 2009;35(5):761–769.
11. Krol M, Brouwer W. How to estimate productivity costs in economic evaluations. *Pharmacoeconomics*. Apr 2014;32(4):335–344.
12. Tang K. Estimating productivity costs in health economic evaluations: a review of instruments and psychometric evidence. *Pharmacoeconomics*. Jan 2014;33(1):31–48.
13. Martin AJ, Glasziou PP, Simes RJ, Lumley T. A comparison of standard gamble, time trade-off, and adjusted time trade-off scores. *Int J Technol Assess Health Care*. Winter 2000;16(1):137–147.
14. Health Utilities Group. Health Utilities Index: Multiattribute Health Status Classification System: Health Utilities Index Mark 3 (HUI3). www.healthutilities.com. Accessed March 14, 2017.
15. The Euroqol Group. Euroqol— what is EQ-5D?. http://www.euroqol.org/contact/contact-information.html. Accessed March 14, 2017.
16. Bell CM, Chapman RH, Stone PW, Sandberg EA, Neumann PJ. An off-the-shelf help list: a comprehensive catalog of preference scores from published cost-utility analyses. *Med Decis Making*. Jul-Aug 2001;21(4):288–294.
17. Sullivan PW, Ghushchyan V. Preference-based EQ-5D index scores for chronic conditions in the United States. *Med Decis Making*. Jul-Aug 2006;26(4):410–420.
18. Sullivan PW, Lawrence WF, Ghushchyan V. A national catalog of preference-based scores for chronic conditions in the United States. *Med Care*. Jul 2005;43(7):736–749.
19. Tengs TO, Wallace A. One thousand health-related quality-of-life estimates. *Med Care*. Jun 2000;38(6):583–637.
20. CDC Diabetes Cost-Effectiveness Study Group. The cost-effectiveness of screening for type 2 diabetes. *JAMA*. Nov 25 1998;2802(20):1757–1763.
21. American Diabetes Association. Screening for diabetes. *Diabetes Care*. 2002;25(S1):S21–S24.
22. Screening for type 2 diabetes mellitus in adults: U.S. Preventive Services Task Force recommendation statement. *Ann Intern Med*. Jun 3 2008;148(11):846–854.

23. Hoerger TJ, Harris R, Hicks KA, Donahue K, Sorensen S, Engelgau M. Screening for type 2 diabetes mellitus: a cost-effectiveness analysis. *Ann Intern Med*. May 4 2004;140(9):689–699.

24. Siu AL. Screening for Abnormal Blood Glucose and Type 2 Diabetes mellitus: U.S. Preventive Services Task Force recommendation statement. *Ann Intern Med*. Dec 1 2015;163(11):861–868.

25. Schad M, John J. Towards a social discount rate for the economic evaluation of health technologies in Germany: an exploratory analysis. *Eur J Health Econ*. Apr 2010;13(2):127–144.

26. Baio G, Dawid AP. Probabilistic sensitivity analysis in health economics. *Stat Methods Med Res*. Dec 2011;24(6):615–634.

27. Neumann PJ, Cohen JT, Weinstein MC. Updating cost-effectiveness: the curious resilience of the $50,000-per-QALY threshold. *N Engl J Med*. Aug 28 2014;371(9):796–797.

28. Eddy D. *Breast Cancer Screening for Medicare Beneficiaries*. Washington, DC: Office of Technology Assessment; 1987.

29. Braithwaite RS, Meltzer DO, King JT, Jr., Leslie D, Roberts MS. What does the value of modern medicine say about the $50,000 per quality-adjusted life-year decision rule? *Med Care*. Apr 2008;46(4):349–356.

30. Garber AM, Phelps CE. Economic foundations of cost-effectiveness analysis. *J Health Econ*. Feb 1997;16(1):1–31.

31. Murray CJ, Evans DB, Acharya A, Baltussen RM. Development of WHO guidelines on generalized cost-effectiveness analysis. *Health Econ*. Apr 2000;9(3):235–251.

32. World Health Organization. *Macroeconomics and Health: Investing in Health for Economic Development*. Geneva: World Health Organization; 2001.

33. McCabe C, Claxton K, Culyer AJ. The NICE cost-effectiveness threshold: what it is and what that means. *Pharmacoeconomics*. 2008;26(9):733–744.

34. Gillick MR. Medicare coverage for technological innovations: time for new criteria? *N Engl J Med*. May 20 2004;350(21):2199–2203.

35. Owens DK. Interpretation of cost-effectiveness analyses. *J Gen Intern Med*. Oct 1998;13(10):716–717.

36. Weinstein MC. How much are Americans willing to pay for a quality-adjusted life year? *Med Care*. Apr 2008;46(4):343–345.

37. Neumann P. *Using Cost-Effectiveness Analysis to Improve Health Care*. New York, NY: Oxford University Press; 2005.

38. Weatherly H, Drummond M, Claxton K, et al. Methods for assessing the cost-effectiveness of public health interventions: key challenges and recommendations. *Health Policy*. Dec 2009;93(2-3):85–92.

39. Zarnke KB, Levine MA, O'Brien BJ. Cost-benefit analyses in the health-care literature: don't judge a study by its label. *Journal of Clinical Epidemiology*. July 1997 1997;50(7):813–822.

40. Drummond MF, Jefferson TO. Guidelines for authors and peer reviewers of economic submissions to the BMJ. The BMJ Economic Evaluation Working Party. *BMJ*. Aug 3 1996;313(7052):275–283.

41. Thiboonboon K, Santatiwongchai B, Chantarastapornchit V, Rattanavipapong W, Teerawattananon Y. A systematic review of economic evaluation methodologies between resource-limited and resource-rich countries: a case of rotavirus vaccines. *Appl Health Econ Health Policy*. Dec 2016;14(6):659–672.

42. Goodrich K, Kaambwa B, Al-Janabi H. The inclusion of informal care in applied economic evaluation: a review. *Value Health*. Sep-Oct 2012;15(6):975–981.

43. Bang H, Zhao H. Cost-effectiveness analysis: a proposal of new reporting standards in statistical analysis. *J Biopharm Stat.* 2014;24(2):443–460.

44. Andronis L, Barton P, Bryan S. Sensitivity analysis in economic evaluation: an audit of NICE current practice and a review of its use and value in decision-making. *Health Technol Assess.* Jun 2009;13(29):iii, ix-xi, 1–61.

45. Gerard K, Mooney G. QALY league tables: handle with care. *Health Econ.* 1993;2(1):59–64.

46. Mauskopf J, Rutten F, Schonfeld W. Cost-effectiveness league tables: valuable guidance for decision makers? *Pharmacoeconomics.* 2003;21(14):991–1000.

47. Al-Janabi H, Flynn TN, Coast J. QALYs and carers. *Pharmacoeconomics.* Dec 2011;29(12):1015–1023.

48. Tsuchiya A. QALYs and ageism: philosophical theories and age weighting. *Health Econ.* Jan 2000;9(1):57–68.

49. Herz-Roiphe D. The young, the old, and the economists: rethinking how agencies account for age in cost-benefit analysis. *Yale J Health Policy Law Ethics.* Summer 2014;14(2):350–375.

50. Tsuchiya A, Williams A. A "fair innings" between the sexes: are men being treated inequitably? *Soc Sci Med.* Jan 2005;60(2):277–286.

51. Groot W. Adaptation and scale of reference bias in self-assessments of quality of life. *J Health Econ.* 2000;19(3):403–420.

52. Menzel P, Dolan P, Richardson J, Olsen JA. The role of adaptation to disability and disease in health state valuation: a preliminary normative analysis. *Soc Sci Med.* Dec 2002;55(12):2149–2158.

53. Gerdtham UG, Johannesson M. Income-related inequality in life-years and quality-adjusted life-years. *J Health Econ.* Nov 2000;19(6):1007–1026.

54. Dolan P. Utilitarianism and the measurement and aggregation of quality-adjusted life years. *Health Care Anal.* 2001;9(1):65–76.

55. Bleichrodt H, Diecidue E, Quiggin J. Equity weights in the allocation of health care: the rank-dependent QALY model. *J Health Econ.* Jan 2004;23(1):157–171.

56. Cookson R, Drummond M, Weatherly H. Explicit incorporation of equity considerations into economic evaluation of public health interventions. *Health Econ Policy Law.* Apr 2009;4(Pt 2):231–245.

57. Ottersen T, Maestad O, Norheim OF. Lifetime QALY prioritarianism in priority setting: quantification of the inherent trade-off. *Cost Eff Resour Alloc.* 2014;12(1):2.

58. Mukherjee M, Stoddart A, Gupta RP, et al. The epidemiology, healthcare and societal burden and costs of asthma in the UK and its member nations: analyses of standalone and linked national databases. *BMC Med.* 2016;14(1):113.

59. American Diabetes Association. Economic costs of diabetes in the U.S. in 2012. *Diabetes Care.* Apr 2013;36(4):1033–1046.

60. Porta M, ed. *A Dictionary of Epidemiology.* 6th ed. New York, NY: Oxford University Press; 2014.

61. Postma MJ, Novak A, Scheijbeler HW, Gyldmark M, van Genugten ML, Wilschut JC. Cost effectiveness of oseltamivir treatment for patients with influenza-like illness who are at increased risk for serious complications of influenza: illustration for the Netherlands. *Pharmacoeconomics.* 2007;25(6):497–509.

62. Alemi F, Gustafson D. *Decision Analysis for Healthcare Managers.* Chicago, IL: Health Administration Press; 2006.

63. Petitti DB. *Meta-analysis, Decision Analysis, and Cost-Effectiveness Analysis: Methods for Quantitative Synthesis in Medicine.* 2nd ed. New York, NY: Oxford University Press; 2000.

64. O'Mara-Eves A, Brunton G, Oliver S, Kavanagh J, Jamal F, Thomas J. The effectiveness of community engagement in public health interventions for disadvantaged groups: a meta-analysis. *BMC Public Health.* 2015;15:129.

65. Cardis E, Vrijheid M, Blettner M, et al. The 15-Country Collaborative Study of Cancer Risk Among Radiation Workers in the Nuclear Industry: estimates of radiation-related cancer risks. *Radiat Res.* Apr 2007;167(4):396–416.

66. Lubin JH, Purdue M, Kelsey K, et al. Total exposure and exposure rate effects for alcohol and smoking and risk of head and neck cancer: a pooled analysis of case-control studies. *Am J Epidemiol.* Oct 15 2009;170(8):937–947.

67. DIPART (Vitamin D Individual Patient Analysis of Randomized Trials) Group. Patient level pooled analysis of 68 500 patients from seven major vitamin D fracture trials in US and Europe. *BMJ.* 2010;340:b5463.

68. National Institutes of Health. NIH Data Sharing Policy and Implementation Guidance. https://grants.nih.gov/grants/policy/data_sharing/data_sharing_guidance.htm. Accessed September 11, 2016.

69. Walport M, Brest P. Sharing research data to improve public health. *Lancet.* Feb 12 2011;377(9765):537–539.

70. McNutt M. Data sharing. *Science.* Mar 4 2016;351(6277):1007.

71. Blettner M, Sauerbrei W, Schlehofer B, Scheuchenpflug T, Friedenreich C. Traditional reviews, meta-analyses and pooled analyses in epidemiology. *Int J Epidemiol.* Feb 1999;28(1):1–9.

72. Samet JM, White RH, Burke TA. Epidemiology and risk assessment. In: Brownson RC, Petitti DB, eds. *Applied Epidemiology: Theory to Practice.* 2nd ed. New York, NY: Oxford University Press; 2006:125–163.

73. World Health Organization. Environmental Burden of Disease Series, World Health Organization. www.who.int/quantifying_ehimpacts/national. Accessed March 14, 2017.

74. US Environmental Protection Agency. Guidelines for Carcinogen Risk Assessment. EPA/630/P-03/001F:https://www.epa.gov/sites/production/files/2013-09/documents/cancer_guidelines_final_3-25-05.pdf. Accessed March 14, 2017.

75. Cole BL, Fielding JE. Health impact assessment: a tool to help policy makers understand health beyond health care. *Annu Rev Public Health.* 2007;28:393–412.

76. Collins J, Koplan JP. Health impact assessment: a step toward health in all policies. *JAMA.* Jul 15 2009;302(3):315–317.

77. World Health Organization. Health Impact Assessment http://www.who.int/hia/en/. Accessed March 14, 2017.

78. Dannenberg AL, Bhatia R, Cole BL, Heaton SK, Feldman JD, Rutt CD. Use of health impact assessment in the U.S.: 27 case studies, 1999-2007. *Am J Prev Med.* Mar 2008;34(3):241–256.

79. Bourcier E, Charbonneau D, Cahill C, Dannenberg AL. An evaluation of health impact assessments in the United States, 2011-2014. *Prev Chronic Dis.* 2015;12:E23.

80. Mueller N, Rojas-Rueda D, Cole-Hunter T, et al. Health impact assessment of active transportation: A systematic review. *Prev Med.* Jul 2015;76:103–114.

81. Cole B, Shimkhada R, Morgenstern H, Kominski G, Fielding J, Wu S. Projected health impact of the Los Angeles City living wage ordinance. *J Epidemiol Commun Health.* 2005;59:645–650.

82. Lhachimi SK, Nusselder WJ, Smit HA, et al. Potential health gains and health losses in eleven EU countries attainable through feasible prevalences of the

life-style related risk factors alcohol, BMI, and smoking: a quantitative health impact assessment. *BMC Public Health*. 2016;16:734.

83. Lhachimi SK, Nusselder WJ, Smit HA, et al. DYNAMO-HIA: a dynamic modeling tool for generic health impact assessments. *PLoS One*. 2012;7(5):e33317.

84. Azimi NA, Welch HG. The effectiveness of cost-effectiveness analysis in containing costs. *J Gen Intern Med*. Oct 1998;13(10):664–669.

85. McDaid D, Needle J. What use has been made of economic evaluation in public health? A systematic review of the literature. In: Dawson S, Morris S, eds. *Future Public Health: Burdens, Challenges and Approaches*. Basingstoke, UK: Palgrave Macmillan; 2009.

86. Grosse SD, Teutsch SM, Haddix AC. Lessons from cost-effectiveness research for United States public health policy. *Annu Rev Public Health*. 2007;28:365–391.

87. Rabarison KM, Bish CL, Massoudi MS, Giles WH. Economic evaluation enhances public health decision making. *Front Public Health*. 2015;3:164.

88. Woolf SH. A closer look at the economic argument for disease prevention. *JAMA*. Feb 4 2009;301(5):536–538.

89. Zhou F, Santoli J, Messonnier ML, et al. Economic evaluation of the 7-vaccine routine childhood immunization schedule in the United States, 2001. *Arch Pediatr Adolesc Med*. Dec 2005;159(12):1136–1144.

90. National Commission on Prevention Priorities. *Preventive Care: A National Profile on Use, Disparities, and Health Benefits*. Washington, DC: Partnership for Prevention; 2007.

91. Tengs TO, Adams ME, Pliskin JS, et al. Five-hundred life-saving interventions and their cost-effectiveness. *Risk Analysis*. 1995;15(3):369–390.

CHAPTER 5

cᴧɔ

Conducting a Community Assessment

The uncreative mind can spot wrong answers. It takes a creative mind to spot wrong questions.

A. Jay

Becoming aware of current conditions through a community assessment is one of the first steps in an evidence-based process. The path to the destination depends very much on the starting point. As noted earlier, evidence-based processes include conducting assessments to identify issues within a community, prioritizing these issues, developing interventions to address these issues based on a review of what has worked effectively in other places, and evaluating the process, impact, and outcome of intervention efforts. Because the determinants of chronic diseases and common risk factors are multilevel (including individual, social, organizational, community, and system level factors), each of these steps will require some engagement of non-health partners across a wide variety of sectors of the community. Their level of engagement in each step may vary.

Community assessments may include efforts to identify morbidity and mortality, environmental and organizational conditions, existing policies, and relationships among key organizations and agencies. In conducting these assessments it is important to attend to not only the needs in the community and problems but also community strengths and assets (similar to the strategic planning considerations outlined in chapter 6).

Although it is ideal to do a complete and thorough assessment, this may not be possible in all instances. Choices about what to assess should be based on what it is that you want to know and who will be using the information. Ideally, assessments should be made with partners who will use the information for decision making about future programs and policies and those who are affected by these decisions. In reality, some of these partners may join at a later stage in the evidence-based process, bringing new perspectives or questions that warrant additional assessments.

This chapter is divided into several sections. The first provides a background on community assessments. The next section describes why a community assessment is critical. The third section discusses a range of partnership models that might be useful in conducting community assessments. The next sections outline who, what, and how to conduct assessments. The final section describes how to disseminate the community assessment findings.

BACKGROUND

Community assessments identify the health concerns in a community, the factors in the community that influence health (i.e., determinants of health), and the assets, resources and challenges that influence these factors.[1,2] Ideally, assessment is a process in which community members and a broad array of medical/health, business, community, faith-based, and governmental organizations become partners in assessing the community and use this information as part of a process to prioritize and develop interventions (programs, policies, or environmental changes) for community improvement.[3] The types of data reviewed are determined within this partnership based on the questions the partnership is interested in answering. After the data are synthesized and provided back to the partnership, they are often then shared with the broader community to inform others' planning efforts.[1]

WHY CONDUCT COMMUNITY ASSESSMENT?

Community assessments are essential to ensure that the right interventions are implemented. This is in part because they can provide insight into the community context so that interventions are designed, planned, and carried out in ways that are acceptable and maximize the benefit to the community. In addition, the assessments can identify (and in some cases build) support for a particular intervention approach. This support is critical for garnering resources and ensuring a successful intervention. Assessments can also provide a baseline measure of a variety of conditions. This baseline, or starting point, is helpful in determining the impact of intervention efforts. In chapter 11, more information will be provided on how to compare baseline measures with measures collected during and after the intervention to identify differences.

Community assessments may be encouraged by local, state or provincial, and national entities as a way to better focus intervention efforts and utilize resources, or they may be conducted as part of a mandatory process for public health agency accreditation or assessment processes for hospitals and health care systems.

ROLE OF PARTNERS IN COMMUNITY ASSESSMENT

The roles of partners, including community members, community-based organizations, governmental or public agencies, private agencies, local businesses, and health practitioners in conducting a community assessment may vary. Although some involvement of each of these groups is important, the assessment may be started by one group, with others joining in at a later time. Alternately, the assessment may be conducted with a small group, with other partners being asked to join only after a specific intervention has been chosen. Some have argued that engagement of community members and these multiple sectors from the beginning and throughout the process is likely to enhance the relevance and accuracy of the overall assessment and increase the effectiveness of the chosen interventions (Box 5.1).[4-7]

Recognizing that solving complex health issues requires that agencies and community leaders work together, public health professionals have worked with existing or created new coalitions. A *coalition* is defined as a group of community members or organizations that join together for a common purpose.[8,9] Some coalitions are focused on categorical issues, such as diabetes prevention or the reduction of infant mortality rates. Other coalitions form to address broader public health issues (e.g., a partnership for prevention).

Coalitions may differ considerably in the roles and responsibilities of each partner and the types of activities in which they wish to engage.[10] This can be thought of as a continuum of integration.[8,9,11,12] At one end of the continuum is the desire of agencies and individuals to work together to identify gaps in services, avoid duplication of services, and exchange information to allow for appropriate client referral. This level is characterized by networking and coordination. The next level of integration involves a higher level of cooperation. Agencies maintain their autonomy, agendas, and resources but begin to share these resources to work on an issue that is identified as common to all. The highest level of integration involves collaboration among the agencies as they work together to develop joint agendas, common goals, and shared resources. Before starting a community assessment it is important for partners to be clear about the level of integration they desire because each requires progressively higher levels of commitment and resources.

Although community coalitions are growing in popularity, their ability to assess their community and create healthful changes depends in part on the

> *Box 5.1*
>
> ## REDUCING DISPARITIES IN DIABETES AMONG AFRICAN-AMERICAN AND LATINO RESIDENTS OF DETROIT: THE ESSENTIAL ROLE OF COMMUNITY PLANNING FOCUS GROUPS
>
> A strong community-academic-health system partnership was created to address long-standing health disparities.[7] The REACH (Racial/Ethnic Approaches to Community Health) Detroit Partnership included community residents, community-based organizations, the health department, a medical care system, and academicians, who worked together to assess the factors influencing diabetes and related risk factors. Partners were involved in all aspects of the development, implementation, and analysis of the data. Community members, including those who were bilingual in Spanish and English, were recruited and trained to moderate the focus groups. Focus groups were held at community sites. All partners worked together to establish a focus group discussion guide and analyze the results. Focus group participants were asked to discuss the challenges as well as the assets in their community, and were provided specific suggestions for strategies to reduce diabetes and related risk factors. The broad-based partnership was able to take these suggested strategies and obtain funding for a wide range of individual, family, health system, social support, and community level interventions.

coalition's ability to move through various stages of development. There are many recent efforts to define and describe these various stages.[8,13,14] Most often, for these groups to be effective, it is essential that they begin by developing a common vision of what they want to accomplish and a common set of skills to engage in the change process together. In addition, it is important that the individuals involved in the coalition build relationships as individuals and as representatives of their respective community organizations. As with other types of community-based health promotion programs, to be effective, coalitions may need to focus on a variety of issues, such as developing a common set of skills and building trust, at different stages. Wolff summarized the unique characteristics that contribute to the development of effective coalitions (Table 5.1).[15] When coalitions have established these processes they are ready to determine what to assess and how to conduct the assessment.

WHO AND WHAT TO ASSESS

What to assess depends very much on the knowledge to be gained and from whom it will be collected. In terms of the "who" question, it is important to

Table 5.1. CHARACTERISTICS OF EFFECTIVE COMMUNITY COALITIONS

Characteristic	Description
1. Holistic and comprehensive	Allows the coalition to address issues that it deems as priorities; well illustrated in the Ottawa Charter for Health Promotion
2. Flexible and responsive	Coalitions address emerging issues and modify their strategies to fit new community needs
3. Build a sense of community	Members frequently report that they value and receive professional and personal support for their participation in the social network of the coalition
4. Build and enhance resident engagement in community life	Provides a structure for renewed civic engagement; coalition becomes a forum where multiple sectors can engage with each other
5. Provide a vehicle for community empowerment	As community coalitions solve local problems, they develop social capital, allowing residents to have an impact on multiple issues
6. Allow diversity to be valued and celebrated	As communities become increasingly diverse, coalitions provide a vehicle for bringing together diverse group to solve common problems
7. Incubators for innovative solutions to large problems	Problem solving occurs not only at local levels but also at regional and national levels; local leaders can become national leaders

Source: Adapted from Wolff.[15]

clearly identify the "community" of interest. The community may be defined as individuals who live within a specified geographic region or as individuals who have a common experience or share a particular social or cultural sense of identity.[16,17] For example, a community might involve members of a particular church, residents of a neighborhood, or individuals connected through social media who share a common bond (e.g., ethnic heritage). In conducting the assessment, it is also important to identify any subgroups within the community of interest (e.g., youth, lower income adults) so that the assessments can adequately reflect the range of community members.

The decision regarding what to assess should be guided by the goal of the assessment. For instance, an assessment focusing on youth would include different elements than an assessment focusing on elderly people. Alternately, some governmental or funding agencies will require that certain things be assessed, and a group will need to decide if it wishes to expand on those requirements. With that in mind, there are some general guidelines that are helpful to consider in planning an assessment. In particular, it is important to assess factors along the full range of the ecological factors that influence population health and well-being, and in doing so include the assets in the community—not just the problems (Figure 5.1).[16, 18–20]

Ecological frameworks (also discussed in chapter 10) suggest that individual, social, and contextual factors influence health.[21] Several variations of an ecological framework have been proposed.[22–25] Based on work conducted by McLeroy and colleagues[22] and Dahlgren and Whitehead,[26] it is useful to consider assessment of factors at five levels:

1. Individual—characteristics of the individual, including biological; knowledge, attitudes, skills, and a person's developmental history; and individual lifestyle behaviors
2. Interpersonal—formal and informal social networks and social support systems, including family and friends

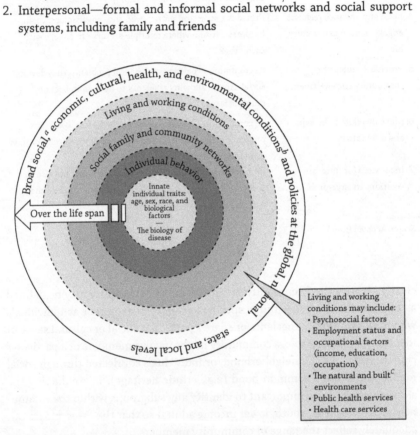

Figure 5.1: Ecological influences on health.

[a]Social conditions include, but are not limited to: economic inequality, urbanization, mobility, cultural values, attitudes and policies related to discrimination and intolerance on the basis of race, gender, and other differences.

[b]Other conditions at the national level might include major sociopolitical shifts, such as recession, war, and governmental collapse.

[c]The built environment includes transportation, water and sanitation, housing, and other dimensions of urban planning.

Source: From the Institute of Medicine.[19]

3. Organizational—living and working conditions, including social institutions, organizational characteristics, and rules or regulations for operation. Assessments of organizational factors may include not only the existence of these institutions but also their organizational capacity and readiness for change (e.g., organizational support, communication within and between organizations, decision-making structures, leadership, resources available[16, 27–29])

4. Community, social, cultural, and environmental conditions—relationships between organizations, economic forces, the physical environment, and cultural factors that shape behavior

5. Governmental and policy—local, state, national, and international laws, rules, and regulations

Using an ecological framework to guide an assessment leads to assessing people in the community (their health and wellness and their behaviors), the organizations and agencies that serve the community, and the environment within which the community members reside.[30] In fact, the most effective interventions act at multiple levels because communities are made up of individuals who interact in a variety of social networks and within a particular context; therefore an assessment needs to provide insight along this wide range of factors. Table 5.2 provides a list of a number of possible indicators for each of these levels of the ecological framework. In addition, the list of resources at the end of the chapter includes a variety of expected indicators for various agencies.

COLLECTING DATA

There are a number of different ways to collect data on each of the indicators listed previously. Too often, community assessment data are collected based on the skills of the individuals collecting the data. If someone knows how to collect survey data, those are the data collected. As noted earlier, for any community assessment process to be effective, it is essential to determine the questions that need answering and from whom data will be collected. Methods should be used that are best suited to answer the questions—obtaining assistance as needed. Some information may be found using existing data, whereas other types of information require new data collection. Data are often classified as either quantitative or qualitative. Quantitative data are expressed in numbers or statistics—they answer the "what" question. Qualitative data are expressed in words or pictures and help to explain quantitative data by answering the "why" question. There are different types and different methods of collecting each. More often than not, it is useful to collect multiple types of

Table 5.2. INDICATORS BY LEVEL OF AN ECOLOGICAL FRAMEWORK

Level	Indicators
Individual: characteristics of the individual such as knowledge, attitudes, skills, and a person's developmental history	• Leading causes of death • Leading causes of hospitalization • Behavioral risk and protective factors • Community member skills and talents
Interpersonal: formal and informal social networks and social support systems, including family and friends	• Social connectedness • Group affiliation (clubs, associations) • Faith communities, churches, and religious organizations • Cultural and community pride
Organizational: social institutions, organizational characteristics, and rules or regulations for operation	• Number of newspaper, local radio or TV, and media • Number of public art projects or access to art exhibits and museums • Presence of food pantries • Number and variety of businesses • Number of faith-based organizations • Number of civic organizations • Supportive services resource list • Public transportation systems • Number of social services (e.g., food assistance, child care providers, senior centers, housing and shelter assistance) • Chamber of Commerce—list of businesses • Number and variety of medical care services: clinics, programs • Number of law enforcement services • Number of nonprofit organizations and types of services performed (e.g., the United Way, Planned Parenthood) • Number of vocational and higher education institutions and fields of study available to students: community college and university • Library
Community and social: relationships between organizations, economic forces, the physical environment, and cultural variables that shape behavior	• Public School System Enrollment numbers • Graduation and drop-out rates • Test scores • Community history • Community values • Opportunities for structured and unstructured involvement in local decision making • Recreational opportunities: green spaces, parks, waterways, gyms, and biking and walking trails • Crosswalks, curb cuts, traffic calming devices • Housing cost, availability

Table 5.2. CONTINUED

Level	Indicators
	• Environmental issues—trash, animals, pollution
	• Existence of local and city-wide strategic planning processes
	• Employment and unemployment rates
	• Area economic data
	• Crime incidence: arrests and convictions, incidence of domestic violence
	• Motor vehicle crashes
	• Informal educational opportunities for children and adults
	• Number and types of existing collaborations among organizations
Governmental and policy: local, state, and national laws, rules, and regulations	• Zoning regulations
	• Housing standards
	• Environmental policies (e.g., air or water standards)
	• Economic policies (e.g., minimum wage, taxes)

data because each has certain advantages and disadvantages. Bringing different types of data together is often called *triangulation*.[31]

Quantitative Data

National, State, and Local Data From Surveillance Systems

These sources of quantitative data are collected through national or statewide initiatives and may include information on morbidity and mortality (cancer registry, death certificates), behavior (Behavioral Risk Factor Surveillance System), or social indicators (European Health for All Database, US Census). The advantage of these data is that they are comparable across geographic regions, allowing comparisons between one community and other communities. The disadvantage of these data is that they may not be a good reflection of a community because of geographic coverage, sampling frames, or method of data collection (e.g., phone interviews). In addition, these data sets may not include data relevant for answering questions related to a particular assessment or the development of a specific intervention.

Surveys or Quantitative Interviews

These data are collected specifically for a particular community and may include information on demographics, social indicators, knowledge, behavior, attitudes, morbidity, and so forth. These data may be collected through phone, mail, face-to-face, or Internet-based interviews. The advantage of this type of data is that one can tailor the survey instrument to specific questions and the community of interest. The disadvantage is that one's ability to compare responses to those of other areas depends on many things, including similarity of questions asked and data collection method. In addition, collecting data of this kind can be quite costly. More information on these approaches can be found in chapter 7.

Community Audits

Community audits are detailed counting of certain factors in a community (e.g., number of recreational centers, supermarkets, fast-food restaurants, schools, places of worship, billboards, number of walkers or bikers, cigarette butts, alcohol bottles, social service and health care facilities).[32-36] Community audits may be conducted using structured checklists or audit tools, or more open-ended processes such as walking or windshield tours of a geographic area.[20] These data are useful in obtaining information about a particular context. However, some data may be influenced by the time of day or time of year (e.g., number of walkers), or observer awareness (e.g., difference between a bottle of soda and a premixed alcohol cocktail).

Qualitative Data

Interviews

Interviews may be individual or group conversations. The conversation may be very structured, using a set of questions that are asked of each individual in exactly the same way, or may be more open, using a general interview protocol that outlines the topics of interest and a variety of probes that may be discussed in the order that seems most appropriate. Group interviews or focus group interviews, as opposed to individual interviews, allow for the influence of social norms to be assessed. The advantages of qualitative data include the potential for enhanced understanding of a particular issue (e.g., not just that someone is inactive but why they are inactive) and participant discussion of the association of various factors with their behavior and health. If a common interview protocol is developed it is possible for interviews to be compared to each other to determine the range of factors influencing behavior and health. It is also possible to conduct several interviews or focus groups so that some comparisons can be made based on different strata (e.g., comparisons across level of physical activity or gender). The disadvantage of qualitative data is that it is often difficult to gather information from as many different individuals and often takes

longer to collect the data. The skills of the interviewer to establish rap-
port with individuals will also have a greater impact in collecting qualitative
compared with quantitative data.

Print Media and Written Documents

Print media also provide a source of qualitative data. For example, newspapers
or newsletters may provide insight into the most salient issues within a community. In addition, more recent technological advances allow for review of
blogs or LISTSERVs as forms of important qualitative data (e.g., the types of
support that a breast cancer LISTSERVs provides or concerns about medical
care within a community). Some have used written diaries as a way to track
and log community events or individual actions.

Observation

Observation is a method of collecting data on a community or an intervention. It entails writing in-depth field notes or descriptions using all of one's
sensory perceptions. By collecting this type of data one can go beyond what a
participant says about the program or the community and can gather information on the local context. The data collected may also be beneficial because
information may be gathered that individuals are uncomfortable talking about
or are not even aware are of interest (like a fish, why talk about the water). In
conducting observations it is important to consider the benefits and drawbacks of participating and the duration of the observation. It is also useful to
recognize that although telling individuals that they are being observed may
alter behavior, not telling them will hinder the development of trusting relationships and may be ethically inappropriate. Observational data are a potentially rich source of information but are highly dependent on the skills and the
abilities of the observer and may take a great deal of time.

Photovoice

Photovoice is a type of qualitative data that uses still or video images to document conditions in a community. These images may be taken by community
members, community-based organization representatives, or professionals. After images are taken they can be used to generate dialogue about the
images.[37] This type of data can be very useful in capturing the salient images
around certain community topics from the community perspective. As they
say, a picture is worth a thousand words. However, it may be difficult to know
what the circumstances surrounding the picture are, when it was taken, or
why it was taken. What an image means is in the "eye of the beholder."

Community Forums or Listening Sessions

Community forums are a method of bringing different segments of the community together to have conversations about the most important issues in their community.[4,38,39] These discussions are larger than focus groups. The community may be presented with a short description of the project and then asked one or two key questions focusing on concerns or visions for how improved population health would look. The community may be given the option of responding verbally or through the creation of visual representations.[13,20] The advantage of bringing the community together to discuss community issues in this way is the ability to engage multiple segments of the community and to create rich and complex dialogue of the issues. The difficulty comes in analyzing the data obtained and in ensuring that the sessions allow for multiple voices to be heard.[38]

ANALYSIS OF DATA

After data has been collected it needs to be analyzed and summarized. Both quantitative and qualitative data analysis requires substantial training far beyond the scope of this book. Chapter 7 will provide an overview of some of the most important analysis considerations when working with quantitative data. Often, in a community assessment the analysis of most interest involves pattern by person, place, and time. Below is an overview of some of the considerations in analyzing qualitative data.

The analysis of qualitative data, whether it is analysis of print media, field notes, photovoice, listening sessions, or interviews, is an iterative process of sorting and synthesizing to develop a set of common concepts or themes that occur in the data in order to discern patterns. The process of analysis often begins during data collection. Similarly, as one collects and analyzes the data there may be interpretations or explanations for patterns seen or linkages among different elements of the data that begin to appear. It is useful to track these as they occur.

There are many different strategies for conducting qualitative data analysis. As with quantitative data, before any analysis it is important to ensure that the data are properly prepared. For example, when analyzing interviews it is important that transcripts (verbatim notes often typed from an audio recording) are accurate and complete. The next step in analysis of qualitative data is the development of a set of codes or categories within which to sort different segments of the data. These codes may be predetermined by the questions driving the inquiry or may be developed in the process of reviewing the data. When the codes are established, the data are reviewed and sorted into the codes or categories, with new codes or categories developed for data that do not fit into established coding schemes. The data within each code are reviewed to ensure that the assignment is accurate and that any subcategories are illuminated. These codes or categories are then reviewed to determine general themes or findings. There are some methods that allow comparison across various groups (e.g., development of matrices that compare findings among men and women or health practitioners and community members). For large data sets there are software packages that can automate parts of this process of data analysis and allow for these types of comparisons (e.g., NVivo, ATLAS.ti). Those interested in further information on qualitative analysis should see additional sources.[31,40] Whenever possible, before finalizing data analysis it is helpful to conduct "member checking." Member checking is a process of going back to the individuals from whom the data were collected and verifying that the themes and concepts derived resonate with participants.[13]

DISSEMINATING COMMUNITY ASSESSMENT FINDINGS

Community assessments within an evidence-based public health decision-making process should be used to understand the community of interest, identify the most important issues for this community, and move toward a collaborative process of developing and implementing interventions. Therefore, after data are collected it is important to summarize and present the data back to all partners, and the community as a whole, in a way that is understandable and integrates the lessons learned from each data source. In doing so it is important to note the advantages and disadvantages of the data collected as well as the parts of the community the data represent. It is also important to share the information in ways that are accessible and useful to the various community audiences.

There are several ways of presenting data. One can provide information in the form of graphs. These graphs can compare rates of morbidity and mortality in one community to those in other communities or can compare subgroups within a particular community. Maps can also be useful in displaying the data collected. For example, maps can be used to highlight areas in a community that have more or less opportunity to access healthy foods or resources for physical activity. One can similarly use maps to identify the density of food outlets, libraries, schools, or even community organizations.[41-43]

In addition to creating materials to document findings from a community assessment, it is important that all partners have an opportunity to reflect on and discuss the findings. This discussion should include dialogue regarding what is surprising and what is expected, what the data represent, and what seems to still be missing. To move toward action the partnership needs to have confidence that the data they have, although never being all the data that could be gathered, are sufficient to move toward action. From there, a full understanding of the data is important in prioritizing the most important issues to work on and developing action plans.

SUMMARY

Community assessments are essential to provide information on existing individual, organizational, and community conditions. Because of the complexity of public health concerns it is important to obtain information at multiple levels of the ecological framework. Involving partners early on in defining what questions need to be asked, and what existing and new data can be used to answer these questions, can save having to wait on action until additional information is gathered and synthesized. Even when partners are involved in the earliest phases, as data are shared the findings inevitably lead to additional questions. It is critical to remember that an assessment is conducted to point the way to action, not as an end in itself. The best way to move effectively to action is to share data in ways that communicate to a wide audience, recognize the strengths and limitations of the data, and provide the opportunity for dialogue regarding findings in ways that lead to prioritization of issues (chapter 9), intervention planning (chapter 10), and evaluation (chapter 11).

KEY CHAPTER POINTS

- Community assessments are essential to provide information on existing individual, organizational, and community conditions.
- Assessments should be conducted at all levels of the ecological framework, using methods that are appropriate for the questions asked.
- Key stakeholders (e.g., community members, community-based organizations, governmental or public agencies) should be involved at the earliest phases possible.
- Triangulated approaches that rely on both quantitative and qualitative data are often the most useful ways of answering key questions.
- Assessments should be conducted in ways that lead to action.
- The best way to move effectively to action is to share data in ways that communicate to a wide audience, recognize the strengths and limitations of the data, and provide the opportunity for dialogue regarding findings in ways that lead to prioritization of issues, intervention planning, and evaluation.

SUGGESTED READINGS AND SELECTED WEBSITES

Suggested Readings

Brennan Ramirez LK, Baker EA, Metzler M. *Promoting Health Equity: A Resource to Help Communities Address Social Determinants of Health.* Atlanta: U.S. Department of Health and Human Services, Centers for Disease Control and Prevention; 2008.

Kretzmann JP, McKnight JL. *Building communities from the inside out: a path toward finding and mobilizing a community's assets.* Chicago, IL: ACTA Publications; 1993.

Miles MB, Huberman AM, Saldana J. *Qualitative Data Analysis: A methods sourcebook.* Thousand Oaks, CA: Sage Publications; 2014.

Plested BA, Edwards RW, Jumper Thurman P. *Community readiness: a handbook for successful change.* Fort Collins, CO: Triethnic Center for Prevention Research; 2005.

Patton, MQ. *Qualitative research and evaluation methods: Integrating theory and practice,* 4th ed. Thousand Oaks, CA: Sage Publications; 2015.

Selected Websites

Centers for Disease Control and Prevention (CDC) Social Determinants of Health Maps <http://www.cdc.gov/dhdsp/maps/social_determinants_maps.htm>. The social determinants of health maps available at the CDC website can be used in conjunction with other data to identify interventions that might positively affect the health of your community of interest.

Centers for Disease Control and Prevention. Community Health Improvement Navigator. http://www.cdc.gov/chinav/tools/assess.html. The Community Health Improvement Navigator provides a series of tools for creating successful community health improvement plans and interventions, including community assessment. The website includes links to lists of indicators and identifying community assets and resources.

Community Commons http://www.communitycommons.org. Community commons provides data, maps, and stories about key community issues related to community health assessment, including economics, education, environment, equity, food, and health.

County Health Rankings & Roadmaps: Building a Culture of Health, County by County. http://www.countyhealthrankings.org Sponsored by the Robert Wood Johnson Foundation, this website provides data and maps on key health factors and health outcomes, as well as policies and programs that communities might want to consider adopting in their communities.

University of California, Los Angeles Center for Health Policy Research, Health DATA Program <http://healthpolicy.ucla.edu/programs/health-data/Pages/overview.aspx>. The Health DATA *(Data. Advocacy. Training. Assistance.)* Program exists to make data understandable to a wide range of health advocates through trainings, workshops, and technical assistance. The site includes instructional videos, Health DATA publications, and links to free online resources in areas such as community-based participatory research, community assessment, data collection (e.g., asset mapping, focus groups, surveys, key informant interviews), and data analysis and presentation.

REFERENCES

1. North Carolina Department of Health and Human Services. *Community Assessment Guide Book: North Carolina Community Health Assessment.* Raleigh, NC: North Carolina Department of Health and Human Services; 2014.

2. Wright J, Williams R, Wilkinson JR. Development and importance of health needs assessment. *BMJ*. Apr 25 1998;316(7140):1310–1313.

3. Eng E, Strazza-Moore K, Rhodes SD, et al. Insiders and outsiders assess who is "the community." In: Israel BA, Eng E, Schulz AJ, Parker EA, eds. *Methods in Community-Based Participatory Research for Health*, 2nd ed. San Francisco, CA: Jossey-Bass Publishers; 2012.

4. Moulton PL, Miller ME, Offutt SM, Gibbens BP. Identifying rural health care needs using community conversations. *J Rural Health*. Winter 2007;23(1):92–96.

5. Green LW, Mercer SL. Can public health researchers and agencies reconcile the push from funding bodies and the pull from communities? *American Journal of Public Health*. Dec 2001;91(12):1926–1929.

6. Clark MJ, Cary S, Diemert G, et al. Involving communities in community assessment. *Public Health Nursing*. Nov-Dec 2003;20(6):456–463.

7. Kieffer EC, Willis SK, Odoms-Young AM, et al. Reducing disparities in diabetes among African-American and Latino residents of Detroit: the essential role of community planning focus groups. *Ethn Dis*. Summer 2004;14(3 Suppl 1):S27–S37.

8. Butterfoss FD, Goodman RM, Wandersman A. Community coalitions for prevention and health promotion. *Health Educ Res*. Sep 1993;8(3):315–330.

9. Parker EA, Eng E, Laraia B, et al. Coalition building for prevention: lessons learned from the North Carolina Community-Based Public Health Initiative. *J Public Health Manag Pract*. Mar 1998;4(2):25–36.

10. World Health Organization. Ottawa Charter for Health Promotion. *International Conference on Health Promotion*. Ontario, Canada; 1986.

11. Alter C, Hage J. *Organizations Working Together: Coordination in Interorganizational Networks*. Newbury Park, CA: Sage Publications; 1992.

12. Himmelman A. *Definitions, decision-making models, roles, and collaboration process guide*. Minneapolis, MN: Himmelman Consulting; 2002.

13. Baker EA, Motton F. Creating understanding and action through group dialogue. In: Israel BA, Eng E, Schultz AJ, Parker EA, eds. *Methods in Community-Based Participatory Research for Health*. San Francisco, CA: Jossey-Bass Publishers; 2005.

14. Cha BS, Lawrence RI, Bliss JC, Wells KB, Chandra A, Eisenman DP. The road to resilience: insights on training community coalitions in the Los Angeles County Community Disaster Resilience Project. *Disaster Med Public Health Prep*. Aug 11 2016:1–10.

15. Wolff T. Community coalition building—contemporary practice and research: introduction. *Am J Community Psychol*. Apr 2001;29(2):165–172; discussion 205–111.

16. Khare MM, Nunez AE, James BF. Coalition for a Healthier Community: lessons learned and implications for future work. *Eval Program Plann*. Aug 2015;51:85–88.

17. Baker EA, Brownson CA. Defining characteristics of community-based health promotion programs. *J Public Health Manag Pract*. Mar 1998;4(2):1–9.

18. Kretzmann JP, Mcknight JL. *Building communities from the inside out: a path toward finding and mobilizing a community's assets*. Chicago, IL: ACTA Publications; 1993.

19. Institute of Medicine. *The Future of the Public's Health in the 21st Century*. Washington, DC: National Academies Press; 2003.

20. Sharpe PA, Greaney ML, Lee PR, Royce SW. Assets-oriented community assessment. *Public Health Reports*. Mar-Jun 2000;115(2-3):205–211.

21. Brownson RC, Baker EA, Leet TL, Gillespie KN, True WR. *Evidence-Based Public Health*. 2nd ed. New York, NY: Oxford University Press; 2011.

22. McLeroy KR, Bibeau D, Steckler A, Glanz K. An ecological perspective on health promotion programs. *Health Educ Q.* Winter 1988;15(4):351–377.

23. Simons-Morton DG, Simons-Morton BG, Parcel GS, Bunker JF. Influencing personal and environmental conditions for community health: a multilevel intervention model. *Fam Community Health.* Aug 1988;11(2):25–35.

24. Breslow L. Social ecological strategies for promoting healthy lifestyles. *American Journal of Health Promotion.* Mar-Apr 1996;10(4):253–257. .

25. Goodman RM, Wandersman A, Chinman M, Imm P, Morrissey E. An ecological assessment of community-based interventions for prevention and health promotion: approaches to measuring community coalitions. *Am J Community Psychol.* Feb 1996;24(1):33–61.

26. Dahlgren G, Whitehead M. *Policies and Strategies to Promote Equity in Health.* Stockholm, Sweden: Institute for Future Studies; 1991.

27. Schulz AJ, Israel BA, Lantz P. Instrument for evaluating dimensions of group dynamics within community-based participatory research partnerships. *Evaluation and Program Planning.* Aug 2003;26(3):249–262.

28. Plested BA, Edwards RW, Jumper Thurman P. *Community Readiness: A Handbook for Successful Change.* Fort Collins, CO: Triethnic Center for Prevention Research; 2005.

29. Baker EA, Brennan Ramirez LK, Claus JM, Land G. Translating and disseminating research- and practice-based criteria to support evidence-based intervention planning. *J Public Health Manag Pract.* Mar-Apr 2008;14(2):124–130.

30. Sallis J, Owen N. Ecological models of health behavior. In: Glanz K, Rimer B, Vishwanath K, eds. *Health Behavior: Theory, Research, and Practice.* 2nd ed. San Francisco, CA: Jossey-Bass Publishers; 2015:43–64.

31. Patton M. *Qualitative Evaluation and Research Methods.* 4th ed. Thousand Oaks, CA: Sage Publications; 2014.

32. Brownson RC, Hoehner CM, Day K, Forsyth A, Sallis JF. Measuring the built environment for physical activity: state of the science. *Am J Prev Med.* Apr 2009;36(4 Suppl):S99–123, e112.

33. Cheadle A, Sterling TD, Schmid TL, Fawcett SB. Promising community-level indicators for evaluating cardiovascular health-promotion programs. *Health Educ Res.* Feb 2000;15(1):109–116.

34. Hausman AJ, Becker J, Brawer R. Identifying value indicators and social capital in community health partnerships. *J Commun Psychol.* 2005;33(6):691–703.

35. McKinnon RA, Reedy J, Morrissette MA, Lytle LA, Yaroch AL. Measures of the food environment: a compilation of the literature, 1990-2007. *Am J Prev Med.* Apr 2009;36(4 Suppl):S124–S133.

36. Glanz K, Sallis JF, Saelens BE. Advances in physical activity and nutrition environment assessment tools and applications: recommendations. *Am J Prev Med.* May 2015;48(5):615–619.

37. Wang C, Burris MA. Photovoice: concept, methodology, and use for participatory needs assessment. *Health Educ Behav.* Jun 1997;24(3):369–387.

38. North Carolina Department of Health and Human Services. *Healthy Carolinas: North Carolina Community Health Assessment Process.* NC Division of Public Office of Healthy Carolinas/Health Education & State Center for Health Statistics; 2008.

39. Minkler M, Hancock. Community driven asset identification and issue selection. In: Minkler M, Wallerstein N, eds. *Community-based Participatory Research for Health: from Process to Outcomes.* San Francisco, CA: Jossey-Bass Publishers; 2008.

40. Huberman M, Miles M. *The Qualitative Researcher's Companion*. London: Sage Publications; 2002.
41. Plescia M, Koontz S, Laurent S. Community assessment in a vertically integrated health care system. *Am J Public Health*. May 2001;91(5):811–814.
42. Zenk SN, Lachance LL, Schulz AJ, Mentz G, Kannan S, Ridella W. Neighborhood retail food environment and fruit and vegetable intake in a multiethnic urban population. *Am J Health Promot*. Mar-Apr 2009;23(4):255–264.
43. Baker EA, Schootman M, Barnidge E, et al. The role of race and poverty in access to foods that enable individuals to adhere to dietary guidelines. *Preventing Chronic Disease*. Jul 2006;3(3):A76.

CHAPTER 6

❦

Developing an Initial Statement
of the Issue

If you don't know where you are going, you will wind up somewhere else.
Yogi Berra

An early step in an evidence-based process is to develop a concise statement of the issue being considered. A clear articulation of the problem at hand will enhance the likelihood that a systematic and focused planning process can be followed, leading to successful outcomes and achievement of objectives. A clear statement of the issue provides a concrete basis for a priority-setting process that is objective, which then leads to better program planning, intervention, and evaluation. A fully articulated issue statement includes a complete description of the problem, potential solutions, data sources, and health-related outcomes. Although this may seem straightforward, developing a sound issue statement can be challenging. In fact, the development of well-stated and answerable clinical questions has been described as the most difficult step in the practice of evidence-based medicine.[1]

Issue statements can be initiated in at least three different ways. They might be part of a section on background and objectives of a grant application for external support of a particular intervention or program. Because this is generally the first portion of a grant application to be viewed by funders, a clear delineation of the issue under consideration is crucial. An issue statement might also be in response to a request from an administrator or an elected official about a particular issue. For example, a governor or minister of health might seek input from agency personnel on a specific problem. Your task might be to develop a politically and scientifically acceptable issue statement within a short time period in response. Or, a program or agency might define issues as a result of a community assessment or as part of a strategic planning process that could take several months to implement and evaluate. Each scenario demonstrates a different set of reasons and circumstances for defining a particular public health issue. In all cases, it is essential that the initial statement of the issue be clear, articulate, and well understood by all members of the public health team, as well as other relevant parties.

This chapter is divided into two major sections. The first examines some lessons and approaches that can be learned from the processes of community assessment and strategic planning. The second describes a systematic approach to developing an issue statement by breaking it into four component parts: background and epidemiologic data; questions about the program or policy; solutions being considered; and potential outcomes. It should be remembered that an initial issue statement is likely to evolve as more information is gathered in the course of program implementation and policy development.

BACKGROUND

Developing a concise and useful issue statement can be informed by the processes of community assessment and strategic planning. In a community assessment, issues emerge and are defined in the process of determining the health needs or desires of a population. In strategic planning, the identification of key strategic issues helps define the priorities and direction for a group or organization. In addition, issue definition is closely linked with the objective-setting steps involved in developing an action plan for a program (chapter 10) and also forms part of the foundation of an effective evaluation strategy (chapter 11).

Important Aspects of Community Assessment

Community (or needs) assessment was discussed in more detail in chapter 5. In brief, a needs assessment is "a systematic set of procedures undertaken for the purpose of setting priorities and making decisions about program or organizational improvement and allocation of resources. The priorities are based on identified needs."[2] A community assessment may involve a variety of different data types, including epidemiologic (quantitative) data, qualitative information, data on health inequalities, and patterns of health resource utilization.[3]

The initial aspects of a community assessment are especially pertinent when defining an issue or problem. A typical community assessment would begin by considering sources of baseline or background data on a health problem or a community. These sources might include primary or secondary data. Primary data involve collection of new information for a particular program or study through such methods as a community survey, interviews, focus groups, and so forth. Collection of primary data often occurs over a relatively long period of time, sometimes years, although a local community assessment survey can be done in 3 to 6 months. Community assessments often rely on secondary data sources—that is, data routinely collected at a local, state, or national level. The biggest advantages of using secondary data rather than collecting primary data are time and cost. Many government, university, and nonprofit agencies spend years and many dollars collecting and maintaining data. These agencies also have the technical expertise that ensures that data are of high quality. Several important sources of secondary data are readily available and are listed with their websites at the end of this chapter. One disadvantage of secondary data is that detailed local information may not be available for smaller or less populous areas. Community health assessments often use a mix of primary and secondary data. In addition to quantitative secondary data on morbidity, mortality, and health behaviors, they may make use of qualitative primary data collected by interviews or focus group methods.

Key Aspects of Strategic Planning

Strategic planning is a disciplined effort to produce decisions and actions that shape and guide what an organization is, what it does, and why it does it.[4] It is a continuous process for identifying intended future outcomes and how success will be measured, often with a 3- to 5-year time horizon. A complete discussion of strategic planning benefits and methods is available elsewhere.[4,5] Rational strategic planning is based on three deceptively simple questions: "Where are we?"; "Where do we want to be?"; and "How do we get there?" In this section, specific aspects that help shape issue definition within an evidence-based public health framework are reviewed.

In many senses, problem definition is similar to the early steps in a strategic planning process, which often involve reaching consensus on the mission and values of the organization, analyzing the internal and external environments, involving people affected by the plan in the process, and creating a common vision for the future. The public health environment is ever-changing and shaped by new science and information, policies, and social forces. In particular, the early phases of a strategic planning process often involve an environmental assessment. This assessment may include an analysis of political, economic, social, and technological (PEST) trends in the larger environment. Such an analysis is important in order to understand the context in which specific problems are embedded and within which they must be addressed. A TOWS analysis (identification of an organization's external Threats, Opportunities, internal Weaknesses, and Strengths) is often prepared as well (Figure 6.1). The TOWS analysis brings the organization into focus and assesses the impact of external forces (threats and opportunities) in relation to the gaps and resources (weaknesses and strengths). As an issue becomes more clearly defined using the methods detailed in the next section, it is important to remember the context in which the issue is being addressed. Some of the questions and areas that may be considered early in an environmental assessment are shown in Table 6.1.[6] Later, when strategies are known, a comprehensive assessment of resources—financial and nonfinancial—is needed. A well-done community assessment or environmental analysis can increase the likelihood of asking the right questions that will later guide an evidence-based process.

DIVIDING AN ISSUE INTO ITS COMPONENT PARTS

When beginning to define an issue, several fundamental questions should be asked and answered[7]:

- What was the basis for the initial statement of the issue? This may include the social, political, or health circumstances at the time the issue was originated, and how it was framed. This provides the context for the issue.
- Who was the originator of the concern? The issue may have developed internally within a community or organization or may be set as an issue by a policy maker or funder.
- Should or could the issue be stated in the epidemiologic context of person (How many people are affected and who are they?), place (What is the

	Negative	Positive
External	Threats	Opportunities
Internal	Weaknesses	Strengths

Figure 6.1: Components of a TOWS (identification of an organization's external Threats, Opportunities, internal Weaknesses, and Strengths) analysis.

Table 6.1. IMPORTANT QUESTIONS TO CONSIDER IN
AN ENVIRONMENTAL ANALYSIS

Area of Interest	Questions to Consider
External assessment	Will the community accept and support addressing this issue?
	Are there government regulations and other legal factors affecting the issue?
	Have the views of each important stakeholder been taken into account?
	Are there other external groups addressing this issue with success or lack of success (both current and in the past)?
Internal assessment	Is this issue relevant to the mission and values of the organization?
	What, if anything, are we already doing to address the issue?
	Does the organization have the desire and ability to address this issue?
	Who in the agency has an interest in seeing the issue addressed?
	If so, how high is the priority of this issue for the organization?

Source: Adapted from Timmreck.[6]

geographic distribution of the issue?), and time (How long has this issue been a problem? What are anticipated changes over time?)?[8]
- What is and what should be occurring?
- Who is affected and how much?
- What could happen if the problem is NOT addressed?
- Is there a consensus among stakeholders that the problem is properly stated?

This section will begin to address these and other questions that one may encounter when developing an initial issue statement. A sound issue statement may draw on multiple disciplines, including biostatistics, epidemiology, health communication, health economics, health education, management, medicine, planning, and policy analysis. An issue statement should be stated as a quantifiable question (or series of questions) leading to an analysis of root causes or likely intervention approaches. It should also be unbiased in its anticipated course of action. Figure 6.2 describes the progression of an issue statement along with some of the questions that are crucial to answer. One question along the way is, "Do we need more information?" The answer to that question is nearly always "yes," so the challenge becomes where to find the most essential information efficiently. It is also essential to remember that the initial issue statement is often the "tip of the iceberg" and that getting to the actual causes of and solutions to the problem takes considerable time and effort. Causal frameworks (also know as analytic frameworks; see chapter 9) are often useful in mapping out an issue.

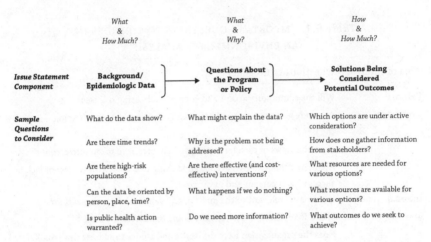

Figure 6.2: A sequential framework for understanding the key steps in developing an issue statement.

Issue Components

The four key components of an issue statement are as follows:

1. Background and epidemiologic data
2. Questions about the program or policy
3. Solutions being considered
4. Potential outcomes

Initially, each of these four components should be framed succinctly, in a maximum of one paragraph each. As intervention approaches are later decided on, these brief initial statements will be refined and expanded into more complete protocols.

An example of the four components of an issue statement, along with potential data sources, is presented in Table 6.2. The section on *background and epidemiologic data* generally presents what is known of the descriptive epidemiology of a public health issue. This includes data on person, place, and time that are often presented as rates or percentage changes over time. It is often useful to present a visual display of the epidemiologic data. For example, Figure 6.3 shows time trends in heart disease mortality in five countries in Europe.[9] These data show large disparities by country; more than a threefold difference is seen in rates in Italy compared with those in the Russian Federation.[9] The variations are significant when comparing Western Europe with Central and Eastern Europe. To show a person-level characteristic, large gender variations are noted for important risk factors such as cigarette smoking (Figure 6.4).[10] If available, qualitative information may also be presented

Table 6.2. EXAMPLES OF AN INITIAL ISSUE STATEMENT
FOR BREAST CANCER CONTROL

Component	Example Statement/Questions	Potential Data Sources
Background and epidemiologic data	Based on data from the Behavioral Risk Factor Surveillance System (BRFSS), only 83% of California women aged 50 years and older are receiving mammography screening each year. Rates of screening have remained constant over the past 5 years and are lowest among lower income women.	CDC WONDER CDC BRFSS data State vital statistics State and local surveillance reports
Questions about the program or policy	Do we understand why screening rates are lower among lower-income women? Why is this a problem? Are there examples in the scientific literature of effective programs to increase the rate of mammography screening among women? Are there similar programs targeted to lower income women? Are there cost-effectiveness studies of these interventions? Have policies been enacted and evaluated that have had a positive impact on mammography screening rates?	MEDLINE/PubMed Professional meetings Guidelines Legislative records
Solutions being considered	Numerous solutions have been proposed, including (1) increased funding for mammography screening among low-income women; (2) a mass media campaign to promote screening; (3) education of health care providers on how to effectively counsel women for mammography screening; and (4) a peer support program that involves the target audience in the delivery of the intervention	Program staff Policymakers Advisory groups or coalitions Women with breast cancer
Potential outcomes	Rate of breast cancer mortality Rate of breast cancer mortality among low-income women Rate of mammography screening Cost of breast cancer treatment Rate of counseling for mammography among primary care providers	CDC WONDER CDC BRFSS data HEDIS data Hospital discharge data Program records

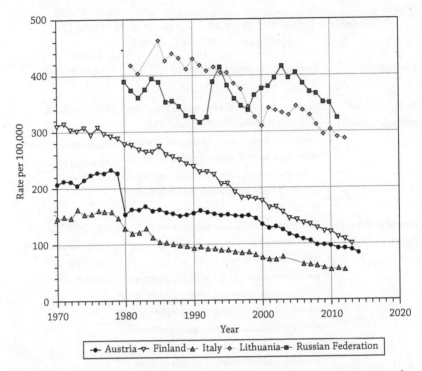

Figure 6.3: Ischemic heart disease deaths in selected European countries, 1970–2014.[9]

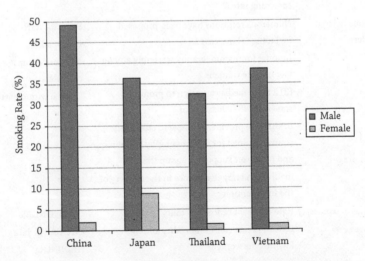

Figure 6.4: Smoking rates among adults in selected Asian countries, by gender.[10]

with the background statement. For example, focus group data may be available that demonstrate a particular attitude or belief toward a public health issue. The concepts presented earlier in this chapter related to community assessment are often useful in assembling background data. In all cases, it is important to specify the source of the data so that the presentation of the problem is credible.

In considering the *questions about the program or policy,* the search for effective intervention options (our Type 2 evidence) begins. You may want to undertake a strategic planning process to generate a set of potentially effective program options that could address the issue. The term *program* is defined broadly to encompass any organized public health action, including direct service interventions, community mobilization efforts, policy development and implementation, outbreak investigations, health communication campaigns, health promotion programs, and applied research initiatives.[8] The programmatic issue being considered may be best presented as a series of questions that a public health team will attempt to answer. It may be stated in the context of an intervention program, a health policy, cost-effectiveness, or managerial challenge. For an intervention, you might ask, "Are there effective intervention programs in the literature to address risk factor X among population Y?" A policy question would consider, "Can you document the positive effects of a health policy that was enacted and enforced in State X?" In the area of cost-effectiveness, it might be, "What is the cost of intervention Z per year of life saved?"[11] And a managerial question would ask, "What are the resources needed to allow us to effectively initiate a program to address issue X?" The questions that ascertain the "how" of program or policy implementation begin to address Type 3 evidence, as described in chapter 1.

As the issue statement develops, it is often useful to consider *potential solutions.* However, several caveats are warranted at this early phase. First, solutions generated at this phase may or may not be evidence based because all the information may not be in hand. Also, the program ultimately implemented is likely to differ from the potential solutions discussed at this stage. Finally, solutions noted in one population or region may or may not be generalizable to other populations (see discussion of external validity in chapter 3). There is a natural tendency to jump too quickly to solutions before the background and programmatic focus of a particular issue are well defined. In Table 6.3, potential solutions are presented that are largely developed from the efforts of the *Guide to Community Preventive Services,* an evidence-based systematic review described in chapter 8.[12]

When framing *potential solutions* of an issue statement, it is useful to consider whether a "high-risk" or population strategy is warranted. The high-risk strategy focuses on individuals who are most at risk for a particular disease or risk factor.[13,14] Focusing an early detection program on lower income individuals who have the least access to screening, for example, is a

Table 6.3. EXAMPLE OF AN INITIAL ISSUE STATEMENT FOR INFLUENZA
VACCINATION AMONG PEOPLE AGED 65 YEARS AND OLDER

Component	Example Statement/Questions	Potential Data Sources
Background/ epidemiologic data	Based on BRFSS data, rates of influenza immunization among people aged 65 years and older have increased nearly 16% among Blacks since 1999. Despite this increase, influenza immunization rates for Black and Hispanic adults aged 65 years and older are lower than those of Whites and below those recommended.	National Health Interview Survey US Administration on Aging State vital statistics State and local surveillance reports
Questions about the program or policy	How effective are vaccinations in reducing hospitalizations and deaths due to influenza? What are historical rates of influenza vaccination among people aged 65 years and older? Are all income and racial/ethnic groups affected equally? Are there public health interventions that have been documented to increase coverage of influenza vaccination among people aged 65 years and older?	PubMed Healthy People 2010, state health plans Professional meetings Guidelines Legislative records
Solutions being considered	Numerous solutions have been proposed, including: (1) educational programs for the target population; (2) client reminder/recall interventions delivered via telephone or letter; (3) home visits for socioeconomically disadvantaged populations; (4) community mass media programs; and (5) programs to expand vaccination access in health care settings.	Program staff Guidelines Policymakers Advisory groups (e.g., AARP)
Potential outcomes	Rates of immunization Rates of influenza incidence (a reportable disease) Rates of influenza vaccination among various Health Maintenance Organizations Rates of mortality due to influenza	CDC WONDER CDC BRFSS data Healthcare Effectiveness Data and Information Set (HEDIS) data Program records

high-risk approach. A population strategy is employed when the risk being considered is widely disseminated across a population. A population strategy might involve conducting a mass media campaign to increase early detection among all persons at risk. In practice, these two approaches are not mutually exclusive. The year 2020 health goals for the United States, for example, call for elimination of health disparities (a high-risk approach) and also target overall improvements in social and physical environments to promote health for all (a population approach).[15] Data and available resources can help in determining whether a population approach, a high-risk strategy, or both are warranted.

Although it may seem premature to consider *potential outcomes* before an intervention approach is decided on, an initial scan of outcomes is often valuable at this stage. It is especially important to consider the answer to the questions, "What outcome do we want to achieve in addressing this issue? What would a good or acceptable outcome look like?" This process allows you to consider potential short- and longer-term outcomes. It also helps shape the choice of possible solutions and determines the level of resources that will be required to address the issue. For many US public health issues (e.g., numerous environmental health exposures), data do not readily exist for community assessment and evaluation at a state or local level. Long-term outcomes (e.g., mortality rates) that are often available are not useful for planning and implementing programs with a time horizon of a few years. A significant challenge to be discussed in later chapters is the need to identify valid and reliable intermediate outcomes for public health programs.

Importance of Stakeholder Input

As the issue definition stage continues, it is often critical to obtain the input of "stakeholders." Stakeholders, or key players, are individuals or agencies with a vested interest in the issue at hand.[3] When addressing a particular health policy, policy makers are especially important stakeholders. Stakeholders can also be individuals who would potentially receive, use, and benefit from the program or policy being considered. In particular, three groups of stakeholders are relevant[8]:

1. Those involved in program operations, such as sponsors, coalition partners, administrators, and staff
2. Those served or affected by the program, including clients, family members, neighborhood organizations, and elected officials
3. Primary users of the evaluation—people who are in a position to do or decide something regarding the program. (These individuals may overlap with the first two categories.)

Table 6.4 shows how the considerations and motivations of various stakeholders can vary.[16] These differences are important to take into account while garnering stakeholder input.

Table 6.4. MAJOR HEALTH POLICY CONSIDERATIONS AMONG
STAKEHOLDERS IN THE UNITED STATES

Stakeholder	Consideration
Politicians	The cost of medical care is high and rising quickly.
	There are many uninsured Americans, and many Americans are at risk for losing their insurance coverage.
	The increasing costs of the Medicaid and Medicare programs strain state and federal budgets.
	Health care providers charge too much.
	There are too many doctors (a rural politician might say the opposite), and too many specialists relative to primary care physicians.
Health care professionals	There is an overutilization of medical services, especially in certain areas of the country, and there is an underutilization of some services in other areas.
	There is an increase in the "intensity" of health services, i.e., technology that results in increased costs.
	The effects of improved health services over time have been decreased death rates and increased life expectancy.
	More efficient health care delivery will reduce health care costs.
Public health advocates	The health of the American public has improved substantially as demonstrated by declining death rates and longer life expectancy.
	Major public health programs have been successful in reducing key risk factors such as cigarette smoking, control of hypertension, and dietary changes.
	There are millions of Americans who lack heath care coverage.
	Environmental monitoring and control have helped decrease morbidity and mortality.
	Prevention is the cornerstone of effective health policy.
Consumers	Personal and out-of-pocket health care costs are too high.
	Quality medical care is often not provided.
	There are substantial risks to the public from "involuntary" environmental hazards such as radiation, chemicals, food additives, and occupational exposures.

Source: Adapted from Kuller.[16]

An example of the need for stakeholder input can be seen in Box 6.1. In this case, there are likely to be individuals and advocacy groups with strong feelings regarding how best to reduce infant mortality. Some of the approaches, such as increasing funding for family planning, may be controversial. As described in other parts of this book, there are several different mechanisms for gaining stakeholder input, including the following:

• Interviews of leaders of various voluntary and nonprofit agencies that have an interest in this issue

---

Box 6.1
REDUCING INFANT MORTALITY IN TEXAS

For the newly hired director of the Maternal and Child Health Bureau at the Texas Department of Health and Human Services, the issue of disparities in infant mortality rates is of high interest. You have been charged with developing a plan for reducing the rate of infant mortality. The plan must be developed within 12 months and implemented within 2 years. The data show that the infant mortality rate in Texas plateaued from 2000 to 2005, but then declined 12% from 2005 to 2015. Significant differences among infant mortality rates of different races continue. The rate among non-Hispanic blacks is currently 10.7 per 1,000 live births, and the rate among non-Hispanic whites is currently 5.1, a relative difference of 110%. Program staff, policy makers, and advisory groups (stakeholders) have proposed numerous intervention options, including (1) increased funding for family planning services; (2) a mass media campaign to encourage women to seek early prenatal care; and (3) global policies that are aimed at increasing health care access for pregnant women. Program personnel face a significant challenge in trying to obtain adequate stakeholder input within the time frame set out by the governor. You have to decide on the methods for obtaining adequate and representative feedback from stakeholders in a short time frame. Some of the issues you need to consider include the following:

- The role of the government and the role of the private sector in reducing infant mortality
- The positions of various religious groups on family planning
- The key barriers facing women of various ethnic backgrounds when obtaining adequate prenatal care
- The views of key policy makers in Texas who will decide the amount of public resources available for your program

- Focus groups with clients who may be served by various interventions
- Newspaper content analysis of clippings that describe previous efforts to enhance health

SUMMARY

This chapter is a transition point to numerous other chapters in this book. It begins a sequential and systematic process for evidence-based decision making in public health. The extent to which a practitioner may undergo a full-fledged baseline community assessment is often dependent on time and resources (see chapters 5 and 11). It should also be remembered that public health is a team sport and that review and refinement of an initial issue statement with one's team are essential.

KEY CHAPTER POINTS

- The extent to which a practitioner may undergo a full-fledged baseline community assessment is often dependent on time and resources.
- There are multiple reasons to draft an issue statement early in an evidence-based process.
- An assessment of the external environment, based on strategic planning methods, will help in understanding the context for a program or policy.
- Breaking an issue into its component parts (background and epidemiologic data, questions about the program or policy, solutions being considered, and potential outcomes) will enhance the assessment process.
- Input from all stakeholders is essential for informing the approaches to solving many public health problems. This can be obtained through a community assessment, which is described in chapter 5.

SUGGESTED READINGS AND SELECTED WEBSITES

Suggested Readings

Bryson JM. *Strategic Planning for Public and Nonprofit Organizations. A Guide to Strengthening and Sustaining Organizational Achievement.* 4th Edition. San Francisco, CA: Jossey-Bass Publishers, 2011.

Ginter PM, Duncan WJ, Swayne LM. *Strategic Management of Health Care Organizations.* 7th ed. West Sussex, UK: John Wiley & Sons Ltd; 2013.

Timmreck TC. *Planning, Program Development, and Evaluation. A Handbook for Health Promotion, Aging and Health Services.* 2nd ed. Boston, MA: Jones and Bartlett Publishers; 2003.

Selected Websites

Behavioral Risk Factor Surveillance System (BRFSS) <http://www.cdc.gov/brfss/>. The BRFSS is the world's largest, ongoing telephone health survey system, tracking health conditions and risk behaviors in the United States yearly since 1984. Currently, data are collected in all 50 states, the District of Columbia, and three US territories. The Centers for Disease Control and Prevention have developed a standard core questionnaire so that data can be compared across various strata. The Selected Metropolitan/Micropolitan Area Risk Trends (SMART) project provides localized data for selected areas. BRFSS data are used to identify emerging health problems, establish and track health objectives, and develop and evaluate public health policies and programs.

Centers for Disease Control and Prevention (CDC). Gateway to Communication and Social Marketing Practice <http://www.cdc.gov/healthcommunication/cdcynergy/problemdescription.html>. CDC's Gateway to Communication and Social

Marketing Practice provides resources to help build your health communication or social marketing campaigns and programs.

CDC Wonder <http://wonder.cdc.gov>. CDC WONDER is an easy-to-use system that provides a single point of access to a wide variety of CDC reports, guidelines, and numeric public health data. It can be valuable in public health research, decision making, priority setting, program evaluation, and resource allocation.

Center for Prevention—Altarum Institute (CFP) <http://altarum.org/research-centers/center-for-prevention>. Working to emphasize disease prevention and health promotion in national policy and practice, the CFP is one of the research centers of the Altarum Institute. The site includes action guides that translate several of the *Community Guide* recommendations into easy-to-follow implementation guidelines on priority health topics such as sexual health, tobacco control, aspirin, and chlamydia.

The Community Health Status Indicators (CHSI) Project <http://wwwn.cdc.gov/communityhealth>. The CHSI Project includes 3,141 county health status profiles representing each county in the United States excluding territories. Each CHSI report includes data on access and utilization of health care services, birth and death measures, Healthy People 2020 targets and US birth and death rates, vulnerable populations, risk-factors for premature deaths, communicable diseases, and environmental health. The goal of CHSI is to give local public health agencies another tool for improving their community's health by identifying resources and setting priorities.

European Health for All Database (HFA-DB) < http://www.euro.who.int/en/data-and-evidence/databases/european-health-for-all-database-hfa-db >. The HFA-DB has been a key source of information on health in the European Region since the World Health Organization (WHO)–Europe launched it in the mid-1980s. It contains time series from 1970. HFA-DB is updated biannually and contains about 600 indicators for the 53 Member States in the Region. The indicators cover basic demographics, health status (mortality, morbidity), health determinants (such as lifestyle and environment), and health care (resources and utilization).

Partners in Information Access for the Public Health Workforce <http://phpartners.org/>. This Workforce is a collaboration of US government agencies, public health organizations, and health sciences libraries that provides timely, convenient access to selected public health resources on the Internet.

WHO Statistical Information System (WHOSIS) <http://www.who.int/whosis/en/>. WHOSIS is an interactive database bringing together core health statistics for the 193 WHO Member States. It comprises more than 100 indicators, which can be accessed by way of a quick search, by major categories, or through user-defined tables. The data can be further filtered, tabulated, charted, and downloaded.

REFERENCES

1. Straus SE, Richardson WS, Glasziou P, Haynes R. *Evidence-Based Medicine. How to Practice and Teach EBM.* 4th ed. Edinburgh, UK: Churchill Livingstone; 2011.
2. Witkin BR, Altschuld JW. *Conducting and Planning Needs Assessments. A Practical Guide.* Thousand Oaks, CA: Sage Publications; 1995.
3. Soriano F. *Conducting Needs Assessments: A Multidisciplinary Approach.* Thousand Oaks, CA: Sage Publications; 2013.

4. Bryson JM. *Strategic Planning for Public and Nonprofit Organizations. A Guide to Strengthening and Sustaining Organizational Achievement.* 4th ed. San Francisco, CA: John Wiley & Sons, Inc.; 2011.
5. Ginter PM, Duncan WJ, Swayne LM. *Strategic Management of Health Care Organizations.* 7th ed. West Sussex, UK: John Wiley & Sons Ltd.; 2013.
6. Timmreck TC. *Planning, Program Development, and Evaluation. A Handbook for Health Promotion, Aging and Health Services.* 2nd ed. Boston, MA: Jones and Bartlett Publishers; 2003.
7. Centers for Disease Control and Prevention. Gateway to communication and social marketing practice. http://www.cdc.gov/healthcommunication/cdcynergy/problemdescription.html. Accessed June 5, 2016.
8. Centers for Disease Control and Prevention. Framework for program evaluation in public health. http://www.cdc.gov/eval/framework/. Accessed June 5, 2016.
9. World Health Organization Regional Office for Europe. European Health for All database http://data.euro.who.int/hfadb/. Accessed June 5, 2016.
10. World Health Organization. Tobacco Free Initiative. http://www.who.int/tobacco/publications/en/. Accessed June 5, 2016.
11. Tengs TO, Adams ME, Pliskin JS, et al. Five-hundred life-saving interventions and their cost-effectiveness. *Risk Anal.* Jun 1995;15(3):369–390.
12. Task Force on Community Preventive Services. Guide to Community Preventive Services. www.thecommunityguide.org. Accessed June 5, 2016.
13. Rose G. Sick individuals and sick populations. *International Journal of Epidemiology.* 1985;14(1):32–38.
14. Rose G. *The Strategy of Preventive Medicine.* Oxford, UK: Oxford University Press; 1992.
15. Koh HK, Piotrowski JJ, Kumanyika S, Fielding JE. Healthy People: a 2020 vision for the social determinants approach. *Health Educ Behav.* Dec 2011;38(6):551–557.
16. Kuller LH. Epidemiology and health policy. *Am J Epidemiol.* 1988;127(1):2–16.

CHAPTER 7

ↄ‎ℳↄ‎

Quantifying the Issue

Everything that can be counted does not necessarily count; everything that counts cannot necessarily be counted.

Albert Einstein

As discussed in chapter 5, the community assessment should include the health condition or risk factor under consideration, the population affected, the size and scope of the problem, prevention opportunities, and potential stakeholders. This task requires basic epidemiologic skills to obtain additional information about the frequency of the health condition or risk factor in an affected population. For example, if there is concern about excess *disease* (a term that will be used as a generic synonym for any health condition or risk factor in this chapter) in a population, we should determine the parameters that define the population at risk. Should we focus on the total population, or restrict the population to males or females of certain ages? After the population is defined, we must estimate the frequency of disease present in the population. Can we determine the number of diseased persons from existing public health surveillance systems, or must we conduct a special survey of the defined population? After disease rates are computed, do we see any patterns of disease that identify or confirm subgroups within the defined population that have the highest disease rates? Finally, can we use this information to develop and evaluate the effectiveness of new public health programs and policies?

This chapter provides an overview of the principles of epidemiology that relate to public health practice. It focuses primarily on methods used to measure and characterize disease frequency in defined populations. It includes information about public health surveillance systems and currently available data sources on the Internet. It also provides an overview of the methods used to evaluate the effectiveness of new public health programs that are designed to reduce the prevalence of risk factors and the disease burden in target populations.

OVERVIEW OF DESCRIPTIVE EPIDEMIOLOGY

Epidemiology is commonly defined as the study of the distribution and determinants of disease frequency in human populations and the application of this study to control health problems.[1] In a more comprehensive definition relevant to public health practice, Terris[2] stated that epidemiology is the study of the health of human populations for the following purposes:

1. To discover the agent, host, and environmental factors that affect health, in order to provide a scientific basis for the prevention of disease and injury and the promotion of health
2. To determine the relative importance of causes of illness, disability, and death, in order to establish priorities for research and action
3. To identify those sections of the population that have the greater risk from specific causes of ill health, in order to direct the indicated action appropriately
4. To evaluate the effectiveness of health programs and services in improving the health of the population

The first two functions provide etiologic (or Type 1) evidence to support causal associations between modifiable and nonmodifiable risk factors and specific diseases, as well as the relative importance of these risk factors when establishing priorities for public health interventions. The third function focuses on the frequency of disease in a defined population and the subgroups within the population to be targeted with public health programs. The last function provides experimental (or Type 2) evidence that supports the relative effectiveness of specific public health interventions to address a particular disease.

The terms *descriptive epidemiology* and *analytic epidemiology* are commonly used when presenting the principles of epidemiology. Descriptive epidemiology encompasses methods for measuring the frequency of disease in defined populations. These methods can be used to compare the frequency of disease within and between populations in order to identify subgroups with the highest frequency of disease and to observe any changes that have occurred over time. Analytic epidemiology focuses on identifying essential factors that influence the prevention, occurrence, control, and outcome of disease. Methods used in analytic epidemiology are necessary for identifying new risk factors for specific diseases and for evaluating the effectiveness of new public health programs designed to reduce the disease risk for target populations.

Estimating Disease Frequency

One way to measure disease frequency is to count the number of diseased persons in a defined population and to report that number of cases. Often newspaper articles from a city will compare the current year's number of cases of sexually transmitted diseases with the number from last year. Yet this case count is not informative for understanding the dynamics of disease in a population. A much better method is to estimate the rate of disease in a defined population over time. This allows us to take into account the size of the population in which disease cases occurred. The rate is computed by dividing the number of persons with the disease of interest by the number of persons at risk for developing the disease during a specified period. For example, 6,550 Texas residents were diagnosed with colon cancer in 2012. Thus, the colon cancer rate equals 6,550 cases divided by 262,060,796 people residing in Texas on July 1, 2012 (or the midpoint of the year). The rate is 0.000251 colon cancers per person, or 25.1 colon cancers per 100,000 people per year. Here, we use data from the Centers for Disease Control and Prevention (CDC) WONDER cancer incidence database to identify newly diagnosed colon cancers that occurred among people residing in Texas during 2012 and data from the US Census Bureau to estimate the number of people residing in Texas on July 1, 2012.

Although a disease rate represents the number of cases of disease that occurs in the population during a specified period, we must realize that the number of people in the population (the denominator in the calculation of the rate) is not static. People can move in and out of the population or can die of another disease, indicating that their time at risk for the disease changes over the specified period. Therefore a more precise way of dealing with persons who move in or out of the population during the surveillance period is to estimate "person-time" for the population at risk, or the amount of time that each person in the population is free from disease during the surveillance period. In our example, every person residing in Texas from January 1 to December 31, 2012 contributes 1 person-year if she or he is not diagnosed with colon cancer during the study period. Each person who is diagnosed with colon cancer during the study period, who moves from the state, or whose colon cancer status is unknown contributes a fraction of a person-year, based on the amount of time that elapsed from January 1, 2012 to the date of diagnosis, departure from the population, or loss to follow-up, respectively. The sum of every person's person-time contribution equals the total number of person-years for this population during the 1-year study period. If we are unable to determine the amount of person-time for each person in the study population, the total person-years (26,060,796 person-years) can be estimated by multiplying the average size of the population at the midpoint of the study period by the duration of the study period. In our previous example, this is the number of people in the state at the midpoint of the year (26,060,796) times the duration of the study period (1 year). Disease rates calculated in this fashion measure the *new occurrence*, or *incidence*, of disease in the population at risk.

This incidence rate should be contrasted with the prevalence rate, which captures the number of *existing* cases of disease among surviving members of the population. Prevalence provides essential information when planning health services for the total number of persons who are living with the disease in the community, whereas incidence reflects the true rate of disease occurrence in the same population. Incidence rates can lead us to hypothesize about factors that are causing disease. Planning for public health services requires a good grasp of the prevalence of the condition in the population, to properly plan for needed personnel, supplies, and even services.

Although incidence rates are ideal for measuring the occurrence of disease in a population for a specified period, they are often not available. In this case, it may be prudent to use cause-specific mortality rates based on the number of deaths from the disease of interest that occurs in the population during the same study period. Mortality rates are often used in lieu of incidence rates, but are only reasonable surrogate measures when the disease is highly fatal. Of course, mortality rates are more appropriate if the goal is to reduce mortality among populations in which screening programs can identify early stages of diseases (e.g., breast cancer or HIV infection) or in which public health programs can reduce the mortality risk for other conditions (e.g., sudden infant death syndrome or alcohol-related motor vehicle collisions).

Globally, there are numerous useful tools for estimating burden based on mortality, life expectancy, disability-adjusted life-years, and other endpoints. Sources include the Global Burden of Disease study that quantifies health loss from hundreds of diseases, injuries, and risk factors so that health systems can be improved and health equity achieved.[3-5] The European Health for All database provides a selection of core health statistics covering basic demographics, health status, health determinants and risk factors, and health care resources, utilization, and expenditure in the 53 countries in the World Health Organization (WHO) European Region.[6]

Using Intermediate Endpoints

Although incidence or mortality rates can be used to evaluate the effectiveness of public health programs, it may not be feasible to wait years to see these effects. On a population basis, these endpoint outcomes actually may be somewhat rare. Instead, the focus should be on identifying and using intermediate biological or behavioral measures as long as there is sufficient Type 1 evidence supporting the relationship between changes in the biological marker or behavior and disease reduction in target populations.[7] If the goal is to reduce breast cancer mortality, then an appropriate intermediate measure is the percentage of women 50 years of age or older who are screened biennially for breast cancer. There is sufficient Type 1 evidence to show that mammography screening reduces the risk for breast cancer mortality among women 50 to 74 years of age, recently confirmed in an updated US Preventive Services Task Force recommendation.[8] Hence, programs designed to increase biennial mammography screening rates in a community should reduce breast cancer mortality rates long-term by providing women, screened and diagnosed with early-stage breast cancer, with more effective treatment options.

Other examples of intermediate measures are the percentage of residents in a community who choose not to smoke cigarettes (to reduce lung cancer risk), who exercise regularly (to reduce cardiovascular disease risk), or who practice safer sex (to reduce HIV infection risk). Furthermore, such measures as changes in knowledge, attitudes, or intentions to change behavior may be very useful for determining the perceived health risk in the general population and whether perceptions differ within subgroups of the population.

Intermediate measures are not readily available for many populations. However, the Behavioral Risk Factor Surveillance System (BRFSS), which provides prevalence data for health behaviors at national and state levels, is a data source that contains a number of intermediate indicators. Recently, the *Morbidity and Mortality Weekly Report (MMWR)* reported on the estimated prevalence of a variety of disease and intermediate measures for states, US territories, 187 Metropolitan/Micropolitan Statistical Areas (MMSAs), and 210 counties for 2012.[9] These rates are based on random samples of residents from each state who complete telephone-based questionnaires each year. For example, we know from this survey that 27.4% of adults in the Baltimore-Columbia-Towson MMSA in Maryland among those interviewed during 2012 were obese. This percentage alone, or combined with that of subsequent years, can be used to establish a baseline rate and to monitor obesity in this population.

Estimating Disease Frequency for Smaller Populations

Disease rates can be estimated if all cases of disease can be enumerated for the population at risk during a specified period and the size of the population at risk (or amount of person-time) can be determined. In many countries, disease rates are routinely computed using birth and death certificate data because existing surveillance systems provide complete enumeration of these events. Although disease rates are commonly computed using national and state data, estimating similar rates for smaller geographically or demo-graphically defined populations may be problematic. The main concern is the reliability of disease rates when there are too few cases of disease occurring in the population. As an example, the US National Center for Health Statistics will not publish or release rates based on fewer than 20 observations. The rea-son behind this practice can be illustrated by examining the relative standard error based on various sample sizes, with rates based on fewer than 20 cases or deaths being very unreliable (Figure 7.1). The relative standard error is the standard error as a percentage of the measure itself.

Several approaches may prove useful to achieve greater representation of so-called low-frequency populations such as recent immigrants or minority populations.[10] These strategies may be related to sampling (e.g., expand the surveillance period by using multiple years to increase the number of cases of disease and person-time units for the target population). Analytic strategies may also be useful, such as aggregating data in a smaller geographical area over several years. Alternate field methods may also be useful (e.g., door-to-door surveys that might increase response rates). Sometimes, "synthetic" esti-mates are useful. These estimates can be generated by using rates from larger geographic regions to estimate the number of cases of disease for smaller geo-graphic or demographically-specific populations. For example, the number of inactive, older persons with diabetes within a particular health status group (homebound, frail, functionally impaired, comorbid conditions, healthy) can be estimated by multiplying the national proportions for the five health status groups stratified into four census regions by the state-specific prevalence of diabetes among adults 50 years or older.[11] These synthetic estimates may then

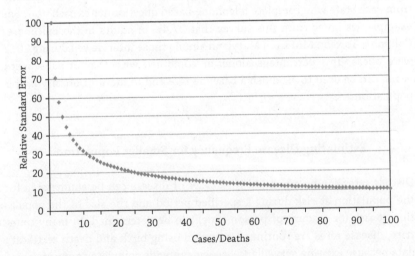

Figure 7.1: Relative standard error of an incidence or mortality rate as a function of the number of cases or deaths.
Source: New York State Department of Health.

allow state-level diabetes control programs to plan physical activity programs for each health status group.

The method of small area estimation has advanced significantly in recent years to meet the needs of public health agencies and others interested in investigating and understanding geographic variation in health conditions and behaviors that affect population health.[12-14] In particular, validated small area estimation methods using regression model approaches allow practitioners to use state level BRFSS data in combination with other datasets such as the National Health Interview Study and the American Community Survey to generate local level estimates that are important for informing policy makers, improving intervention planning and implementation, and allocating sufficient public health resources.[12-15] Although not all state or local health agencies might have the statistical capacity to generate small area estimates using these methods for all indicators, the National Cancer Institute has a website for small area estimates for states, counties, and health service areas for a limited number of cancer risk factors and screening behaviors (http://www.sae.cancer.gov). State and county level estimates can also be queried on the State Cancer Profiles website (https://statecancerprofiles.cancer.gov/data-topics/screening-risk-factors.html)

Rosen and colleagues have provided guidance for analyzing regional data that take into account seven factors.[16] The factors include (1) when available, the importance of the health problem for a community; (2) the regional pattern of the descriptive data; (3) the (tested or anticipated) quality of the data; (4) the consistency of the data with other health indicators; (5) the consistency of the data with known risk factors; (6) trends in the data; and (7) the consistency of the data with other independent studies and with the experiences of local health personnel. Using several of these principles, researchers were able to analyze national data from Sweden over a 35-year time period to determine that cancer patients have a greater risk for committing suicide than the general population.[17] The approach also showed that alcohol-related mortality among men in a specific county in Sweden was lower but increasing faster than the national rate. Their step-by-step analysis dealt with many problems that are crucial in regional health analysis by looking closely at the quality of the data for their analysis and by examining trends using other factors associated with alcohol-related mortality.

CHARACTERIZING THE ISSUE BY PERSON, PLACE, AND TIME

Stratifying Rates by Person

Rates are routinely computed for specific diseases using data from public health surveillance systems. These rates, if computed for the total population (e.g., state or county populations) are crude (or unadjusted) rates because they represent the actual frequency of disease in the defined population for a specified period. Category-specific rates, which are "crude rates" for subgroups of the defined population, provide more information than crude rates about the patterns of disease. Category-specific rates are commonly used to characterize disease frequency by person, place, and time for a defined population (see example in Box 7.1[18]). In most public health surveillance systems, demographic variables (e.g., age, sex, and race or ethnicity) are routinely collected for all members of the defined population. Some surveillance systems (e.g., BRFSS) also collect other demographic characteristics, including years of formal education, income level, and health insurance status. Using category-specific rates to look at disease patterns will identify subgroups within the population with the highest disease rates, thereby identifying groups in need of intervention and even permitting hypotheses about why the rates may be higher for some subgroups.

Box 7.1

SUICIDE RATES BY PERSON, PLACE, AND TIME

In 2013, suicide was the 10th leading cause of death in the United States. There were more than 2.5 times as many deaths due to suicide as homicide (41,149 vs. 16,121 deaths).[36] Overall, the crude suicide rate was 13.0 deaths per 100,000 population. Suicide rates by person, place, and time revealed the following trends:

- Suicide rates were highest for people who were 45–54 years old (19.7/100,000), followed by those who were older than 85 years (18.6/100,000).
- Age-adjusted suicide rates were four times higher for males (20.3/100,000) than females (5.5/100,000), although females are more likely to attempt suicide.
- Age-adjusted suicide rates for whites (14.2/100,000) and Native Americans (11.7/100,000) were more than twice as high as for other racial or ethnic groups.
- Age-adjusted suicide rates for non-Hispanic whites (15.9/100,000) were almost three times the rates for Hispanics (5.7/100,000) and non-Hispanic blacks (5.6/100,000).
- Age-adjusted suicide rates were highest in Montana (23.7/100,000) and lowest in the District of Columbia (5.7/100,000).
- Age-adjusted suicide rates have increased from 10.8 deaths per 100,000 in 2003 to 12.6 deaths per 100,000 in 2013.
- More than half of all suicides in 2013 were committed with a firearm.[18]

Stratifying Rates by Place

Category-specific rates are often computed to show patterns of disease by place of residence for the defined population. This information is routinely collected in most public health surveillance systems and can be used to identify areas with the highest disease rates. Figure 7.2 shows breast cancer mortality rates by county in Missouri. These data provide useful information for determining whether to implement new breast cancer mortality reduction programs statewide or selectively in those counties where the mortality rates are highest. Data can also be used to highlight country-wide variations in major public health issues (e.g., see Figure 7.3). All six countries show improvement in rates between 2000 and 2012. Despite apparent similarities among these populations we see very different rates, with Finland having higher rates throughout the period and France consistently having the lowest rates among these countries. Further uncovering of evidence may reveal differences in baseline demographic characteristics, lifestyle or dietary behaviors, prevention program differences, or health care access, and organization of medical services.

For larger metropolitan areas, zip codes, census tracts, and neighborhoods can be used to stratify disease rates geographically if the number of diseased persons and the size of the defined population are large enough to provide precise rates. This may provide additional information to pinpoint areas where HIV infection, homicide, or infant mortality rates are highest for a community. Other important variables (e.g., population density and migration patterns)

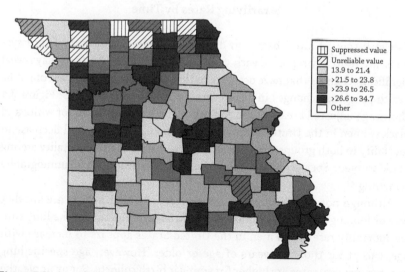

Figure 7.2: Age-adjusted breast cancer mortality rates by county for Missouri women, 1999–2014.
Source: CDC WONDER, Compressed Mortality 1999–2014.

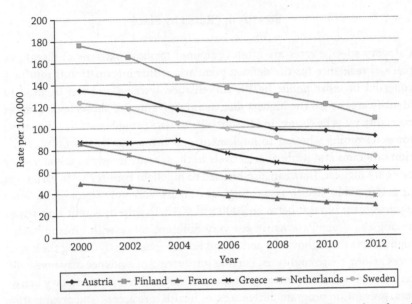

Figure 7.3: Age-adjusted ischemic heart disease mortality rates for all ages for selected European countries 2000–2012.
Source: European Health for All database.

can also be used to stratify disease rates, but are not usually collected in public health surveillance systems.

Stratifying Rates by Time

Category-specific rates, based on data from public health surveillance systems, are routinely reported each year. Looking at rates over time may reveal significant changes that have occurred in the population as the result of public health programs, changes in health care policies, or other events. Figure 7.4 shows age-adjusted breast cancer incidence and mortality rates for white and black women in the United States for 1976 to 2012.[19] An overall decrease in mortality in both groups of women is observed, with higher mortality among black women. Socioeconomic disparities have increased in mammography screening.[20]

Although not often computed, disease rates by birth cohort are another way of looking at patterns of disease over time. In Figure 7.5, the lung cancer mortality rate for all men in the United States appears to increase with age, except for those 85 years of age or older. However, age-specific lung cancer mortality rates are higher for younger birth cohorts. For example, the lung cancer mortality rate for 65- to 74-year-old men is approximately 200

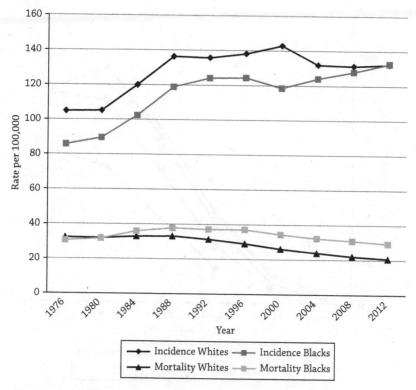

Figure 7.4: Age-adjusted breast cancer incidence and mortality rates by year and race for US women, 1976–2012.
Source: SEER Cancer Statistics Review 1975–2013.

deaths per 100,000 men for those born between 1896 and 1905. The mortality rate for the same age group continues to increase in subsequent birth cohorts, with the highest rate of approximately 430 deaths per 100,000 for the cohort born between 1916 and 1925. The most logical explanation for this pattern is differences in cumulative lifetime exposure to cigarette smoke seen in the birth cohorts that are represented in this population during 2000. In other words, members of the population born after 1905 were more likely to smoke cigarettes and to smoke for longer periods than those born before 1905. Hence, the increasing age-specific lung cancer mortality rates reflect the increasing prevalence of cigarette smokers in the population for subsequent birth cohorts. An example of cohort effect is clearer for the generations shown because of the marked historical change in smoking patterns. At the present time, with increased awareness of the dangers of smoking, the prevalence of smoking is declining, but these changes will not manifest in present age cohorts for some time.

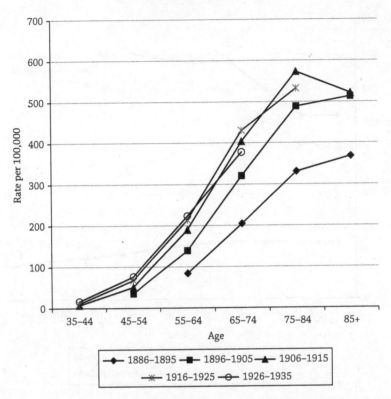

Figure 7.5: Mortality rates due to trachea, bronchus, and lung cancer by birth cohort for US men. Each line represents age-specific rates for birth cohorts denoted by labels in boxes.

Adjusting Rates

Although category-specific rates are commonly used to characterize patterns of disease for defined populations, it is sometimes necessary to adjust rates. Crude rates are often adjusted when the objective is to compare the disease rates between populations or within the same population over time. Rate adjustment is a technique for "removing" the effects of age (or any other factor) from crude rates so as to allow meaningful comparisons across populations with different age structures or distributions. For example, comparing the crude bronchus and lung cancer mortality rate in Florida (63.8 deaths per 100,000 persons) to that of Alaska (35.1 deaths per 100,000 persons) for the years 2004 to 2014 is misleading because the relatively older population in Florida will lead to a higher crude death rate, even if the age-specific bronchus and lung cancer mortality rates in Florida and Alaska are similar. For such a comparison, age-adjusted rates are preferable.

The calculations required to compute age-adjusted rates are reasonably straightforward (Table 7.1). First, age-specific bronchus or lung cancer mortality rates are generated for each state. Second, the age-specific bronchus or lung cancer mortality rates for each state are multiplied by the number of persons in the corresponding age groups from the 2000 US standard population (which have been prorated to equal 1,000,000). This produces the number of "expected" deaths in each age group if the numbers of persons at risk for dying in each age group were the same for the state and US populations. The total number of expected deaths in each state is then divided by the total number of persons in the US standard population to compute the age-adjusted bronchus or lung cancer mortality rate for Florida (47.5 deaths per 100,000) and Alaska (50.0 deaths per 100,000) residents. Thus after adjusting the lung cancer mortality rates for each state we find that the age-adjusted rates are about the same, indicating that differences in the crude rates are due to differences in the age distributions of the two state populations and not necessarily other factors that may increase lung cancer mortality.

Table 7.1. DIRECT ADJUSTMENT OF LUNG CANCER MORTALITY RATES FOR FLORIDA AND ALASKA RESIDENTS (2004–2014)

Age (years)	FLORIDA[a]			ALASKA[b]		
	Lung Cancer Mortality Rate/100,000	2000 Standard US Population	Expected Number of Deaths	Lung Cancer Mortality Rate/100,000	2000 Standard US Population	Expected Number of Deaths
<5	0.0	110,589	0.0	0.0	110,589	0.0
5–14	0.0	145,565	0.0	0.0	145,565	0.0
15–24	0.0	138,646	0.0	0.0	138,646	0.0
25–34	0.3	135,573	0.4	0.0	135,573	0.0
35–44	4.3	162,613	7.0	2.6	162,613	4.2
45–54	30.9	134,834	41.7	21.2	134,834	28.6
55–64	95.4	87,247	83.2	73.9	87,247	64.5
65–74	212.3	66,037	140.2	235.3	66,037	155.4
75–84	329.8	44,842	147.9	417.0	44,842	187.0
85+	348.9	15,508	54.1	387.5	15,508	60.1
Total		1,000,000	474.5		1,000,000	499.8

[a]Age-adjusted lung cancer mortality rate for Florida residents = 474.5 deaths/1,000,000 persons = 47.5 deaths/100,000 persons.
[b]Age-adjusted lung cancer mortality rate for Alaska residents = 499.8 deaths/1,000,000 persons = 50.0 deaths/100,000 persons

PUBLIC HEALTH SURVEILLANCE SYSTEMS

A tried and true public health adage is, "what gets measured, gets done."[21] This measurement often begins with public health surveillance—the ongoing systematic collection, analysis, interpretation, and dissemination of health data for the purpose of preventing and controlling disease, injury, and other health problems.[22] Surveillance systems are maintained at federal, state, and local levels and can be used to estimate the frequency of diseases and other health conditions for defined populations. At least five major purposes for surveillance systems can be described: (1) assessing and monitoring health status and health risks; (2) following disease-specific events and trends; (3) planning, implementing, monitoring, and evaluating health programs and policies; (4) conducting financial management and monitoring information; and (5) conducting public health research.[23] The surveillance systems that currently exist can provide information on births, deaths, infectious diseases, cancers, birth defects, and health behaviors. Each system usually contains sufficient information to estimate prevalence or incidence rates and to describe the frequency of diseases or health condition by person, place, and time. Although data from surveillance systems can be used to obtain baseline and follow-up measurements for target populations, there may be limitations when using the data to evaluate intervention effectiveness for narrowly defined populations. In this case, it may be necessary to estimate the frequency of disease or other health condition for the target population by using special surveys or one of the study designs described later in this chapter. This section focuses primarily on US data sources. There are similar data sources for many countries and regions; some of these resources are noted in the list at the end of the chapter.

Vital Statistics

Vital statistics are based on data from birth and death certificates and are used to monitor disease patterns within and across defined populations. Birth certificates include information about maternal, paternal, and newborn demographics, lifestyle exposures during pregnancy, medical history, obstetric procedures, and labor and delivery complications for all live births. Fetal death certificates include the same data, in addition to the cause of death, for all fetal deaths that exceed a minimum gestational age or birth weight. The data collected on birth and fetal death certificates are similar for many states and territories since the designs of the certificates were modified, based on standard federal recommendations issued in 1989. The reliability of the data has also improved since changing from a write-in to a check-box format, although some variables are more reliable than others. Birth-related outcomes—maternal smoking, preterm delivery, and fetal death rates—are routinely monitored, using data from birth and fetal death certificates.

Like birth certificates, death certificates provide complete enumeration of all events in a defined population. Death certificates include demographic and cause-of-death data that are used to compute disease and injury-specific mortality rates. Mortality rates can be estimated for local populations if the number of deaths and the size of the defined population are large enough to provide precise rates. Birth and death certificates are generated locally and maintained at state health departments. Data from birth and death certificates are analyzed at state and national levels and electronically stored at state health departments and the National Center for Health Statistics. Country-specific mortality data are also available in data systems such as the European Health for All database, maintained by the WHO.[6]

Reportable Diseases

In addition to vital statistics, all states and territories mandate the reporting of some diseases. Although the type of reportable diseases may differ by state or territory, they usually include specific childhood, foodborne, sexually transmitted, and other infectious diseases. These diseases are reported by physicians and other health care providers to local public health authorities and are monitored for early signs of epidemics in the community. The data are maintained by local and state health departments and are submitted weekly to the CDC for national surveillance and reporting. Disease frequencies are stratified by age, gender, race or ethnicity, and place of residence and are reported routinely in the *MMWR*. However, reporting is influenced by disease severity, availability of public health measures, public concern, ease of reporting, and physician appreciation of public health practice in the community.[23, 24]

Registries

Disease registries routinely monitor defined populations, thereby providing very reliable estimates of disease frequency. All 50 states have active cancer registries supported by the state or federal government. These registries provide data that can be used to compute site-specific cancer incidence rates for a community, if the number of cancers and the size of the defined population are large enough to provide precise rates. Since 1973, the federally sponsored Surveillance, Epidemiology, and End Results (SEER) program of the National Cancer Institute has provided estimates of national cancer rates based on 10% to 15% of the total population.[25] Along with state-based cancer registries, this surveillance system can provide rates for specific types of cancer, characterized by person, place, and time. All invasive cancers that occur among residents within the geographic catchment area of the registry are confirmed pathologically and recorded electronically for surveillance and research purposes. They are also linked with death certificates to provide additional information about disease-specific survival rates.

In 1998, the US Congress passed the Birth Defects Prevention Act that authorized the CDC to collect, analyze, and make available data on birth defects; operate regional centers for applied epidemiologic research on the prevention of birth defects; and inform and educate the public about the prevention of birth defects. Subsequently, the CDC awarded cooperative agreements to specific states to address major problems that hinder the surveillance of birth defects and the use of data for prevention and intervention programs. The states were awarded funding to initiate new surveillance systems where none existed, to support new systems, or to improve existing surveillance systems. Birth defects registries are either active or passive, reporting surveillance systems designed to identify birth defects diagnosed for all stillborn and live-born infants. Active reporting surveillance systems provide more reliable estimates of the prevalence of specific birth defects, if staff and resources are available to search medical records from hospitals, laboratories, and other medical sources for all diagnosed birth defects in a defined population. Passive reporting surveillance systems are designed to estimate the prevalence of birth defects that can be identified using computer algorithms to link and search birth certificates, death certificates, patient abstract systems, and other readily available electronic databases.

Surveys

There are several federally sponsored surveys, including the National Health Interview Survey (NHIS), National Health and Nutrition Examination Survey (NHANES), and BRFSS, that have been designed to monitor the nation's health. These surveys are designed to measure numerous health indexes, including acute and chronic diseases, injuries, disabilities, and other health-related outcomes. Some surveys are ongoing annual surveillance systems, whereas others are conducted periodically. These surveys usually provide prevalence estimates for specific diseases among adults and children in the United States. Although the surveys can also provide prevalence estimates for regions and individual states, they cannot currently be used to produce estimates for smaller geographically defined populations.

USING NATIONAL AND STATE-BASED SURVEILLANCE SYSTEMS AND OTHER READILY AVAILABLE ONLINE TOOLS

Several of the large US surveillance datasets such as the BRFSS and CDC WONDER allow users to access national as well as state-level data. State health agencies are increasingly making their health data available in user-friendly data query systems that allow the estimation of baseline and follow-up rates for needs assessment and for evaluating the effectiveness of new public health interventions. Examples of the international, national, and state-based query systems described in this chapter are provided at the end of the chapter under "Selected Websites."

OVERVIEW OF DESIGNS IN ANALYTIC EPIDEMIOLOGY

As stated earlier, descriptive epidemiology provides information about the patterns of disease within defined populations that can be used to generate etiologic or intervention-based hypotheses. These hypotheses can be evaluated using study designs and analytic methods that encompass the principles of analytic epidemiology. Most study designs can be used to provide Type 1 evidence to support causal associations between modifiable (and nonmodifiable) risk factors and specific diseases. Figure 7.6 provides a schematic for determining the type of study design that is most appropriate for the question under study. When there is sufficient Type 1 evidence, additional work is needed to determine the effectiveness of public health programs designed to reduce the prevalence of these risk factors in the population. Experimental and quasi-experimental study designs are generally used, depending on available resources and timing, to evaluate the effectiveness of new public health programs. Issues related to program and policy evaluation are also covered in chapter 11.

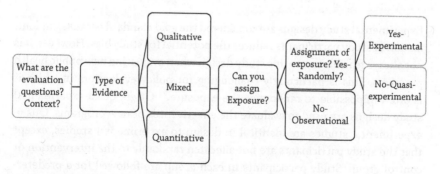

Figure 7.6 Schematic of key study design decision points in epidemiology.

Experimental Study Designs

Experimental study designs provide the most convincing evidence that new public health programs are effective. If study participants are randomized into groups (or arms), the study design is commonly called a randomized controlled trial. When two groups are created, the study participants allocated randomly to one group are given the new intervention (or treatment), and those allocated to the other group serve as controls. The study participants in both groups are followed prospectively, and disease (or health-related outcome) rates are computed for each group at the end of the observation period. Because both groups are identical in all aspects, except for the intervention, a lower disease rate in the intervention group implies that the intervention is effective.

The same study design can also be used to randomize groups instead of individuals to evaluate the effectiveness of health behavior interventions for communities. Referred to as a group-randomized trial, groups of study participants (e.g., schools within a school system or communities within a state) are randomized to receive the intervention or to serve as controls for the study. Initially, the groups may be paired, based on similar characteristics. Then, each group within each pair is allocated randomly to the intervention or control group. This helps to balance the distribution of characteristics of the study participants for both study groups and to reduce potential study bias. The intervention is applied to all individuals in the intervention group and is withheld or delayed for the control group. Measurements are taken at baseline and at the end of the observation period to determine whether there are significant differences between the disease rates for the intervention and control groups. The group-randomized design has been used to evaluate the effectiveness of public health interventions designed to increase immunization coverage, reduce tobacco use, and increase physical activity.[26]

Quasi-Experimental Study Designs

Experimental study designs are considered the gold standard because randomization of study participants reduces the potential for study bias. However, it is not always feasible to use this study design when evaluating new public health programs. This is particularly challenging for policy evaluation, in which it is often impossible to randomize the exposure.[27] Often, quasi-experimental study designs are used to evaluate the effectiveness of new programs. Quasi-experimental studies are identical in design to experimental studies, except that the study participants are not allocated randomly to the intervention or control group. Study participants in each group are followed for a predetermined period, and outcomes (e.g., disease rates, behavioral risk factors) are computed for each group to determine whether the intervention is effective. As is the case for experimental study designs, baseline (or preintervention) measurements are crucial because the investigator must determine how similar the intervention and control groups are before the intervention. Ideally, outcomes should be identical at baseline and for the period prior to the execution of the study. Examining the characteristics of the study groups by person, place, and time will reduce the probability of concluding that the intervention is effective when actually there are other factors historically affecting the risk factors in the community.

If a comparable control group is not available, quasi-experimental study designs can still be used to measure the impact of public health interventions on a particular health outcome in the same population. Actually, quasi-experimental study designs are commonly used when comparing new public health initiatives that affect the total population.

Reichardt and Mark have described four prototypical quasi-experimental study designs: (1) before-after; (2) interrupted time-series; (3) nonequivalent group; and (4) regression-discontinuity designs.[28] Each of these designs can be altered with a variety of design features to make them more complex (e.g., multiple control groups, variations in treatments, multiple outcome variables).[28,29] In a before-after design, a participant is measured before (pretest) and after a treatment (posttest) is introduced. The treatment effect is the difference between pretest and posttest. The interrupted time-series design is an extension of the before-after approach in that it adds further measurements over time. The outcome of interest is measured at multiple points before and after a treatment is introduced (see example in Box 7.2[30-32] and Figure 7.7). In nonequivalent group designs, comparisons are made among participants who receive different treatments but have been assigned to the treatments nonrandomly. This may arise when participants select a treatment condition based on personal preferences.[28] Therefore the primary threat to internal validity involves selection bias among treatment groups. In the regression-discontinuity design, participants are ordered on a quantitative assignment variable (QAV) and allotted to a treatment condition according to a cutoff score on that variable.[28] Therefore, the treatment effect is estimated using a statistical technique (multiple regression) to relate the outcome of interest to the QAV in each treatment group. See Table 7.2 for a description of the strengths and weaknesses of these designs.

Observational Study Designs

Because it may not be ethical to use experimental or quasi-experimental study designs in all research settings, investigators can use observational study designs to evaluate hypotheses that prior exposures increase the risk

Box 7.2

HEALTH IN ALL POLICIES—THE NORTH KARELIA PROJECT

In the 1960s, Finland had the world's highest coronary heart disease mortality rates with the highest rates in the eastern province of North Karelia. In 1971, representatives of the province appealed to national authorities for help to reduce the burden of cardiovascular disease in the area. In 1972, the North Karelia Project was launched with the idea to carry out and evaluate a comprehensive prevention intervention aimed at changing the area's social, physical, and policy environment to reduce the main behavioral risk factors for cardiovascular disease. The community-based approach of the intervention was a novel approach at the time. After the initial evaluation period, the interventions were extended nationally to promote cardiovascular disease prevention through Finland. By 2006, cardiovascular mortality in Finland decreased by 80% among working-age adults and by 85% in North Karelia (Figure 7.7).[30-32] Life expectancy has increased by 10 years, and other improvements in health and well-being have also been observed. "North Karelia demonstrated the dramatic impact of low-resource, community-based interventions that target general lifestyles."[31] This project and ultimately the national impact of this comprehensive prevention intervention have led to a greater understanding of the importance of considering a variety of social determinants across different public and private sectors to affect health outcomes and to the Finnish Health in All Policies initiative.

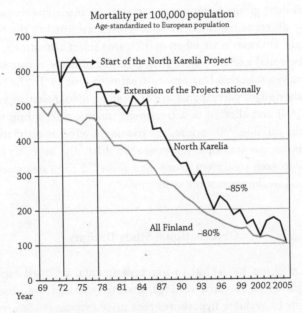

Mortality per 100,000 population
Age-standardized to European population

Figure 7.7: Time-series analysis of age-adjusted coronary heart disease mortality rates in North Karelia and Finland among males 35–64 years of age, 1969–2006.[32]

Table 7.2. COMPARISON OF QUASI-EXPERIMENTAL STUDY DESIGNS

Design	Schematic	Strengths	Weaknesses
1. Before-after	O X O	Simplest measure; quick outcome; demonstrates feasibility of implementing intervention; may indicate value of a more systematic evaluation	Threats to validity: history, maturation, seasonality, testing, instrumentation, attrition, regression to mean
2. Interrupted time-series	O O O O O X O O O O O O	Removes some threats to validity of #1 (maturation, seasonality, regression to mean) and inferentially stronger; no control group necessary; can use multiple interventions, groups, outcomes	Multiple observations require resources; permutations of design can require sophisticated statistical procedures; autocorrelation must be addressed
3. Nonequivalent group	X O O	Easy to implement observations; little disruption to services; opportunistic natural experiments easy to capture; design permutations allow flexibility of measurement, comparisons, and interventions	Allocation to groups may be influenced by motivation; comparability of groups difficult to assess; pretest and posttest assessments of groups complex; complex statistical procedures necessary for assessing comparability
4. Regression-discontinuity	(see diagram)	Split into groups accomplished by statistical criteria; group assignment relatively clean statistically with usual threats to validity removed; results statistically more credible	Requires almost three times the sample of an experimental design; may be useful when an experimental design not feasible

Treatment 1   Treatment 2

O = Observation; X = implementation of treatment.

Source: Reichardt and Mark.[28]

for specific diseases. Generally, observational study designs are used to provide Type 1 evidence, for which the exposure has already occurred and disease patterns can be studied for those with and without the exposure of interest. A good historical example is the association between cigarette use and lung cancer. Because people choose whether or not to smoke cigarettes (one would not assign this exposure), we can evaluate the hypothesis that cigarette smokers are at increased risk for developing lung cancer by following smokers and nonsmokers over time to assess their lung cancer rates.

Cohort and case-control studies are two observational study designs that can be used to evaluate the strength of the association between prior exposure and risk for disease in the study population. Cohort studies compare the disease rates of exposed and unexposed study participants who are free of disease at baseline and followed over time to estimate the disease rates in both groups. Cohort studies are often conducted when the exposure of interest can be identified and followed to determine whether the disease rate is significantly higher (or lower) than the rates for unexposed individuals from the same population. Studies that have focused on the effects of diet or exercise on specific diseases or health-related outcome[33] are good examples of cohort studies.

Case-control studies compare the frequency of prior exposures for study participants who have been diagnosed recently with the disease (cases) with those who have not developed the disease (controls). Case-control studies are the preferred study design when the disease is rare, and they are efficient when studying diseases with long latency. As is true for all study designs, selecting appropriate controls and obtaining reliable exposure estimates are crucial when evaluating any hypothesis that a prior exposure increases (or decreases) the risk for a specific disease. A recent study provides an example of an unusually large case-control study conducted examining lung cancer cases in Italy for differences in history of occupations.[34] Public health professionals operating in typical settings may find much more modest case-control designs useful for exploring possible exposures for health issues encountered.

Cross-sectional studies, a third type of observational study design, can be completed relatively quickly and inexpensively to look at associations between exposure and disease. Because information regarding potential exposures and existing diseases for the study participants is measured simultaneously when the study is conducted, cross-sectional studies are unable to ascertain whether the exposure preceded the development of the disease among the study participants. Hence, cross-sectional studies are used primarily to generate hypotheses. Nevertheless, cross-sectional studies are used for public health planning and evaluation. For example, if a public health administrator wants to know how many women of reproductive age smoked cigarettes while pregnant, knowledge about the prevalence of maternal smoking in the community is important. Knowing the maternal smoking rates for subgroups of this population will help target interventions, if needed, for each subgroup. Cross-sectional studies are also used to help set research priorities based on consideration of the disease burden. A cross-sectional study in China was able to establish, for example, that a rapid screening test for detecting 14 high-risk types of human papillomavirus was effective in two county hospitals in rural China.[35]

SUMMARY

As they develop, implement, and evaluate new public health intervention programs, public health professionals need a core set of epidemiologic skills to quantify the frequency of a variety of health outcomes in target populations.

KEY CHAPTER POINTS

- Knowing the frequency of disease in the population before implementing any new public health program is crucial and can help focus efforts toward reducing the disease burden by targeting high-risk groups in the population.
- Public health surveillance systems provide the necessary data to measure the frequency of some health outcomes, but special surveys are often needed to obtain baseline data for other health outcomes in defined populations.
- Public health surveillance data are currently available on the Internet for some health outcomes and can be used to look interactively at disease or behavior patterns by person, place, and time.
- Understanding the trade-offs of various study designs will improve how we evaluate the effects of various public health programs and policies.

SUGGESTED READINGS AND SELECTED WEBSITES
Suggested Readings

Bauman A, Keopsell T. Epidemiologic issues in community interventions. In: Brownson RC, Petitti DB, eds. *Applied Epidemiology: Theory to Practice.* 2nd ed. New York, NY: Oxford University Press; 2006:164–206.

Friis RH, Sellers TA. *Epidemiology for Public Health Practice.* 5th ed. Gaithersburg, MD: Aspen Publishers, Inc.; 2014.

Gordis L. *Epidemiology.* 5th ed. Philadelphia, PA: Saunders Elsevier; 2014.

Shadish W, Cook T, Campbell D. *Experimental and Quasi-Experimental Designs for Generalized Causal Inference.* Boston, MA: Houghton Mifflin; 2002.

Newcomer K, Hatry H, Wholey J eds. *Handbook of Practical Program Evaluation.* San Francisco, CA: Jossey-Bass Publishers, 2015.

Lee LM, Teutsch SM, Thacker SB, St. Louis ME, eds. *Principles and Practice of Public Health Surveillance.* 3rd ed. New York, NY: Oxford University Press, 2010.

Selected Websites

American Community Survey https://www.census.gov/programs-surveys/acs/about. html. The American Community Survey is an ongoing annual survey that is conducted by the US Census Bureau and includes questions on a variety of demographic, housing, economic, and social factors. Data are provided at the level of census tracts and in some cases block groups. Though this survey does not contain health status or behavior data, it provides a rich source of information about the population and can be an integral part of a needs assessment process.

Centers for Disease Control and Prevention Behavioral Risk Factor Surveillance System (BRFSS) http://www.cdc.gov/nccdphp/brfss. The BRFSS, an ongoing, reliable and valid data collection program conducted in all states, the District of Columbia, and three US territories, and the world's largest telephone survey, tracks health risks in the United States. Information from the survey is used to improve the health of the American people. The CDC has developed a standard core questionnaire so that data can be compared across various strata.

CDC WONDER http://wonder.cdc.gov. CDC WONDER is an easy-to-use query system that provides a single point of access to a wide variety of CDC reports, guidelines, and public health data. It can be valuable in public health research, decision making, priority setting, program evaluation, and resource allocation.

Community Commons http://www.communitycommons.org/maps-data/. Community Commons is a platform for data, tools, and stories to improve communities and inspire change. Topic areas include equity, economy, education, environment, food, and health. The creative and dynamic site allows users to create and share data visualizations and provides a variety of resources that can be used in program development and public health decision making.

County Health Rankings http://www.countyhealthrankings.org/. The County Health Rankings are being developed by the University of Wisconsin Population Health Institute through a grant from the Robert Wood Johnson Foundation. This website seeks to increase awareness of the many factors—clinical care access and quality, health-promoting behaviors, social and economic factors, and the physical environment—that contribute to the health of communities; foster engagement among public and private decision makers to improve community health; and develop incentives to encourage coordination across sectors for community health improvement.

European Health for All database (HFA-DB) http://www.euro.who.int/en/data-and-evidence/databases/european-health-for-all-database-hfa-db. The HFA-DB provides statistics for demographic characteristics, health status, risk factors, health care resources and utilization, and health expenditures for the 53 countries in the World Health Organization European Region.

Global Burden of Disease (GBD) data http://www.healthdata.org/gbd/data. The GBD houses all global, regional, and country-level estimates for mortality, disability, disease burden, life expectancy, and risk factors, which can be downloaded from the Global Health Data Exchange, a catalog of the world's health and demographic data. The tool allows users to explore the input sources to GBD based on various criteria and to export the results. The GBD also includes many useful data visualization tools.

National Center for Health Statistics http://www.cdc.gov/nchs/. The National Center for Health Statistics is the principal vital and health statistics agency for the US government. NCHS data systems include information on vital events as well as information on health status, lifestyle, and exposure to unhealthy influences, the onset and diagnosis of illness and disability, and the use of health care. NCHS has two major types of data systems: systems based on populations, containing data collected through personal interviews or examinations (e.g., National Health Interview Survey and National Health and Nutrition Examination Survey), and systems based on records, containing data collected from vital and medical records. These data are used by policymakers in Congress and the administration, by medical researchers, and by others in the health community.

Organization for Economic Cooperation and Development (OECD) <www.oecd.org>. The OECD provides data for its 35 member countries on a wide variety of demographic, economic, and health indicators. The mission of the OECD is to promote policies that will improve the economic and social well-being of people around the world.

PH Partners https://phpartners.org/. Partners in Information Access for the Public Health Workforce (PH Partners) is a collaboration between US government agencies, public health organizations, and health science libraries to provide access to a variety of public health resources, including national, state, and local data.

World Bank Group <www.worldbank.org>. The World Bank Group has two goals: to end extreme poverty within a generation and to boost shared prosperity. In support of these goals the World Bank Group website provides information at the country level on numerous demographic, economic, and health indicators for dozens of countries worldwide.

World Health Organization (WHO) Global Health Observatory (GHO) data <www.who.int/gho/en/>. The GHO is the WHO gateway to health-related statistics for more than 1,000 indicators for its 194 member countries.

REFERENCES

1. Porta M, ed. *A Dictionary of Epidemiology*. 6th ed. New York, NY: Oxford University Press; 2014.
2. Terris M. The Society for Epidemiologic Research (SER) and the future of epidemiology. *Am J Epidemiol*. Oct 15 1992;136(8):909–915.
3. GBD 2015 Mortality and Causes of Death Collaborators. Global, regional, and national disability-adjusted life-years (DALYs) for 315 diseases and injuries and healthy life expectancy (HALE), 1990-2015: a systematic analysis for the Global Burden of Disease Study 2015. *Lancet*. Oct 8 2016;388(10053):1603–1658.
4. GBD 2015 Mortality and Causes of Death Collaborators. Global, regional, and national incidence, prevalence, and years lived with disability for 310 diseases and injuries, 1990-2015: a systematic analysis for the Global Burden of Disease Study 2015. *Lancet*. Oct 8 2016;388(10053):1545–1602.
5. GBD 2015 Mortality and Causes of Death Collaborators. Global, regional, and national life expectancy, all-cause mortality, and cause-specific mortality for 249 causes of death, 1980-2015: a systematic analysis for the Global Burden of Disease Study 2015. *Lancet*. Oct 8 2016;388(10053):1459–1544.
6. World Health Organization Regional Office for Europe. European Health for All database http://data.euro.who.int/hfadb/. Accessed June 5, 2016.
7. Brownson RC, Seiler R, Eyler AA. Measuring the impact of public health policy. *Prev Chronic Dis*. Jul 2010;7(4):A77.

8. US Preventive Services Task Force. Final Recommendation Statement: Breast Cancer: Screening. 3rd. http://www.uspreventiveservicestaskforce.org/Page/Document/RecommendationStatementFinal/breast-cancer-screening1. Accessed September 2, 2016.

9. Chowdhury PP, Mawokomatanda T, Xu F, et al. Surveillance for Certain Health Behaviors, Chronic Diseases, and Conditions, Access to Health Care, and Use of Preventive Health Services Among States and Selected Local Areas—Behavioral Risk Factor Surveillance System, United States, 2012. *MMWR Surveill Summ.* 2016;65(4):1–142.

10. Andresen EM, Diehr PH, Luke DA. Public health surveillance of low-frequency populations. *Annu Rev Public Health.* 2004;25:25–52.

11. Kirtland KA, Zack MM, Caspersen CJ. State-specific synthetic estimates of health status groups among inactive older adults with self-reported diabetes, 2000-2009. *Prev Chronic Dis.* 2012;9:E89.

12. Goodman MS. Comparison of small-area analysis techniques for estimating prevalence by race. *Prev Chronic Dis.* Mar 2010;7(2):A33.

13. Pierannunzi C, Xu F, Wallace RC, et al. A Methodological Approach to Small Area Estimation for the Behavioral Risk Factor Surveillance System. *Prev Chronic Dis.* 2016;13:E91.

14. Zhang X, Holt JB, Lu H, et al. Multilevel regression and poststratification for small-area estimation of population health outcomes: a case study of chronic obstructive pulmonary disease prevalence using the behavioral risk factor surveillance system. *Am J Epidemiol.* Apr 15 2014;179(8):1025–1033.

15. Zhang X, Holt JB, Yun S, Lu H, Greenlund KJ, Croft JB. Validation of multilevel regression and poststratification methodology for small area estimation of health indicators from the behavioral risk factor surveillance system. *Am J Epidemiol.* Jul 15 2015;182(2):127–137.

16. Rosen M, Nystrom L, Wall S. Guidelines for regional mortality analysis: an epidemiological approach to health planning. *Int J Epidemiol.* Jun 1985;14(2):293–299.

17. Bjorkenstam C, Edberg A, Ayoubi S, Rosen M. Are cancer patients at higher suicide risk than the general population? *Scand J Public Health.* 2005;33(3):208–214.

18. Xu J, Murphy SL, Kochanek KD, Bastian BA. Deaths: final data for 2013. *Natl Vital Stat Rep.* Feb 16 2016;64(2):1–119.

19. Howlader N, Noone A, Krapcho M, et al. *SEER Cancer Statistics Review, 1975-2013.* Bethesda, MD: National Cancer Institute; 2016.

20. Harper S, Lynch J, Meersman SC, Breen N, Davis WW, Reichman MC. Trends in area-socioeconomic and race-ethnic disparities in breast cancer incidence, stage at diagnosis, screening, mortality, and survival among women ages 50 years and over (1987-2005). *Cancer Epidemiol Biomarkers Prev.* Jan 2009;18(1):121–131.

21. Thacker SB. Public health surveillance and the prevention of injuries in sports: what gets measured gets done. *J Athl Train.* Apr-Jun 2007;42(2):171–172.

22. Thacker S. Historical developments. In: Teutsch S, Churchill R, eds. *Principles and Practice of Public Health Surveillance.* 2nd ed. New York, NY: Oxford University Press; 2000:1–16.

23. Teutsch S, Churchill R, eds. *Principles and Practice of Public Health Surveillance.* 2nd ed. New York, NY: Oxford University Press; 2000.

24. Thacker SB, Stroup DF. Future directions for comprehensive public health surveillance and health information systems in the United States. *Am J Epidemiol.* Sep 1 1994;140(5):383–397.

25. Jemal A, Siegel R, Ward E, Murray T, Xu J, Thun MJ. Cancer statistics, 2007. *CA Cancer J Clin*. Jan-Feb 2007;57(1):43–66.
26. Zaza S, Briss PA, Harris KW, eds. *The Guide to Community Preventive Services: What Works to Promote Health?* New York, NY: Oxford University Press; 2005.
27. Brownson RC, Diez Roux AV, Swartz K. Commentary: Generating rigorous evidence for public health: the need for new thinking to improve research and practice. *Annu Rev Public Health*. 2014;35:1–7.
28. Reichardt C, Mark M. Quasi-experimentation. In: Wholey J, Hatry H, Newcomer K, eds. *Handbook of Practical Program Evaluation*. 2nd ed. San Francisco, CA: Jossey-Bass Publishers; 2004:126–149.
29. Shadish W, Cook T, Campbell D. *Experimental and Quasi-Experimental Designs for Generalized Causal Inference*. Boston, MA: Houghton Mifflin; 2002.
30. Puska P. Health in all policies. *Eur J Public Health*. Aug 2007;17(4):328.
31. Puska P. The North Karelia Project: 30 years successfully preventing chronic diseases. *Diabetes Voice*. 2008;53:26–29.
32. Puska P, Stahl T. Health in all policies—the Finnish initiative: background, principles, and current issues. *Annu Rev Public Health*. 2010;31:315–328 313 p following 328.
33. Hu FB, Manson JE, Stampfer MJ, et al. Diet, lifestyle, and the risk of type 2 diabetes mellitus in women. *N Engl J Med*. Sep 13 2001;345(11):790–797.
34. Consonni D, De Matteis S, Lubin JH, et al. Lung cancer and occupation in a population-based case-control study. *Am J Epidemiol*. Feb 1 2010;171(3):323–333.
35. Qiao YL, Sellors JW, Eder PS, et al. A new HPV-DNA test for cervical-cancer screening in developing regions: a cross-sectional study of clinical accuracy in rural China. *Lancet Oncol*. Oct 2008;9(10):929–936.
36. Heron M, Hoyert D, Murphy S, Xu J, Kochanek K, Tejada-Vera B. *Deaths: Final data for 2006. National vital statistics reports*. Hyattsville, MD: National Center for Health Statistics; 2009.

CHAPTER 8

 ⟨⁊⟩

Searching the Scientific Literature
and Using Systematic Reviews

Where is the wisdom we have lost in knowledge? Where is the knowledge we have lost in information?

T.S. Eliot

As you develop an issue statement and begin to understand the epidemiologic nature of a particular public health issue along with the intervention options, the scientific literature is a crucial source of information on what works. Because of the considerable growth in the amount of information available to public health practitioners, it is essential to follow a systematic approach to literature searching. The underpinnings of an evidence-based process rest largely on one's ability to find credible, high-quality evidence as efficiently and exhaustively as possible. A systematic searching process also helps ensure that others can replicate the same results. With modern information technologies, virtually all public health workers have an excellent opportunity to find valuable information quickly. Published information resources are now increasingly available for anyone with an Internet connection, enabling professionals outside major institutions to perform professional and thorough searches for needed resources.

This chapter provides guidance on how to identify existing evidence of effective interventions using systematic reviews and online resources, and if necessary how to conduct a primary search of the scientific literature. It focuses on the importance of a literature search, where to search, how to find evidence, and how to organize the results of a search. Evaluation of the quality of the evidence is covered in other chapters (primarily chapters 3 and 11).

BACKGROUND

As noted in chapter 1, there are many types and sources of evidence on public health programs and policies. Scientific information (the "scientific literature") on theory and practice can be found in textbooks, government reports, scientific journals, and policy statements and at scientific meetings. Three levels of reading the scientific literature have been described: (1) browsing—skimming through actual books and articles, looking for anything of interest, and browsing topic-related sites on the Internet; (2) reading for information—approaching the literature in search of an answer to a specific question; and (3) reading for research—reading to obtain a comprehensive view of the existing state of knowledge on a specific topic.[1] In practice, most of us obtain most of our information through browsing.[2,3] However, to conduct a literature review for building evidence-based programs efficiently, it is important to take a more structured approach. We focus primarily on journal publications here because they have gone through a process of peer review to enhance the quality of the information and are the closest thing to a gold standard that is available (see chapter 3).

When conducting a search of the scientific literature, there are four broad categories of publications to consider for evidence-based decision making (Figure 8.1):

1. *Original research articles:* These are the papers written by the authors who conducted the original research studies. These articles provide details on the methods used, results, and implications of results. A thorough and comprehensive summary of a body of literature will consist of careful reading of original research articles, particularly when a topic area is changing rapidly or there are too few original articles to conduct a review.

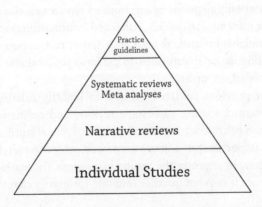

Figure 8.1: Hierarchy of scientific evidence for evidence-based decision making.

2. *Narrative review articles:* These provide a descriptive summary of what is known on a particular topic. A narrative review article presents a summary of original research articles. The *Annual Review of Public Health* is an excellent source of review articles on a variety of topics (http://arjournals.annualreviews.org/loi/publhealth). A limitation of narrative review articles is that they do not always follow systematic approaches, a practice that sometimes leads to selection bias and inconsistent results.[4]

3. *Systematic review articles:* These review articles involve a detailed, structured, and exhaustive search of original research articles with the goal of reducing selection bias and synthesizing all relevant articles on a particular topic.[4-6] Systematic reviews often feature a quantitative synthesis of results, or meta-analysis, to produce a summary statistical estimate of the measure of association or effect. For example, the Cochrane Collaboration, an international organization of clinicians, epidemiologists, and others, has produced quantitative reviews on the effectiveness of various health care interventions and practices covering a wide range of subjects (www.cochrane.org). A more detailed discussion of finding evidence of effective interventions using systematic reviews is provided later in this chapter.

4. *Guidelines:* Practice guidelines are formal statements that offer advice to clinicians, public health practitioners, managed-care organizations, and the public on how to improve the effectiveness and impact of clinical and public health interventions. Guidelines translate the findings of research and demonstration projects into accessible and usable information for public health practice. There are several examples of useful guidelines. The terminology used within them differs across the globe. Thus, in the European Community, directives are stronger than recommendations, which are stronger than guidelines.[7] No such hierarchy exists in North America.

Review articles and guidelines often present a useful shortcut for many busy practitioners who do not have the time to master the literature on multiple public health topics.

In addition to the type of publication, timeliness of scientific information is an important consideration. To find the best-quality evidence for medical decision making, Sackett and colleagues recommended that practitioners burn their (traditional) textbooks.[8-10] Although this approach may seem radical, it brings to light the limitations of textbooks for providing information on the cause, diagnosis, prognosis, or treatment of a disorder. To stay up to date in clinical practice, a textbook may need to be revised on a yearly basis. Though considered to provide more timely scientific findings, research and publication of results in a journal are a deliberative process that often takes years from the germination of an idea, to obtaining funding, carrying out the study, analyzing data, writing up results, submitting to a journal, and waiting out the peer-review process and publication lag for a journal.

The number of scientific publications has increased dramatically since the 1940s.[11] In Medline alone in 2015, there were 806,326 new citations, 5,618 journal titles indexed, and 2.8 billion searches conducted.[12] There are an estimated 25,000 to 40,000 scientific journals in the world, publishing approximately 1.4 million new research papers each year. About 8% to 10% of these are published in open access journals, and only about 20% of scientific articles are available free of charge.[13] To assimilate even a fraction of this large body of evidence, the practitioner needs to find ways to take advantage of the vast amount of scientific information available and to find information quickly. Of increasing interest to health professionals is the ease with which this literature may be accessed by those not directly supported by major library resources. Consequently, there is interest in open access availability of scientific publications. A recent study reported that in 2011, 12% of articles became immediately available, and an additional 5% become available within 12 months of publication.[14] Therefore nearly 20% of articles may be readily accessible, and professionals may also use the PubMed author information to obtain the author's email address for direct requests of articles. With easy access to abstracts and an increasing ability to obtain research articles, public health professionals—regardless of their institutional resources—may be able to actively work with the scientific literature in their areas of concern.

Methods for searching the literature have changed dramatically. Thirty years ago, a practitioner wishing to find information on a particular topic would speak with a librarian and inform him or her of the type of information being sought, perhaps provide a sample article, and help in selecting some key words. The librarian would run the search, consult with the practitioner as to whether it captured the desired types of articles, modify the search as needed, rerun it, consult with the practitioner again, and so forth. This whole iterative process could take weeks. Current practitioners with an Internet connection can now search for relevant information from the world's scientific literature and, with training and experience, can discern relevance and quality so as to improve the practice of public health. There also are numerous online training modules on how to search the literature, such as those at www.ebbp.org or www.nlm.nih.gov.

FINDING EVIDENCE FOR EFFECTIVE INTERVENTIONS USING SYSTEMATIC REVIEWS AND ONLINE RESOURCES

Systematic Reviews

As noted earlier, systematic reviews are syntheses of comprehensive collections of information on a particular topic. Given the huge number of new scientific articles published each year and the fact that no single study could provide a conclusive answer with regard to an intervention's effectiveness, there is an increased call to shift the focus in our decision making from single studies to the larger body of scientific evidence.[5,15] By focusing on the body of scientific evidence, practitioners can have greater confidence in the magnitude and consistency of results after careful consideration of the influence of methodological and publication biases. General methods used in a systematic review, as well as several types of reviews and their practical applications, are described here; more detailed descriptions of these methods are available elsewhere.[16–18] Several checklists, tools, and recommendations can be useful in assessing the methodological quality of a systematic review,[19–23] including AMSTAR[23] and PRISMA[24] protocols.

Methods for Conducting a Systematic Review

The goal of this section is not to teach readers how to conduct a systematic review but to provide a basic understanding of the six common steps in conducting a systematic review. Each is briefly summarized, and some selected differences in approaches are discussed.

Identify the Problem

The first step in a systematic review is the identification of the problem. Reviewing the literature, considering the practical aspects of the problem, and talking to experts in the area are all ways to begin to develop a concise statement of the problem (see chapter 6). Systematic reviews focusing on effectiveness typically begin with a formal statement of the issue to be addressed. This usually includes statements of the intervention under study, the population in which it might be used, the outcomes being considered, and the relevant comparison. For example, the problem might be to determine the effectiveness of screening for Type 2 diabetes in adult black men to reduce the occurrence of macrovascular and microvascular complications of diabetes compared with usual care. Problem identification should also include a description of where the information for the systematic review will be obtained (e.g., information will come from a search of the literature over the last 10 years in three specific databases).

Search the Literature

There are numerous electronic databases available, and one or more of these should be systematically searched. Several of these are excellent sources of hard or electronic copies of published literature as well. For a variety of reasons, however, limiting searching to electronic databases can have drawbacks:

- Most systematic reviews use the peer-reviewed, published literature as the source of their data. Databases, however, may not include technical or final reports. If these are thought to be important relative to the intervention being considered, then a source for these documents should be identified and searched.
- Published studies may be subject to publication bias—the tendency of research with statistically significant results to be submitted and published over results that are not statistically significant or null.[6] To reduce the likelihood of publication bias, some reviews go to considerable lengths to find additional unpublished studies[25-27] (see chapter 3, section on publication bias).
- Even the best database searches typically find only one-half to two-thirds of the available literature. Reviews of reference lists and consultations with experts are very helpful in finding additional sources. Often, advice from experts in the field, national organizations, and governmental public health agencies can be very helpful.

Apply Inclusion and Exclusion Criteria

The third step is to develop inclusion and exclusion criteria for those studies to be reviewed. This step often leads to revision and further specification of the problem statement. Common issues include the study design, the level of analysis, the type of analysis, and the sources and time frame for study retrieval. The inclusion and exclusion criteria should be selected so as to yield those studies most relevant to the purpose of the systematic review. If the purpose of the systematic review is to assess the effectiveness of interventions to increase physical activity rates among schoolchildren, for example, then interventions aimed at representative populations (e.g., those including adults) would be excluded. Ideally, as the inclusion and exclusion criteria are applied, at least a portion of the data retrieval should be repeated by a second person, and results should be compared. If discrepancies are found, the inclusion and exclusion criteria are probably not sufficiently specific or clear. They should be reviewed and revised as needed.

Study Design

The first issue to consider is the type of study. Should only randomized controlled trials be included? Some would answer "yes" because randomized controlled trials are said to provide the most reliable data and to be specially suited for supporting causal inference. Others would argue that randomized controlled trials also have their limitations, such as contamination or questionable external validity, and that including a broader range of designs could increase the aggregate internal and external validity of the entire body of evidence. An additional problem with limiting public health systematic reviews to randomized trials is that there are many public health areas in which this would result in no studies being possible (because trials would be unethical or infeasible). Observational and quasi-experimental studies are appropriate designs for many intervention topics. There may also be characteristics of a study that are necessary for inclusion, such as that baseline and follow-up assessment be made in conjunction with the intervention or that a comparison group be used.

Level of Analysis

The inclusion and exclusion criteria for level of analysis should match the purpose of the systematic review. The most salient feature for public health is whether studies are at the individual or the community level. A potentially confusing problem, especially if one is interested in assessing community-based interventions, is what to do with "mixed" studies—those that include interventions aimed at both the community and the individual. A good strategy in that case is to include all related studies in the data searching and then use the data abstraction form (described later) to determine whether the study should remain in the data set.

Type of Analysis

Evaluations of interventions can use several methods. Some, like the use of focus groups, are more qualitative; others, such as regression modeling, are more quantitative. Often, the specification of the question will make some types of analysis relevant and others off-topic. Some questions can be addressed in varied ways, and when this is true, broad inclusiveness might give more complete answers. However, the more disparate the methodologies included, the more difficult it is to combine and consolidate the results. A qualitative approach to the review tends to be more inclusive, collecting information from all types of analysis. Meta-analysis, because it consolidates results using a statistical methodology, requires quantitative analysis.

Data Sources and Time Frame

The final items to be specified are where a search for studies will be conducted and the time period to be covered. The natural history of the intervention should help determine the time frame. A major change in the delivery of an intervention, for example, makes it difficult to compare results from studies before and after the new delivery method. In this case, one might limit the time to the "after" period. An additional factor influencing time frame is the likely applicability of the results. Sometimes, substantial changes in context have occurred over time. For example, results from the 1980s may be of questionable relevance to the current situation. In that case, one might limit the review to more recent data. A pragmatic factor influencing the selection of a time frame is the availability of electronic databases.

Conduct Data Abstraction

After the inclusion and exclusion criteria have been specified, the next step is to find the studies that fit the framework, and then to extract a common set of information from them. In general, a data abstraction form should be used. This form should direct the systematic extraction of key information about the elements of the study so that they can be consolidated and assessed. Typical elements include the number of participants, the type of study, a precise description of the intervention, and the results of the study. If the data abstraction form is well designed, the data consolidation and assessment can proceed using only the forms. The exact format and content of the abstraction form depend on the intervention and the type of analysis being used in the systematic review. An excellent and comprehensive example of an abstraction form is provided by the Task Force on Community Preventive Services.[28]

Consolidate the Evidence

The next step in a systematic review is an assessment of whether data from the various studies can be combined. (Often they should not if, for example, all of the available studies have serious flaws or if the interventions or outcomes are too disparate.) If data can be combined to reach an overall conclusion, it may be done either qualitatively or quantitatively.

Assess Data to Draw a Conclusion

After the evidence has been consolidated, the final step is to assess it and reach a conclusion. For example, suppose that the intervention being reviewed is the launching of mass media campaigns to increase physical activity rates among adults. Further, assume that a meta-analysis of this topic reveals that a majority of studies find that community-based interventions improve physical activity rates. However, the effect size is small. What should the review conclude?

The review should consider both the strength and weight of the evidence and the substantive importance of the effect. This assessment can be done by the reviewer using his or her own internal criteria, or by using explicit criteria that were set before the review was conducted. An example of the latter approach is the method employed by the US Preventive Services Task Force (USPSTF).[29] The USPSTF looks at the quality and weight of the evidence (rated good, fair, or poor), and the net benefit, or effect size, of the preventive service (rated substantial, moderate, small, or zero/negative). Their overall rating and recommendation reflect a combination of these two factors. For example, if a systematic review of a preventive service finds "fair" evidence of a "substantial" effect, the Task Force gives it a recommendation of "B," or a recommendation that clinicians routinely provide the service to eligible patients.

If no formal process for combining the weight of the evidence and the substantive importance of the findings has been specified beforehand, and the systematic review yields mixed findings, then it is useful to seek help with assessing the evidence and drawing a conclusion. The analyst might ask experts in the field to review the evidence and reach a conclusion or make a recommendation.

After completing the systematic review, the final step is to write up a report and disseminate the findings. The report should include a description of all of the previous steps.[23,24] In fact protocols currently exist for writing up and evaluating systematic reviews. Ideally, the systematic review should be disseminated to the potential users of the recommendations. The method of dissemination should be targeted to the desired audience. Increasingly, this means putting reports on the Internet so that they are freely accessible or presenting the findings to a community planning board. However, it is also important to submit reviews for publication in peer-reviewed journals. This provides one final quality check. Various methods for disseminating the results of systematic reviews are described later in this chapter.

Meta-Analysis

Over the past three decades, meta-analysis has been increasingly used to synthesize the findings of multiple research studies. Meta-analysis, a type of systematic review, was originally developed in the social sciences in the 1970s when hundreds of studies existed on the same topics.[6] Meta-analysis uses a quantitative approach to summarize evidence, in which results from separate studies are pooled to obtain a weighted average summary result.[6] Its use has appeal because of its potential to pool a group of smaller studies, enhancing statistical power. Meta-analysis studies can increase the statistical and scientific credibility of a scientific finding because they summarize effects across sites and methodologies. They also may allow researchers to test subgroup effects (e.g., by gender or racial or ethnic group) that are sometimes difficult to assess in a single, smaller study. Finally, reviews that summarize various intervention trials are an extremely efficient method for obtaining the "bottom line" about what works and what does not.[4] Suppose there were several studies examining the effects of exercise on cholesterol levels, with each reporting the average change in cholesterol levels, the standard deviation of that change, and the number of study participants. These average changes could be weighted by sample size and pooled to obtain an average of the average changes in cholesterol levels. If this grand mean showed a significant decline in cholesterol levels among exercisers, then the meta-analyst would conclude that the evidence supported exercise as a way to lower cholesterol levels.

Similar to the method described previously for conducting a systematic review, Petitti notes four essential steps in conducting a meta-analysis: (1) identifying relevant studies; (2) deciding on inclusion and exclusion criteria for studies under consideration; (3) abstracting the data; and (4) conducting the statistical analysis, including exploration of heterogeneity.[6]

Meta-analysis includes several different statistical methods for aggregating the results from multiple studies. The method chosen depends on the type of analysis used in the original studies, which, in turn, is related to the type of data analyzed. For example, continuous data, such as cholesterol levels, can be analyzed by comparing the means of different groups. Continuous data could also be analyzed with multiple linear regression. Discrete (dichotomous) data are often analyzed with relative risks or odds ratios, although a range of other options also exists.

An important issue for meta-analysis is the similarity of studies to be combined. This similarity, or homogeneity, is assessed using various statistical tests. If studies are too dissimilar (high heterogeneity), then combining their results is problematic. One approach is to combine only homogenous subsets of studies. Although statistically appealing, this to some extent defeats the purpose of the systematic review because a single summary assessment of the evidence is not reported. An alternative approach is to use meta-analytic methods that allow the addition of control variables that measure the differences among studies. For example, studies may differ by type of study design. If so, then a new variable could be created to code different study design types, such as observational and randomized controlled trials.

The statistical issue of the similarity of studies is related to the inclusion and exclusion criteria. These criteria are selected to identify a group of studies for review that are similar in a substantive way. If the meta-analysis finds that the studies are not statistically homogeneous, then the source of heterogeneity should be investigated. Measures of inconsistency describe the variation across studies that is due to heterogeneity rather than chance.[18] This kind of measure can describe heterogeneity across methodological and clinical subgroups as well. A careful search for the sources of heterogeneity and a consideration of their substantive importance can improve the overall systematic review.

Meta-analysis has generated a fair amount of controversy, particularly when it is used to combine results of observational studies. However, the quality of meta-analyses has improved, perhaps owing to the dissemination and adoption of guidelines for their conduct.[24] Journal articles based on meta-analysis need to be read in the same critical manner as articles based on original research. Despite its limitations, a properly done meta-analysis provides a rigorous way of integrating the findings of several studies. Because it follows a set of specified guidelines, it can be less subjective than the usual qualitative review that weights and combines studies, based on the expert opinion of the authors.

The *Community Guide* and Other Online Resources for Systematic Reviews in Public Health

In 2000, an expert panel (the Task Force on Community Preventive Services), supported by the Centers for Disease Control and Prevention, began publishing the *Guide to Community Preventive Services: Systematic Reviews and Evidence-Based Recommendations* (the *Community Guide*).[28] The underlying reasons for developing the *Community Guide* were as follows: (1) practitioners and policy makers value scientific knowledge as a basis for decision making; (2) the scientific literature on a given topic is often vast, uneven in quality, and inaccessible to busy practitioners; and (3) an experienced and objective panel of experts is seldom locally available to public health officials on a wide range of topics.[30] This effort evaluates evidence related to community, or "population-based," interventions and is intended as a complement to the *Guide to Clinical Preventive Services*. It summarizes what is known about the effectiveness and cost-effectiveness of population-based interventions designed to promote health and to prevent disease, injury, disability, and premature death as well as reduce exposure to environmental hazards.

Sets of related systematic reviews and recommendations are conducted for interventions in broad health topics, organized by behavior (e.g., tobacco product use prevention), environment (e.g., the sociocultural environment), or specific diseases, injuries, or impairment (e.g., vaccine-preventable diseases, asthma). A systematic process is followed that includes forming a review development team, developing a conceptual approach focused around an analytic framework, selecting interventions to evaluate, searching for and retrieving evidence, abstracting information on each relevant study, and assessing the quality of the evidence of effectiveness. Information on each intervention is then translated into a recommendation for or against the intervention or a finding of insufficient evidence. For interventions for which there is insufficient evidence of effectiveness, the *Community Guide* provides guidance for further prevention research. In addition, the *Community Guide* takes a systematic approach to economic evaluation, seeking cost-effectiveness information for those programs and policies deemed effective.[31] A number of systematic economic evaluations have been published as companions to effectiveness reviews found in the *Community Guide*.[32-35]

As of November 2016, evidence reviews and recommendations were available for 20 different public health topics, including reducing risk factors (e.g., tobacco use, excessive alcohol consumption, obesity), promoting prevention (e.g., diabetes, HIV/AIDS), early detection (e.g., cancer screening), management of health conditions (e.g., mental health, asthma), addressing sociocultural determinants (e.g., housing, social environment), and promoting health in settings (e.g., emergency preparedness, worksites). Based on dissemination of evidence reviews in the *Community Guide*, health policy has already been positively influenced at the national and state levels (Box 8.1).

In addition to the *Community Guide,* there are a number of resources available to identify evidence-based interventions that have undergone systematic review. Using these reputable resources reduces the likelihood of making decisions based on the growing number of flawed and misleading systematic reviews and meta-analyses present is the literature.[36] In Table 8.1, we have summarized key attributes of several online resources for identifying evidence-based public health interventions. These sites vary in the topics covered, the rating continuum that is used, whether they include economic evaluations or not, and so forth. Some sites still index new studies, whereas

---

Box 8.1

THE COMMUNITY GUIDE IN ACTION – NEBRASKA'S BLUEPRINT FOR SUCCESS IN REDUCING TOBACCO USE

In 2009–2010 in Nebraska, tobacco use claimed 2,200 lives and cost the state $537 million in health care. It was projected that 36,000 Nebraskans younger than 18 years would die prematurely from smoking. Charlotte Burke, manager of the Lincoln-Lancaster County Health Department's Division of Health Promotion and Outreach, was alarmed by these statistics. They made reducing tobacco use and prevention of exposure to secondhand smoke in the city of Lincoln and the surrounding county a priority. The Lincoln-Lancaster County Health Department partnered with the Tobacco Free Lincoln Coalition, the local Board of Health, and local health organizations and experts to identify resources to decrease tobacco use. Using recommendations from the *Community Guide* they built a plan that started with local education efforts and ultimately led to statewide policy changes. By working with local partners and organizations and educating the public and policymakers, they could make changes that ultimately led to a higher state tobacco tax, a statewide indoor smoking ban, and lower county smoking rates among adults and youth.

Details for this effort and other community initiatives across the United States that used evidence-based recommendations from the *Community Guide* to make communities healthier and safer can be found at http://www.thecommunityguide.org/CG-in-Action/.

Table 8.1 RECOMMENDED ONLINE RESOURCES FOR COMPILED EVIDENCE REVIEWS FOR PUBLIC HEALTH INTERVENTIONS

Start with Searching Syntheses or Predigested Information

Resource	Source	What	User Notes
The Community Guide http://www. thecommunityguide.org	Centers for Disease Control and Prevention	Resource to help you choose programs and policies to improve health and prevent disease in your community. Systematic reviews are used to answer these questions: • Which program and policy interventions have been proved effective? • Are there effective interventions that are right for my community? • What might effective interventions cost; what is the likely return on investment?	Credible source based on scientific review process, complements other decision support tools, such as Healthy People 2020 and the Guide to Clinical Preventive Services. Some topic areas missing or are less comprehensive, length of time to complete review means emerging prevention methods may be ahead of the Community Guide. Topic areas (continuously updated): *Adolescent Health, Alcohol—Excessive Consumption, Asthma, Birth Defects, Cancer, Cardiovascular Disease, Diabetes, Emergency Preparedness, Health Communication, Health Equity, HIV/AIDS, Sexually Transmitted Infections, Pregnancy, Mental Health, Motor Vehicle Injury, Nutrition, Obesity, Oral Health, Physical Activity, Social, Environment, Tobacco, Vaccination, Violence, Worksite*
PH Partners (Partners in Information Access for the Public Health Workforce) **http://phpartners.org/ index.html**	Collaboration of US government agencies, public health organizations, and health sciences libraries	• Homepage provides a dashboard for public health professionals, including news, links to data, jobs, and upcoming conferences and trainings. • Also includes link to Healthy People 2020 Structured Evidence Queries—a topical list of HP2020 goals that link directly to preformed PubMed searches on the literature evidence for each.	Easy way to access/search high-quality, peer-reviewed scientific literature to identify research evidence for selected Healthy People 2020 objectives. Queries are "live" and update as new research is added. Some HP2020 topic areas are still in "beta" status (including heart disease), which means the query has not yet been reviewed by subject experts. The query itself is quite complex and would be hard to replicate outside of the PH partners evidence queries.

(continued)

Table 8.1. CONTINUED

Resource	Source	What	User Notes
RTIPS (Research-Tested Intervention Programs) http://rtips.cancer.gov/rtips/index.do	National Cancer Institute	Searchable database of 159 cancer control interventions and program materials; designed to provide program planners and public health practitioners easy and immediate access to research-tested materials.	Can search by topic, setting, or target population. Topics cover early prevention, such as healthy eating/physical activity, and other areas that overlap with other chronic disease program areas. Does not cover all topic areas in public health (e.g., environmental health, communicable disease).
TRIP (Turning Research Into Practice) https://www.tripdatabase.com	Incorporated enterprise: Jon Brassey and Dr. Chris Price	Clinical search engine (includes population-based interventions) designed to allow users to quickly and easily find and use high-quality research evidence to support their practice and/or care.	Can also search images, videos, patient information leaflets, educational courses, and news. Research from PubMed updates every 2 weeks, and other content updates once per month.
Cochrane Collaboration http://www.cochrane.org/ http://ph.cochrane.org/	A global independent network of researchers, professionals, patients, carers, and people interested in health, based in London	Cochrane contributors—37,000 from more than 130 countries—work together to produce credible, accessible health information that is free from commercial sponsorship and other conflicts of interest. Cochrane exists so that health care decisions get better. Contributors gather and summarize the best health evidence from research to help you make informed choices about treatment.	Although the Cochrane Collaboration is primarily clinical in focus, public health is one of 34 subject areas in which there are systematic reviews. http://www.cochranelibrary.com/topic/Public%20health/

Health Evidence http://www.healthevidence.org	McMaster University Ontario, Canada	Contains nearly 4,500 quality-rated systematic reviews evaluating the effectiveness of public health interventions.	Houses systematic reviews evaluating the effectiveness of public health interventions, particularly in the areas of prevention, health protection, and health promotion. Must sign up to search, but it's free.
What Works for Health http://www.countyhealthrankings.org/roadmaps/what-works-for-health	University of Wisconsin Population Health Institute	Searches systematic reviews, individual peer-reviewed studies, private organizations, and gray literature to find evidence. Useful for topic areas that have not undergone extensive systematic review	Easy way to access/search high-quality literature for topic areas not yet included in the Community Guide or for which there is growing but not yet complete literature. For each included topic area, there are implementation examples and resources that communities can use to move forward with their chosen strategies.

others are no longer including new studies or interventions. It is advisable that practitioners consider several sites together to identify possible intervention solutions, which would lead to more inclusive and informed decision making.

UNDERTAKING A PRIMARY SEARCH OF THE SCIENTIFIC LITERATURE WHEN THERE ARE FEW STUDIES OR REVIEWS

Though for many topic areas in public health, systematic reviews are often available and there are fairly clear recommendations on what works, there are topic areas that are less studied or advances in technology, for example, that have not yet been evaluated. Therefore practitioners may need to conduct a primary search of the scientific literature to identify original research studies or evaluations in their topic area or population of interest. Though not as rigorous as the process of conducting a systematic review, a systematic approach to literature searching can increase the chances of finding pertinent information. Figure 8.2 describes a process for searching the literature and organizing the findings of a search. The following sections provide a step-by-step breakdown of this process.[11]

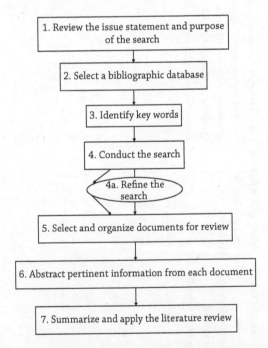

Figure 8.2: Flow chart for organizing a search of the scientific literature. (The later stages [especially steps 5 and 6] of the process are based largely on the Matrix Method, developed by Garrard.[11])

We focus mainly on the use of PubMed because it is the largest and most widely available bibliographic database, with coverage of more than 25 million articles from MEDLINE and life sciences journals. We also focus our search for evidence on peer-reviewed programs and studies and on data that have been reviewed by other researchers and practitioners.

Review the Issue Statement and Purpose of the Search

Based on the issue statement described in chapter 6, the purpose of the search should be well outlined. Keep in mind that searching is an iterative process, and a key is the ability to ask one or more answerable questions. Though the goal of a search is to identify all relevant material and nothing else, in practice, this is difficult to achieve.[6] The overarching questions include, "Which evidence is relevant to my questions?" and "What conclusions can be drawn regarding effective intervention approaches based on the literature assembled?"[37]

Select a Bibliographic Database

Numerous bibliographic databases are now available online (Table 8.2). We recommend that readers become familiar with one or more of them. Some of the databases in Table 8.2 require a fee, but if an individual has access to a library, a global fee may already cover the cost. These resources are available at PubMed (http://www.ncbi.nlm.nih.gov/sites/entrez), a database that is widely used by scholars and the public for searching the biomedical literature in the United States. It is maintained by the National Library of Medicine and has several advantages over other databases—it is free to users, updated frequently, and relatively user-friendly. MEDLINE does not provide the full text of articles, but rather lists the title, authors, source of the publication, the authors' abstract (if one is available), key word subject headings, and a number of other "tags" that provide information about each publication. For some journals (e.g., the *British Medical Journal*), the full text of articles can be accessed by a link on the search results page. Numerous other evidence databases exist for a variety of health care specialties and subspecialties. Subspecialty databases do not currently exist for public health, so it is recommended that practitioners become familiar with MEDLINE and similar databases listed in Table 8.2.

Identify Key Words

Key words are terms that describe the characteristics of the subject being reviewed. A useful search strategy is dependent on the sensitivity and

Table 8.2. RECOMMENDED BIBLIOGRAPHIC DATABASES

Database	Dates	Subjects Covered	Free	Website
PubMed	1966–present	The premier source for bibliographic coverage of biomedical literature; includes references and abstracts from more than 5,600 journals	No	www.ncbi.nlm.nih.gov/pubmed
Google Scholar		Provides access to scholarly literature across many formats, including peer-reviewed journal articles, books, conference papers, theses and dissertations, technical reports, patents, etc.	No	https://scholar.google.com/
Web of Science™	1900–present	Provides access to seven online databases covering science, social sciences, arts and humanities. Contains more than 90 million records.	Yes	https://apps.webofknowledge.com
PsycINFO®	1887–present	The world's most comprehensive source for bibliographic coverage of psychology and behavioral sciences literature; with special subset files ClinPSYC; databases contain more than 1.5 million records. Available to nonmembers of the American Psychological Association for a fee.	Yes	http://www.apa.org/psycinfo/

precision of the key words used. "Sensitivity" is the ability to identify all relevant material, and "precision" is the amount of relevant material among the information retrieved by the search.[38] Thus, sensitivity addresses the question, "Will relevant articles be missed?" whereas precision addresses the question, "Will irrelevant articles be included?" Most bibliographic databases require the use of standardized key words. These key words are often found in the list of Medical Subject Heading (MeSH) terms. There are a number of tutorials on the PubMed site about using the database, including information about identifying and selecting MeSH terms. There are two small screens on the right of the search page of PubMed that are helpful. One, named "Titles with your search terms," will permit the user to consult other published articles similar to what is being searched in order to check the search terms used. Looking at these titles may suggest additional search terms to include. There is also a screen "Search details," which includes MeSH terms. This screen may be helpful when entering open text on a search and noting that an indicated MeSH term may be a better choice. For a literature search in MEDLINE, these sources of key words are useful (Figure 8.2):

1. Identify two scientific papers that cover the topic of interest—one more recent and one less recent. These papers can be pulled up on PubMed. In the MEDLINE abstract, a list of MeSH terms will be provided. These can, in turn, be used in subsequent searches.
2. Key words can be found within the alphabetical list of MeSH terms, available online at <http://www.nlm.nih.gov/mesh/meshhome.html>. Alternatively, the MeSH list can be searched through PubMed by selecting it as the database to search from the dropdown box to the left of the main search box.
3. MEDLINE and Google Scholar do not require users to use standardized key words. Therefore, you can select your own key words—these are searched for in article titles and abstracts. Generally, using nonstandardized key words provides a less precise literature search than does using standardized terms. However, the MEDLINE interface between standardized and nonstandardized key words allows complete searching without a detailed knowledge of MeSH terms.

Conduct the Search

After the databases and initial key words are identified, it is time to run the search. After the initial search is run, the number of publications returned will likely be large and include many irrelevant articles. Several features of PubMed can assist searchers in limiting the scope of the search to the most relevant articles.

- Searches can also be limited to English-language publications, to a certain date of publication, or to certain demographics of the participants, such as age and gender. These tags are found by clicking the "Limits" icon.
- Specific designations such as "editorial," "letter," or "comment" can be excluded, or the search can be limited to "journal article." An initial search can focus on review articles by selecting the publication type. This allows a search of the citation list of review articles to identify original research articles of particular interest.

- PubMed will allow you to link to other "related articles" by simply clicking an icon on the right side of each citation.
- If a particularly useful article is found, the author's name can be searched for other similar studies. The same author will often have multiple publications on the same subject. To avoid irrelevant retrievals, you should use the author's last name and first and middle initials in the search.
- In nearly every case, it is necessary to refine the search approach. As articles are identified, the key word and search strategy will be refined and improved through a "snowballing" technique that allows users to gain familiarity with the literature and gather more useful articles.[11] Articles that may be useful can be saved during each session by clicking "send to" within PubMed.
- Searches may be refined using Boolean operators, words that relate search terms to each other, thus increasing the reach of the search. Help screens of different databases will provide more information, but the most common Boolean operators are (used in CAPS): AND, NOT, OR, NEAR, and " ". The word AND searches for the terms before and after the AND, yielding only articles that include both terms. An example would be: asthma AND adolescents, which would find all articles about asthma in adolescents. An example of the operator NOT would be: accidents NOT automobiles, which would find articles about nonautomobile accidents. (A caution: automobiles is a MeSH term, so this search will exclude cars but not trucks or other vehicles. Using the more general MeSH term Motor vehicles would exclude more articles.) The operator OR permits coupling two search terms that may tap a similar domain. For example, adolescents OR teenagers will find articles that used either term. The operator NEAR will define two search terms that must appear within 10 words of each other to select an article. For example, elevated NEAR lead will find articles discussing elevated blood lead levels. Use of quotation marks "..." will define a search term that must appear as listed. For example, the search term "school clinic" must appear as that phrase to be identified, rather than identifying articles that contain the words "school" and "clinic" separately. Boolean terms are highly useful in specifying a search and can be used to facilitate a search more efficiently.

Select and Organize Documents for Review

Once a set of articles has been located, it is time to organize the documents.[11] This will set the stage for abstracting the pertinent information. Generally, it is helpful to organize the documents by the type of study (original research, review article, review article with quantitative synthesis, guideline). It is often useful to enter documents into a reference management database such as EndNote (http://www.endnote.com) or RefWorks (www.refworks.com), which require a paid subscription, or Mendeley (https://www.mendeley.com/) or Zotero (www.zotero.org), which are free packages. These software applications allow users to switch from one reference format to another when producing reports and grant applications and to download journal citations directly from the Internet, eliminating the chance for typing errors. They also have helpful search and sort capabilities. Choosing the reference management system that is best for you will depend on several factors, including whether you can afford it, will be working without Internet access, want to store PDFs of articles, want to be able to share your reference database with other authors and colleagues, and will be pulling in large files from multiple databases (e.g., if you are doing a systematic review). A systematic method of organizing the articles themselves is essential. A limited number of articles on a certain topic can be kept in a three-ring binder, but larger bodies of evidence may be entered in a reference management database by key word; articles can then be filed alphabetically by the last name of the first author of each article or simply with an identification number. This allows users to search a database by key word later in the research process.

Abstract Pertinent Information From Each Document

When a group of articles has been assembled, the next step is to create an evidence matrix—a spreadsheet with rows and columns that allows users to abstract the key information from each article.[11] Creating a matrix provides a structure for putting the information in order. In developing a matrix, the choice of column topics is a key consideration. It is often useful to consider both methodological characteristics and content-specific results as column headings. A sample review matrix is shown in Table 8.3 (using physical activity studies for illustration[39-43]). In this example, studies were also organized within rows by an ecological framework, described in detail in chapter 5.

Summarize and Apply the Literature Review

After a body of studies has been abstracted into a matrix, the literature may be summarized for various purposes. For example, you may need to provide background information for a new budget item that is being presented to the administrator of an agency. Knowing the best intervention science and determining the best way to transfer that knowledge to key policy makers should increase the chances of convincing these policy makers of the need for a particular program or policy.[44] You may also need to summarize the literature in

Table 8.3. EXAMPLE EVIDENCE MATRIX FOR LITERATURE ON PHYSICAL ACTIVITY PROMOTION AT VARIOUS LEVELS OF AN ECOLOGICAL FRAMEWORK

Lead author, article title, journal citation	Year	Methodologic Characteristics				Content-Specific Findings		Other Comments
		Study Design	Study Population	Sample Size	Intervention Characteristics	Results	Conclusions	
Individual Level								
Ory et al.[39] Social and environmental predictors of walking among older adults. United States	2016	Cross-sectional	Community-dwelling older adults (>=60y) from a healthcare system in Texas	272	N/A—not an intervention	Factors associated with not meeting PA recommendations included being 60-69 y, poor mental health in past month, and lack of social support for walking	Physicians must communicate the importance of PA to older patients and discuss strategies to overcome barriers to walking.	
Interpersonal Level								
Dowda et al.[40] Family support for physical activity in girls from 8th to 12th grade in South Carolina. United States	2007	Longi-tudinal	Adolescent girls in 8th grade in South Carolina in 1998	421	Perceived family support for PA, perceived behavioral control, self-efficacy	Family support was independently associated with age-related changes in PA which more rapid declines in PA among those with low family support for PA	Support of PA from family members may reduce the decline in PA in adolescent girls independent of self-efficacy and perceived behavioral control.	PA was assessed using a 3 day activity recall and then converted to METs per day at each measurement time point (8th, 9th, 12th grades)

Gilson et al.[41] Walking towards health in a university community. United Kingdom	2007	Randomized controlled trial (feasibility study)	Employees at Leeds Metropolitan University UK	64	1 control group which received no intervention and 2 intervention groups: a) walking routes-followed prescribed walks around campus with a goal of at least 15 minutes of brisk walking during the work day; b) walking within tasks-encouraged the accumulation of steps in and around the office during usual activities.	Differences in step counts between groups	Significant mean differences between groups with an average decrease in steps in the control groups and increases in steps in both walking groups.

Kamada et al.[42] A community-wide campaign to promote physical activity in middle-aged and elderly people: a cluster randomized controlled trial. Japan	2013	Cluster Randomized controlled trial	12 communities within Unnan city in Shimane, Japan—9 intervention (3 levels of PA) and 3 comparison	4414	Community-wide campaign to promote PA as a public health project at the cluster level	Short term changes in knowledge and awareness but no changes in PA at 1 year	The CWC did not change PA beliefs, intention or behavior though there were short term changes in knowledge and awareness.

(continued)

Table 8.3. CONTINUED

Lead author, article title, journal citation	Year	Methodologic Characteristics				Content-Specific Findings		
		Study Design	Study Population	Sample Size	Intervention Characteristics	Results	Conclusions	Other Comments
					Health Policy Level			
Slater et al.[43] The impact of state laws and district policies on physical education and recess practices in a nationally representative sample of US public elementary schools. United States	2012	Panel study	47 states, 690 school districts and 1761 schools assessed during the 2006-2007, 2007-2008, and 2008-2009 school years		Examine the association of state and school district policies on the prevalence of physical education and recess	Schools in states or school districts that had a law/policy requiring 150 min/wk of PE were more likely to have 150 min/wk of PE and schools in states with laws encouraging recess were more likely to have 20 minutes of recess daily. No association with district policies and prevalence of recess.	Mandating only increased PE or recess does not result in greater overall PA as schools/districts compensate to manage daily time. To increase school PA, policy makers need to mandate both PE and recess time.	

order to build the case for a grant application that seeks external support for a particular program.

SEEKING SOURCES OUTSIDE THE SEARCHABLE LITERATURE

A great deal of important evidence on public health topics is not found in published journal articles and books.[6] Reasons for the limitations of searching the published literature include the following: (1) many researchers and practitioners fail to write up their research because of competing projects and other time demands; (2) journal editors are faced with difficult decisions on what to publish, and there is a tendency toward publishing studies showing a significant effect of an intervention (publication bias); and (3) in some areas of the world, lack of resources precludes systematic empirical research. The following approaches should prove useful in finding evidence beyond the scientific literature.

The "Fugitive" Literature

The "fugitive" or "gray" literature includes government reports, book chapters, conference proceedings, and other materials that are not found in online databases such as MEDLINE. These are particularly important in attempting a summary of the literature involving meta-analysis or cost-effectiveness analysis (see chapter 4). It can be difficult to locate the fugitive literature. Experts on the topic of interest are probably the best source of information—you can write or email key informants asking them to provide information on relevant publications that would not be identified through database searching. More broad-based searches can be conducted of the Internet using search engines such as Google (www.google.com) or Google Scholar (https://scholar. google.com/). The advantage of these search engines is their ability to find a large number of sources inside and outside of the peer-reviewed scientific literature, such as unpublished reports, meeting abstracts, and government or foundation publications. The main disadvantage is the user's lack of control over the quality of the information returned. Information collected from a wide search of the Internet must be viewed with a critical eye.[45,46] Resources also exist to see what current research is being conducted in the United States and beyond. The RePORTER (Research Portfolio Online Reporting Tool) database, maintained by the US National Institutes of Health, provides summaries of funded research projects that can be useful in finding information before its appearance in the peer-reviewed literature (http://projectreporter. nih.gov/reporter.cfm). Similarly, the Community Research and Development

Information Service (CORDIS) is the European Union (EU) primary public repository and portal to disseminate information on EU-funded research projects since 1990.

Key Informant Interviews

Often a public health practitioner wants to understand not only the outcomes of a program or policy but also the process of developing and carrying out an intervention (see chapter 10). Many process issues are difficult to glean from the scientific literature because the methods sections in published articles may not be comprehensive enough to show all aspects of the intervention. A program may evolve over time, and what is in the published literature may differ from what is currently being done. In addition, many good program and policy evaluations go unpublished.

In these cases, key informant interviews may be useful. Key informants are experts on a certain topic and may include a university researcher who has years of experience in a particular intervention area or a local program manager who has the field experience to know what works when it comes to designing and implementing effective interventions. There are several steps in carrying out a "key informant" process:

1. Identify the key informants who might be useful for gathering information. They can be found in the literature, through professional networks, and increasingly, on the Internet (see <http://www.profnet.com>, a site that puts journalists and interested persons in touch with scientific experts who are willing to share their expertise).
2. Determine the types of information needed. It is often helpful to write out a short list of open-ended questions that are of particular interest. This can help in framing a conversation and making the most efficient use of time. Before a conversation with an expert, it is useful to email him or her questions to allow thinking about replies.
3. Collect the data. This often can be accomplished through a 15- to 30-minute phone conversation if the questions of interest are well framed ahead of time.
4. Summarize the data collected. Conversations can be recorded and transcribed using formative research techniques. More often, good notes are taken and conversations recorded to end up with a series of bullet points from each key informant conversation.
5. Conduct follow-up, as needed. As with literature searching, key informant interviews often result in a snowballing effect in which one expert

identifies another who is also knowledgeable. As information becomes repetitious, the data collector can decide when enough information has been collected.

Professional Meetings

Annually, there are dozens of relevant and helpful professional meetings in public health, ranging from large conventions such as that of the American Public Health Association to smaller, specialty meetings such as the annual meeting on diabetes prevention and control. Important intervention research is often presented at these meetings. There are regional public health associations that hold meetings and are a rich source for networking and developing resources. The smaller venues allow one to talk informally with the researcher to learn details of his or her work and how it might apply in a particular setting. Practitioners should seek out meetings that use a peer-review process for abstract review, helping to ensure that high-quality research is presented. Meetings generally provide a list of presenters and abstracts of presentations before or during the meeting. The main limitation for many practitioners is the inability to attend a variety of professional meetings because of limited travel funds.

SUMMARY

Literature searching can be an inexact science because of the wide scope of public health and inconsistencies in search strategies.[47] But a systematic search of the literature is a key for evidence-based decision making. Although this chapter attempts to provide the essential information for locating scientific information quickly, there is no substitute for trying out these approaches and customizing procedures to your own needs.

KEY CHAPTER POINTS

- It is important to understand the various uses of different types of scientific literature (i.e., original research articles, review articles, systematic reviews, reviews with quantitative synthesis, and guidelines).
- Whenever available, start with "predigested" literature such as systematic reviews available through the *Community Guide* and other online resources to identify evidence of what works.

- A step-by-step approach to literature searching will improve the sensitivity and precision of the search process.
- Other valuable sources of scientific information can include the gray literature, key informant interviews, and professional meetings.

SUGGESTED READINGS AND WEBSITES
Suggested Readings

Bambra C. Real world reviews: a beginner's guide to undertaking systematic reviews of public health policy interventions. *Journal of Epidemiology and Community Health.* January 1, 2011 2011;65(1):14–19.

Briss PA, Zaza S, Pappaioanou M, et al. Developing an evidence-based Guide to Community Preventive Services—methods. The Task Force on Community Preventive Services. *Am J Prev Med.* 2000;18(1 Suppl):35–43.

Carande-Kulis VG, Maciosek MV, Briss PA, et al. Methods for systematic reviews of economic evaluations for the Guide to Community Preventive Services. Task Force on Community Preventive Services. *Am J Prev Med.* Jan 2000;18(1 Suppl):75–91.

Harris RP, Helfand M, Woolf SH, et al. Current methods of the U.S. Preventive Services Task Force. A review of the process. *Am J Prev Med.* 2001;20(3 Suppl):21–35.

Higgins J, Green S. *Cochrane Handbook for Systematic Review of Interventions: Cochrane Book Series.* Chichester, England: John Wiley & Sons Ltd; 2008.

Lefebvre C, Glanville J, Wieland LS, Coles B, Weightman AL. Methodological developments in searching for studies for systematic reviews: past, present and future? *Systematic Reviews.* 2013;2(1):1–9.

Mahood Q, Van Eerd D, Irvin E. Searching for grey literature for systematic reviews: challenges and benefits. *Res Synth Methods.* Sep 2014;5(3):221–234.

Truman BI, Smith-Akin CK, Hinman AR, et al. Developing the guide to community preventive services—overview and rationale. *American Journal of Preventive Medicine.* 2000;18(1S):18–26.

Uman LS. Systematic reviews and meta-analyses. *Journal of the Canadian Academy of Child and Adolescent Psychiatry.* 2011;20(1):57–59.

Selected Websites

Agency for Healthcare Research and Quality (AHRQ) <http://www.ahrq.gov/>. The AHRQ mission is to improve the quality, safety, efficiency, and effectiveness of health care for all Americans. Information from AHRQ research helps people make more informed decisions and improve the quality of health care services.

Annual Review of Public Health <http://publhealth.annualreviews.org/>. The mission of Annual Reviews is to provide systematic, periodic examinations of scholarly advances in a number of scientific fields through critical authoritative reviews. The comprehensive critical review not only summarizes a topic but also roots out errors of fact or concept and provokes discussion that will lead to new research activity. The critical review is an essential part of the scientific method.

Evidence-based behavioral practice (EBBP) <http://www.ebbp.org/>. The EBBP.org project creates training resources to bridge the gap between behavioral health research and practice. An interactive website offers modules covering topics such as the EBBP process, systematic reviews, searching for evidence, critical appraisal, and randomized controlled trials. This site is ideal for practitioners, researchers, and educators.

National Academy of Sciences Institute of Medicine (IOM) <http://www.iom.edu/>. The IOM is an independent, nonprofit organization that works outside of government to provide unbiased and authoritative advice to government, the private sector, and the public. This site includes IOM reports published after 1998. All reports from the IOM and the National Academies, including those published before 1998, are available from the National Academies Press.

National Registry of Evidence-based Programs and Practices (NREPP) <http://nrepp.samhsa.gov/>. This is the Substance Abuse and Mental Health Services Administration (SAMHSA) searchable online registry of evidence-based interventions focused on mental health and substance abuse. Similar to other resources described here, the interventions must meet specific minimal requirements for review, and each program is independently assessed and rated by certified reviewers. This repository is intended to increase access to evidence-based interventions and reduce the lag time between scientific discovery and application in the field.

See Table 8.1 for additional websites.

REFERENCES

1. Jones R, Kinmonth A-L. *Critical Reading for Primary Care.* Oxford, UK: Oxford University Press; 1995.
2. Greenhalgh T. How to read a paper. Getting your bearings (deciding what the paper is about). *British Medical Journal.* 1997;315:243–246.
3. Makela M, Witt K. How to read a paper: critical appraisal of studies for application in healthcare. *Singapore Med J.* Mar 2005;46(3):108–114; quiz 115.
4. Uman LS. Systematic Reviews and Meta-Analyses. *Journal of the Canadian Academy of Child and Adolescent Psychiatry.* 2011;20(1):57–59.
5. Garg AX, Hackam D, Tonelli M. Systematic review and meta-analysis: when one study is just not enough. *Clinical Journal of the American Society of Nephrology.* January 1, 2008 2008;3(1):253–260.
6. Petitti DB. *Meta-analysis, Decision Analysis, and Cost-Effectiveness Analysis: Methods for Quantitative Synthesis in Medicine.* 2nd ed. New York, NY: Oxford University Press; 2000.
7. Porta M, ed. *A Dictionary of Epidemiology.* 6th ed. New York, NY: Oxford University Press; 2014.
8. Sackett DL, Rosenberg WMC. The need for evidence-based medicine. *Journal of the Royal Society of Medicine.* 1995;88:620–624.
9. Sackett DL, Rosenberg WMC, Gray JAM, Haynes RB, Richardson WS. Evidence based medicine: what it is and what it isn't. *British Medical Journal.* 1996;312:71–72.
10. Straus SE, Richardson WS, Glasziou P, Haynes R. *Evidence-Based Medicine. How to Practice and Teach EBM.* 4th ed. Edinburgh, UK: Churchill Livingston; 2011.
11. Garrard J. *Health Sciences Literature Review Made Easy. The Matrix Method.* 2nd ed. Sudbury, MA: Jones and Bartlett Publishers; 2006.
12. US National Library of Medicine. Key Medline Indicators *Medline statistics* [http://www.nlm.nih.gov/bsd/bsd_key.html. Accessed October 2, 2016.
13. Science Intelligence and InfoPros. How many science journals? https://scienceintelligence.wordpress.com/2012/01/23/how-many-science-journals/. Accessed October 2, 2016.

14. Laakso M, Björk B-C. Anatomy of open access publishing: a study of longitudinal development and internal structure. *BMC Medicine*. 2012;10(1):1–9.

15. Murad MH, Montori VM. Synthesizing evidence: shifting the focus from individual studies to the body of evidence. *JAMA*. Jun 5 2013;309(21):2217–2218.

16. Bambra C. Real world reviews: a beginner's guide to undertaking systematic reviews of public health policy interventions. *Journal of Epidemiology and Community Health*. January 1, 2011 2011;65(1):14–19.

17. Guyatt G, Rennie D, Meade M, Cook D, eds. *Users' Guides to the Medical Literature. A Manual for Evidence-Based Clinical Practice*. 3rd ed. Chicago, IL: American Medical Association Press; 2015.

18. Higgins J, Green S. *Cochrane Handbook for Systematic Review of Interventions: Cochrane Book Series*. Chichester, England: John Wiley & Sons Ltd; 2008.

19. Briss PA, Zaza S, Pappaioanou M, et al. Developing an evidence-based *Guide to Community Preventive Services*—methods. The Task Force on Community Preventive Services. *Am J Prev Med*. 2000;18(1 Suppl):35–43.

20. Liberati A, Altman DG, Tetzlaff J, et al. The PRISMA statement for reporting systematic reviews and meta-analyses of studies that evaluate healthcare interventions: explanation and elaboration. *BMJ*. 2009;339:b2700.

21. Moher D, Simera I, Schulz KF, Hoey J, Altman DG. Helping editors, peer reviewers and authors improve the clarity, completeness and transparency of reporting health research. *BMC Med*. 2008;6:13.

22. Page MJ, Shamseer L, Altman DG, et al. Epidemiology and reporting characteristics of systematic reviews of biomedical research: a cross-sectional study. *PLoS Med*. 2016;13(5):e1002028.

23. Shea BJ, Grimshaw JM, Wells GA, et al. Development of AMSTAR: a measurement tool to assess the methodological quality of systematic reviews. *BMC Medical Research Methodology*. 2007;7(1):10–16.

24. Moher D, Shamseer L, Clarke M, et al. Preferred reporting items for systematic review and meta-analysis protocols (PRISMA-P) 2015 statement. *Systematic Reviews*. 2015;4(1):1–9.

25. Blackhall K. Finding studies for inclusion in systematic reviews of interventions for injury prevention the importance of grey and unpublished literature. *Inj Prev*. Oct 2007;13(5):359.

26. Hopewell S, McDonald S, Clarke M, Egger M. Grey literature in meta-analyses of randomized trials of health care interventions. *Cochrane Database Syst Rev*. 2007;(2):Mr000010.

27. Mahood Q, Van Eerd D, Irvin E. Searching for grey literature for systematic reviews: challenges and benefits. *Res Synth Methods*. Sep 2014;5(3):221–234.

28. Task Force on Community Preventive Services. Guide to Community Preventive Services. www.thecommunityguide.org. Accessed June 5, 2016.

29. Harris RP, Helfand M, Woolf SH, et al. Current methods of the U.S. Preventive Services Task Force. A review of the process. *Am J Prev Med*. 2001;20(3 Suppl):21–35.

30. Truman BI, Smith-Akin CK, Hinman AR, al e. Developing the *Guide to Community Preventive Services*—overview and rationale. *American Journal of Preventive Medicine*. 2000;18(1S):18–26.

31. Carande-Kulis VG, Maciosek MV, Briss PA, et al. Methods for systematic reviews of economic evaluations for the *Guide to Community Preventive Services*. Task Force on Community Preventive Services. *Am J Prev Med*. Jan 2000;18(1 Suppl):75–91.

32. Li R, Qu S, Zhang P, et al. Economic evaluation of combined diet and physical activity promotion programs to prevent type 2 diabetes among persons at increased risk: a systematic review for the Community Preventive Services Task Force. *Ann Intern Med.* Sep 15 2015;163(6):452–460.

33. Patel M, Pabst L, Chattopadhyay S, et al. Economic review of immunization information systems to increase vaccination rates: a community guide systematic review. *J Public Health Manag Pract.* May-Jun 2015;21(3):1–10.

34. Ran T, Chattopadhyay SK. Economic evaluation of community water fluoridation: a *Community Guide* systematic review. *Am J Prev Med.* Jun 2016;50(6):790–796.

35. Ran T, Chattopadhyay SK, Hahn RA. Economic evaluation of school-based health centers: a *Community Guide* systematic review. *Am J Prev Med.* Jul 2016;51(1):129–138.

36. Ioannidis JP. The mass production of redundant, misleading, and conflicted systematic reviews and meta-analyses. *Milbank Q.* Sep 2016;94(3):485–514.

37. Bartholomew L, Parcel G, Kok G, Gottlieb N, Fernandez M. *Planning Health Promotion Programs: An Intervention Mapping Approach.* 3rd ed. San Francisco, CA: Jossey-Bass Publishers; 2011.

38. Lefebvre C, Glanville J, Wieland LS, Coles B, Weightman AL. Methodological developments in searching for studies for systematic reviews: past, present and future? *Systematic Reviews.* 2013;2(1):1–9.

39. Ory MG, Towne SD, Won J, Forjuoh SN, Lee C. Social and environmental predictors of walking among older adults. *BMC Geriatrics.* 2016;16(1):155–167.

40. Dowda M, Dishman RK, Pfeiffer KA, Pate RR. Family support for physical activity in girls from 8th to 12th grade in South Carolina. *Prev Med.* Feb 2007;44(2):153–159.

41. Gilson N, McKenna J, Cooke C, Brown W. Walking towards health in a university community: a feasibility study. *Prev Med.* Feb 2007;44(2):167–169.

42. Kamada M, Kitayuguchi J, Inoue S, et al. A community-wide campaign to promote physical activity in middle-aged and elderly people: a cluster randomized controlled trial. *Int J Behav Nutr Phys Act.* 2013;10:44.

43. Slater SJ, Nicholson L, Chriqui J, Turner L, Chaloupka F. The impact of state laws and district policies on physical education and recess practices in a nationally representative sample of US public elementary schools. *Arch Pediatr Adolesc Med.* Apr 2012;166(4):311–316.

44. Oliver K, Innvar S, Lorenc T, Woodman J, Thomas J. A systematic review of barriers to and facilitators of the use of evidence by policymakers. *BMC Health Serv Res.* 2014;14:2.

45. Boeker M, Vach W, Motschall E. Google Scholar as replacement for systematic literature searches: good relative recall and precision are not enough. *BMC Med Res Methodol.* 2013;13:131.

46. Shultz M. Comparing test searches in PubMed and Google Scholar. *Journal of the Medical Library Association: JMLA.* 2007;95(4):442–445.

47. Rimer BK, Glanz DK, Rasband G. Searching for evidence about health education and health behavior interventions. *Health Educ Behav.* 2001;28(2):231–248.

CHAPTER 9

✧

Developing and Prioritizing
Intervention Options

For every complex problem, there is a solution that is simple, neat, and wrong.
H. L. Mencken

A central challenge for public health is to articulate and act on a broad definition of public health—one that incorporates a multidisciplinary approach to the underlying causes of premature death and disability.[1] When implementing an evidence-based process within this framework, there are a large number of possible program and policy options. Identifying and choosing among these options is not a simple, straightforward task. The preceding chapters were designed to help readers define a problem and develop a broad array of choices. For example, methods from descriptive epidemiology and public health surveillance can be used to characterize the magnitude of a particular issue, and tools such as economic evaluation are useful in assessing the benefits of an intervention compared with the costs.

After options are identified, priorities need to be set among various alternatives. In general, methods for setting priorities are better developed for clinical interventions than for community approaches,[2] in part because there is a larger body of evidence on the effectiveness of clinical interventions than on that of community-based studies. There is also a larger base of cost-effectiveness studies of clinical interventions. However, it is unlikely that even the most conscientious and well-intentioned clinician will incorporate all recommended preventive services during each visit by a patient, given competing demands. Decisions about which clinical services to deliver are driven in part by patient demands, recent news stories, medical education, and adequacy of reimbursement.[3] A patient in a clinical setting might have several health issues, so part of the evidence-based medicine process is deciding which to address first. Similarly, communities have many public health challenges, and a systematic process helps to prioritize these. In community settings many of the tools and approaches for identifying and prioritizing interventions are still being developed and tested.

This chapter is divided into four main sections. The first describes some broad-based considerations to take into account when examining options and priorities. The next section outlines analytic methods and processes that have been applied when setting clinical and community priorities in promoting health. The third part is an overview of the concepts of innovation and creativity in option selection and prioritization. And the final portion describes the development and uses of analytic frameworks in developing and prioritizing options. This chapter focuses on Type 1 evidence (etiology, burden) and its role in identifying and prioritizing public health issues. It also introduces issues related to Types 2 and 3 evidence (selecting, adapting, and applying specific interventions), which are expanded on in later chapters.

BACKGROUND

Resources are always limited in public health. This stems from the funding priorities in which public health receives only a small percentage of the total health spending in the United States, making funding for public health programs a "zero-sum game" in many settings.[4,5] That is, the total available resources for public health programs and services are not likely to increase substantially from year to year. Only rarely are there exceptions to this scenario, such as the investments several US states have made in tobacco control, resulting in substantial public health benefits.[6] Therefore, careful, evidence-based examination of program options is necessary to ensure that the most effective approaches to improving the public's health are taken. The key is to follow a process that is both systematic, objective, and time-efficient, combining science with the realities of the environment.[7]

At a macrolevel, part of the goal in setting priorities carefully is to shift from resource-based decision making to a population-based process. To varying degrees this occurred in the United States over the past century. In the resource-based planning cycle, the spiral of increased resources and increased demand for resources helped to drive the cost of health care services continually higher, even as the health status of some population groups declined.[8] In contrast, the population-based planning cycle gives greater attention to population needs and outcomes, including quality of life, and has been described as the starting point in decision making.[8] On a global scale, the Sustainable Development Goals[9] offer insights into the need to set a broad range of priorities and the need to involve many sectors (e.g., economics, education) outside of health to achieve progress (Box 9.1). This population-based, intersectoral planning cycle is the framework that is either implicitly or explicitly followed throughout this chapter.

When one is examining intervention options, there are several different sources of information, including several that have been discussed in earlier

---

Box 9.1
HEALTH IN THE SUSTAINABLE DEVELOPMENT GOALS

Focus
1. End poverty in all its forms everywhere
2. End hunger, achieve food security and improved nutrition, and promote sustainable agriculture
3. Ensure healthy lives and promote well-being for all at all ages
4. Ensure inclusive and equitable quality education and promote life-long learning opportunities for all
5. Achieve gender equality and empower all women and girls
6. Ensure availability and sustainable management of water and sanitation for all
7. Ensure access to affordable, reliable, sustainable, and modern energy for all
8. Promote sustained, inclusive, and sustainable economic growth, full and productive employment, and decent work for all
9. Build resilient infrastructure, promote inclusive and sustainable industrialization, and foster innovation
10. Reduce inequality within and among countries
11. Make cities and human settlements inclusive, safe, resilient, and sustainable
12. Ensure sustainable consumption and production patterns
13. Take urgent action to combat climate change and its impacts (in line with the United Nations Framework Convention on Climate Change)
14. Conserve and sustainably use the oceans, seas, and marine resources for sustainable development
15. Protect, restore, and promote sustainable use of terrestrial ecosystems, sustainably manage forests, combat desertification, and halt and reverse land degradation and halt biodiversity loss
16. Promote peaceful and inclusive societies for sustainable development, provide access to justice for all and build effective, accountable, and inclusive institutions at all levels
17. Strengthen the means of implementation and revitalize the global partnership for sustainable development

chapters. These sources can be grouped in two broad categories: scientific information and "other expert" information. Among scientific sources, the practitioner might seek program options derived from peer-reviewed sources; this might include journal articles or evidence-based summary documents such as clinical or community guidelines. Within the broad group of "other expert" information, one might seek input from professional colleagues in the workplace, at professional meetings, or through key stakeholders (see chapters 5 and 6). Overarching all of these categories is the process for identifying intervention options. Electronic mechanisms such as the Internet can be promising in this regard for busy practitioners. Using the Internet, program options can be rapidly scanned. Some excellent examples of useful Internet sites are provided at the end of this chapter.

As options are being considered and a course of action determined, it is important to distinguish decision making from problem solving. Problem solving involves the determination of one correct solution, for example, when one solves a mathematical problem. In contrast, decision making in organizations is the process of making a choice from among a set of rational alternatives. In choosing a public health intervention approach, there is often not one "correct" answer but rather a set of options to be identified and prioritized. Decision making in public health settings always occurs in the context of uncertainty. Epidemiologic uncertainty in study design and interpretation was discussed in chapters 3 and 7. Other influences on the decision-making process include politics, legal issues, economic forces, and societal values. Modern decision-making theory also recognizes that individual decision makers are influenced by their values, unconscious reflexes, skills, and habits.[10] Key elements for effective decision making in the context of uncertainty include the following:

- Acquiring sufficient evidence on all plausible alternatives
- Approaching the problem in a rational and systematic fashion
- Relying on experience, intuition, and judgment

It is also important to understand that decision making often involves some element of risk and that these risks can occur at various levels. At the program level, the program option chosen may not be the optimal choice or may not be implemented properly, thus limiting the ability to reach objectives. Within an organization, program staff may be hesitant to provide objective data on various options, especially when a negative outcome could lead to political pushback or program discontinuation (and loss of jobs). But an organization and leaders who support creativity and innovation will encourage new ideas even when risk is present (e.g., an innovative new program may bring political baggage).

ANALYTIC METHODS FOR PRIORITIZING HEALTH ISSUES AND PROGRAM AND POLICY OPTIONS

There are many different ways of prioritizing program and policy issues in public health practice. Although it is unlikely that "one size fits all," several tools and resources have proved useful for practitioners in a variety of settings. In addition to using various analytic methods, priority setting will occur at different geographic and political levels. An entire country may establish broad health priorities. In the Netherlands, a comprehensive approach was applied to health services delivery that included an investment in health technology assessment, use of guidelines, and development of criteria to determine priority on waiting lists. Underlying this approach was the belief that excluding certain health care services was necessary to ensure access of all citizens to essential health care.[11] In Croatia, a participatory, "bottom up" approach combined quantitative and qualitative approaches to allow each county to set its priorities based on local population health needs.[12] The Croatian example also provides an example of how a country can avoid a centralized, one-size-fits-all approach that may be ineffective.

In other instances, an individual state or province may conduct a priority-setting process. Based on the recommendations of a group of consumers and health care professionals, Oregon was one of the first US states to rank public health services covered under its Medicaid program, using cost-effectiveness analysis and various qualitative measures, to extend coverage for high-priority services to a greater number of the state's poor residents.[13,14] The Oregon Health Evidence Review Commission (created by HB 2100 in 2011) leads efforts to develop a prioritized list of health services based on methods that place a significant emphasis on preventive services and chronic disease management. The process determines a benefit package designed to keep a population healthy rather focusing on health care services that treat illness. Prioritization of health services relates to a set of variables that are entered into a formula; variables include impact on healthy life-years, impact on suffering, effects on population, vulnerability of population affected, effectiveness, need for service, and net cost.[15]

Experience in New Zealand and Australia shows that stakeholder input can be valuable in priority setting and developing community action plans (Box 9.2).[16,17] The team developed the ANGELO (Analysis Grid for Elements Linked to Obesity) model that has been used to prioritize a set of core issues related to obesity prevention. The ANGELO framework is generalizable to other regions across the globe.[18,19] Many of the same approaches that have been applied at a macrolevel can be used to prioritize programs or policies within a public health or voluntary health agency, within a health care organization, or at a city or county level.

Box 9.2
PRIORITIZING ENVIRONMENTAL INTERVENTIONS TO PREVENT OBESITY

Obesity is increasing at such a rate that some now consider it a pandemic. Researchers from New Zealand and Australia proposed an ecological framework for understanding obesity that included influences of biology, individual behavior, and the environment.[16] With this framework, they developed the ANGELO (Analysis Grid for Elements Linked to Obesity) model that has been used to prioritize the settings and sectors for interventions to address obesity. The ANGELO method utilizes a grid that includes two sizes of environments on one axis (i.e., microsettings, such as neighborhoods and schools, and macrosectors, such as transportation systems and health care systems). On the other axis, four types of environments (physical, economic, political, and sociocultural) are mapped. This framework has been used in six diverse obesity prevention projects in Australia, New Zealand, Fiji, and Tonga, where data were collected from group and individual (stakeholder) interviews among local residents and health workers.[17] Stakeholders generated a long list of potential "obesogenic" elements and ranked each according to the perceived relevance to their community and their potential changeability. The ANGELO framework has proved to be a flexible and efficient tool for action planning and setting priorities that is responsive to community needs and the latest scientific knowledge.[16] It has been applied successfully in various areas of the world (e.g., Mediterranean and Pacific regions) to identify effective and sustainable change strategies.[18, 19]

Prioritizing Clinical Preventive Services

There have been few systematic attempts to develop and apply objective criteria for prioritizing clinical preventive services. As noted in chapter 8, prioritization of clinical interventions tends to benefit from the development of guidelines for primary care providers. Some of the earliest efforts included the Canadian Task Force on the Periodic Health Examination[20] and the US Preventive Services Task Force.[21]

An approach to prioritizing clinical preventive services was first proposed by Coffield and colleagues.[3,22,23] This method was developed in conjunction with the publication of the third edition of the *Guide to Clinical Preventive Services*. With analytic methods, clinical interventions were ranked according to two dimensions: burden of disease prevented by each service and average cost-effectiveness. Burden was described by the clinically preventable burden (CPB): the amount of disease that would be prevented by a particular service in usual practice if the service were delivered to 100%

of the target population. CPB was measured in quality-adjusted life-years (QALYs), as defined in chapter 4. Cost-effectiveness (CE) was the ratio of net costs to burden of disease prevented, that is, (costs of prevention – costs averted)/QALYs saved. Each service was assigned CPB and CE scores from 1 to 5 (according to quintile), with 5 being the best possible score. The rankings were added so that each service ended up with a final score from 1 to 10 (Table 9.1).[24] It is worth noting that scores are not proportionate;

Table 9.1. RANKING OF CLINICAL PREVENTIVE SERVICES FOR THE US POPULATION

Clinical Preventive Service	CPB	CE	Total
Discuss daily aspirin use: men 40+, women 50+	5	5	10
Childhood immunizations	5	5	10
Smoking cessation advice and help to quit: adults	5	5	10
Alcohol screening and brief counseling: adults	4	5	9
Colorectal cancer screening: adults 50+	4	4	8
Hypertension screening and treatment: adults 18+	5	3	8
Influenza immunization: adults 50+	4	4	8
Vision screening: adults 65+	3	5	8
Cervical cancer screening: women	4	3	7
Cholesterol screening and treatment: men 35+, women 45+	5	2	7
Pneumococcal immunization: adults 65+	3	4	7
Breast cancer screening: women 40+	4	2	6
Chlamydia screening: sexually active women <25	2	4	6
Discuss calcium supplementation: women	3	3	6
Vision screening: preschool children	2	4	6
Folic acid chemoprophylaxis: women of childbearing age	2	3	5
Obesity screening: adults	3	2	5
Depression screening: adults	3	1	4
Hearing screening: adults 65+	2	2	4
Injury-prevention counseling: parents of child 0–4	1	3	4
Osteoporosis screening: women 65+	2	2	4
Cholesterol screening: men <35, women <45 at high risk	1	1	2
Diabetes screening: adults at risk	1	1	2
Diet counseling: adults at risk	1	1	2
Tetanus-diphtheria booster: adults	1	1	1

CE = cost-effectiveness; CPB = clinically preventable burden.
Maciosek et al.,[23] Maciosek et al.,[3] and the Partnership for Prevention.[24]

for example, a total score of 8 is more valuable but not necessarily twice as valuable as a total score of 4.[25] With this method, the three interventions with the highest priority rankings were discussion of daily aspirin use with men 40 years and older and women 50 years and older, vaccination of children to prevent a variety of infectious diseases, and smoking cessation advice for adults.

Prioritizing Public Health Issues at the Community Level

There are both qualitative and quantitative approaches to setting public health priorities for communities. Although many and diverse definitions of "community" have been offered, we define it as a group of individuals who share attributes of place, social interaction, and social and political responsibility.[26] In practice, many data systems are organized geographically, and therefore communities are often defined by place. A sound priority-setting process can help generate widespread support for public health issues when it is well documented and endorsed by communities.

The prioritization approach, based on comparison of a population health problem with the "ideal" or "achievable" population health status, is sometimes used to advance the policy decision-making process by singling out an objective, limited set of health problems. It usually involves identifying desirable or achievable levels for an epidemiologic measure such as mortality, incidence, or prevalence. One such approach used the lowest achieved mortality rate, calculated from mortality rates that actually have been achieved by some population or population segment at some time and place, and risk-eliminated mortality rates, estimated by mortality levels that would have been achieved with elimination of known-risk factors.[27] A variation of this approach can be used to identify disparities related to race and ethnicity, gender, or other groupings of populations. Similar approaches have been applied in states in the United States,[28-30] in Japan,[31] and in Spain.[32] Another approach used a comparison of observed and expected deaths to estimate the number of potentially preventable deaths per year in each state in the United States for the five leading causes of death.[33]

Multiple groups of researchers and practitioners have proposed standardized, quantitative criteria for prioritizing public health issues at the community level.[5,34-41] Each of these methods differs, but they have some combination of three common elements (similar to those for clinical priorities noted previously). First, each relies on some measure of burden, whether measured in mortality, morbidity, or years of potential life lost. Some methods also attempt to quantify preventability (i.e., the potential effects of intervention).

And finally, resource issues are often addressed in the decision-making process, in terms of both costs of intervention and the capacity of an organization to carry out a particular program or policy. Two analytic methods frequently used as auxiliary in the prioritization process are economic appraisal and an approach based on comparison with "ideal" or "achievable" population health status.[27] Several approaches to categorizing and prioritizing various interventions that use the three common elements are discussed briefly here, as well as one example each of the approaches based on economic data and achievable population health status.

Specific Methods for Prioritizing Public Health Issues

In most areas of public health, important and creative decisions are enhanced by group decision-making processes. Often in a group process, a consensus is reached on some topics. There are advantages and disadvantages to group decision-making processes (Table 9.2), but the former generally outweigh the latter.[42] Probably, the biggest advantage is that more and better information is available to inform a decision when a group is used. Additional advantages include better acceptance of the final decision, enhanced communication, and more accurate decisions. The biggest disadvantage of group decision making is that the process takes longer. However, the management literature shows that, in general, the more "person-hours" that go into a decision, the more likely it will be that the correct one emerges, and the more likely that the decision will be implemented.[43,44] Other potential disadvantages include the potential for indecisiveness, compromise decisions, and domination by one individual. In addition, an outcome known as "groupthink" may result,

Table 9.2. ADVANTAGES AND DISADVANTAGES OF GROUP DECISION MAKING

Advantages	Disadvantages
More information and knowledge are available	The process takes longer and may be costlier
More alternatives are likely to be generated	Compromise decisions resulting from indecisiveness may emerge
Better acceptance of the final decision is likely, often among those who will carry out the decision	One person may dominate the group
Enhanced communication of the decision may result	"Groupthink" may occur
More accurate and creative decisions often emerge	

in which the group's desire for consensus and cohesiveness overwhelms its desire to reach the best possible decision.[43,45] One way to offset groupthink is by rotating new members into a decision-making group, ensuring that leaders speak less and listen more (the 80/20 rule), and encouraging principled dissent.[46]

The following sections briefly outline several popular brainstorming techniques that are useful in developing and managing an effective group process for prioritization. Other techniques for gathering information from groups and individuals (e.g., focus groups, key informant interviews) are described in chapters 5 and 11. The methods that follow are both

---

Box 9.3

A MIXED-METHOD APPROACH FOR PRIORITIZING ISSUES AT THE COMMUNITY LEVEL

The most effective approaches for improving the health of the public are likely to involve a merger of scientific evidence with community preferences. In three communities in Massachusetts, Ramanadhan and Viswanath worked with community-based organizations (CBOs) to implement an evidence-based decision-making process.[47] The team sought to better understand the drivers of priority setting and the ways in which data influence the prioritization process. The overall goal of their efforts was to build capacity among CBOs to adopt and sustain evidence-based practices. Their approach involved qualitative methods (focus groups with 31 staff members) and quantitative data collection (a survey of 214 staff members). In the focus groups, participants were asked to describe their use of local or state data for priority setting. In the quantitative survey, respondents were queried about the resources they use in setting priorities (multiple options, including community needs assessment, academic journals, provider observations, and many others). Their team found that the top drivers of priority setting included findings from needs assessment, existing data, organizational mission, partnerships, and funding. They also found that drivers sometimes compete (e.g., funding streams pushing one way and community needs another). Several key barriers for using data in priority settings were identified. These included out-of-date information, lack of local data, and challenges in accessing data. Overall, the project showed the value of mixed-methods approaches for establishing a data-driven approach to priority setting among CBOs. By building capacity among CBOs and taking a systematic approach to priority setting, it is likely that programs can be developed with greater impact and ability to address health equity.

quantitative and qualitative. In practice, the most effective approaches to prioritization often mix quantitative approaches with qualitative methods (Box 9.3).[47]

The Diamond Model of Prioritization

Using a process that relies on existing data, the diamond model of prioritization considers two quantitative dimensions: the magnitude of rates and the trends in rates. It classifies each of these two dimensions into three groups resulting in a grid of 9 cells (3 × 3).[48] In Figure 9.1, the diamond model was applied for 30 causes of death in Taiwan. The diamond model permits country, state, and local comparisons of various endpoints, based on morbidity and mortality rates. This initial prioritization is based solely on quantitative data and does not include qualitative factors. One of its major advantages is that it is based on existing data sets and is therefore relatively easy to carry out. A disadvantage is that it is often based on mortality rates, which are not highly explanatory for some causes of morbidity (e.g., arthritis, mental health).

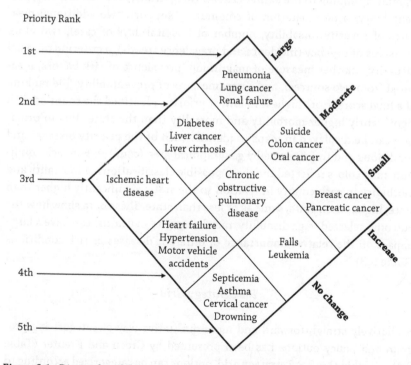

Figure 9.1: Diamond model for major causes of death, Taiwan, 1991–2008.
Source: Adapted from Lu et al.[48]

The Hanlon Method

An approach to prioritization, largely based on quantitative methods, was proposed by Hanlon and Pickett[34] and further elaborated by Vilnius and Dandoy[41] and Simoes and colleagues (in the United States and in Europe).[37,49] The model, the Basic Priority Rating (BPR), is based on the following formula:

$$BPR = [(A + B) \bullet C] / 3 \times D,$$

where A is the size of the problem, B the seriousness of the problem, C the effectiveness of the intervention, and D the propriety, economics, acceptability, resources, and legality (known as PEARL). Values for each part of the formula are converted from rates and ratings to scores. Finer details of these quantitative rating systems are available in the original publications.[34, 37, 41]

As an illustration, the Missouri Department of Health and Senior Services applied a prioritization method using surveillance-derived data (the Priority MICA).[37] The Priority MICA extends the work of Vilnius and Dandoy by adding to the earlier criteria (magnitude, severity, urgency, preventability) a new criterion of community support, two additional measures of severity (disability, number of hospital days of care), two more measures of urgency (incidence and prevalence trends), a criterion of racial disparity, another measure of magnitude (prevalence of risk factors, measured from two sources), and a new measure of preventability. The ranking of a final score, from highest to lowest priority, identified the counties with significantly higher morbidity and mortality than the state. This information can be displayed in maps to identify each of the priority diseases and conditions and to prioritize by geographical area (county). For each condition, map colors reflected the three possible classifications of mortality and morbidity in each county in relation to the state: significantly higher than state, higher than state, same as or less than state. These data show how the outcome selected (e.g., disability, racial disparity in deaths) can have a large impact on the relative importance of different diseases or risk conditions (Table 9.3).[50]

The Strategy Grid

A relatively straightforward and more qualitative way of categorizing program and policy options has been presented by Green and Kreuter (Table 9.4).[51] Within this 2 × 2 strategy grid, options can be categorized according to their importance and changeability. Importance might be based on burden of disease, injury, impairment, or exposure. Changeability is synonymous with

Table 9.3. RANKING OF DISEASES ON THE BASIS OF DIFFERENT CRITERIA, MISSOURI, 2016

Ranking	All Measures	Specific Criteria		
		Deaths for People Younger Than 65 Years	Disability burden	Racial Disparity for Deaths
1	Diabetes	Heart disease	Affective disorder	Sickle cell anemia
2	Heart disease	Lung cancer	Alzheimer's disease, dementia, senility	Assaults, homicides
3	Alcohol- and substance-related diseases	Alcohol- and substance-related diseases	Arthritis, lupus	HIV/AIDS
4	Arthritis, lupus	Motor vehicle injuries	Alcohol- and substance-related diseases	Burns (fire and flames)
5	COPD*	Suicides, self-inflicted injuries	COPD	Syphilis
6	Pregnancy complications	Infant health problems	Diabetes	Salmonella
7	Infant health problems	COPD	Stroke, other cerebrovascular disease	Pregnancy complications
8	Assaults, homicides	Stroke, other cerebrovascular disease	Asthma, anxiety-related mental disorder	Tuberculosis
9	Motor vehicle injuries	Diabetes	Schizophrenia and psychosis	Asthma
10	Sickle cell anemia	Assaults, homicides	Heart disease	Abuse, neglect

COPD = chronic obstructive pulmonary disease.
Missouri Department of Health and Senior Services.[50]

preventability. Within this framework, options in the upper left and lower right cells are relatively easy to prioritize. Those in the lower left and upper right are more difficult to assess. A highly important issue but one about which little is known from a preventive standpoint should be the focus of innovation in program development. A strong focus on evaluation should be maintained in this category so that new programs can be assessed for effectiveness. A program or policy in the upper right corner might be initiated for political, social, or cultural reasons. The Strategy Grid method can be varied by changing the labels for the X and Y axes; for example, need and feasibility might be substituted for importance and changeability.[52]

Table 9.4. CONSIDERATIONS IN SETTING PROGRAM PRIORITIES

	More Important	Less Important
More changeable	Highest priority for program focus *Example:* Program to improve vaccination coverage in children, adolescents, and adults	Low priority except to demonstrate change for political or other purpose *Example:* Program to prevent work-related pneumoconiosis
Less changeable	Priority for innovative program with evaluation essential *Example:* Program to prevent mental impairment and disability	No intervention program *Example:* Program to prevent Hodgkin's disease

Source: Adapted from Green and Kreuter.[51]

The Delphi Method

The Delphi method was developed by the Rand Corporation in the 1950s. It is named after the oracle of Delphi from Ancient Greece, who could offer advice on the right course of action in many situations.[53] It is a judgment tool for prediction and forecast, involving a panel of anonymous experts to whom intensive questionnaires and feedback were given in order to obtain consensus on a particular topic.[54,55] Although the method has been modified and used in various ways over the years, it remains a useful way to solicit and refine expert opinion. The Delphi method is most appropriate for broad, long-range issues such as strategic planning and environmental assessments. It is not feasible for routine decisions. It can be especially useful for a geographically dispersed group of experts. There are three types of Delphi: classical, policy, and decision.[56] The decision Delphi is most relevant here because it provides a forum for decisions. Panel members are not anonymous (although responses are), and the goal is a defined and supported outcome. Another important characteristic of the Delphi method is that it is iterative and responses are refined over rounds of sampling.

The first step in a Delphi process involves the selection of an expert panel. This panel should generally include a range of experts across the public health field, including practitioners, researchers, and funders. A panel of 30 or fewer members is often used.[57] The Delphi method may involve a series of questionnaires (by mail or email) that begin more generally and, through iteration, become more specific over several weeks or months. Open-ended questions may be used in early drafts, with multiple-choice responses in later versions. A flow chart for a typical Delphi process is shown in Figure 9.2.[58]

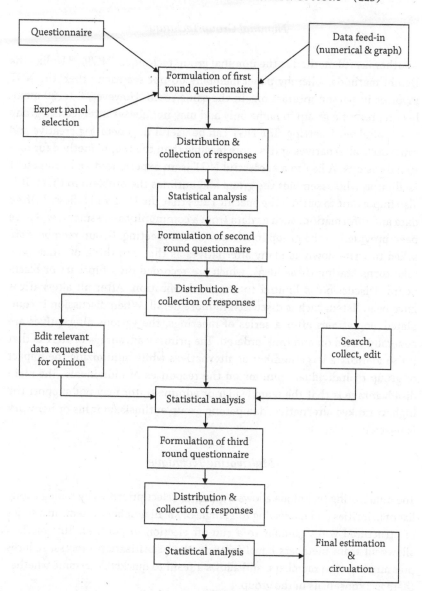

Figure 9.2: Flow chart of the Delphi methods.
Source: Krueger and Casey.[58]

Definitions of consensus within a Delphi method vary—from full consensus to majority rule—and should be specified at the outset. The critical elements of a successful Delphi process include identifying an appropriate panel of experts, designing a useful set of questions, and summarizing individual input.[58]

Nominal Group Technique

Another useful method is the nominal group technique (NGT).[59] Unlike the Delphi methods, whereby panel members do not see each other, the NGT involves in-person interactions in the same room. However, 6 to 10 members represent a group in name only and may not always interact as a group in a typical work setting. The NGT can be useful in generating creative and innovative alternatives and is more feasible than the Delphi method for routine decisions. A key to a successful NGT is an experienced and competent facilitator, who assembles the group and outlines the problem to them. It is also important to outline the specific rules that the NGT will follow.[57] Often data and information, such as data from a community assessment, will have been provided to the group in advance of the meeting. Group members are asked to write down as many alternatives as they can think of. They then take turns stating these ideas, which are recorded on a flipchart or blackboard. Discussion is limited to simple clarification. After all alternatives have been listed, each is discussed in more detail. When discussion is completed, sometimes after a series of meetings, the various alternatives are generally voted on and rank-ordered. The primary advantage of NGT is that it can identify a large number of alternatives while minimizing the impact of group or individual opinions on the responses of individuals. The main disadvantage is that the team leader or administrator may not support the highest ranked alternative, dampening group enthusiasm if his or her work is rejected.

Multivoting Technique

The multivoting technique allows a group to select priorities by taking a long list of priorities and narrowing to a single or small number of items in a series of structured votes (similar to a run-off election in politics). This method allows all team members equal input in the prioritization process, reduces pressure between members, and allows a team to quickly determine whether there is a consensus in the group.

The multivoting technique begins with brainstorming or a review of the literature to develop a list of health problems for prioritization. The list is reviewed among the group to be sure each person understands the options and to merge any similar ideas. The round 1 voting allows each participant to vote for as many ideas as he or she wishes. In some cases, depending on the number of items on the list, a maximum number of votes per person can be established. The list is next updated based on the top vote-getters. Issues with a vote count equivalent to about half the number of participants remain on the list. Next, a second round of voting occurs. In this round, participants can only vote a number of times equivalent to half the number of items on the list. The group continues voting and narrowing down the list until the desired number of priorities are determined. Often this is a range of three to five items. The group can then discuss the pros and cons of remaining items, either in small groups or among the group as a whole.

Other Considerations and Caveats

Regardless of the method used, the first major stage in setting community priorities is to decide on the criteria. The framework might include one of those described previously or may be a composite of various approaches. After criteria are determined, the next steps include forming a working team or advisory group, assembling the necessary data to conduct the prioritization process, establishing a process for stakeholder input and review, and determining a process for revisiting priorities at regular intervals. Vilnius and Dandoy recommend that a six- to eight-member group be assembled to guide the BPR process.[41] This group should include members within and outside the agency. A generic priority-setting worksheet is provided in Table 9.5.[40] This worksheet provides some guidance on the types of information that would typically need to be collected and summarized before a work group begins its activity.

In setting priorities within public health, it important to consider several issues related to leadership and measurement. No determination of public health priorities should be reduced solely to numbers; values, social justice, and the political climate all play roles. Changes in public health leadership present a unique challenge. The median tenure for a US state public health officer is only 1.8 years,[60] whereas for city and county health officers the median tenure is longer (about 6 years).[61] Because each new leader is likely to bring new ideas, this turnover in leadership often results in a lack of long-term focus on public health priorities that require years or decades to accomplish. Each analytic method for prioritization has particular strengths and weaknesses. Some methods rely heavily on quantitative data, but valid and usable data can be difficult to come by, especially for smaller geographic areas such as cities or neighborhoods. It can also be difficult to identify the proper metrics for comparison of various health conditions. For example, using mortality alone would ignore the disabling burden of arthritis when it is compared with other chronic diseases. Utility-based measures (e.g., QALYs) are advantageous because they are comparable across diseases and risk factors. Rankings, especially close ranks, should be assessed with caution. One useful approach is to divide a distribution of health issues into quartiles or quintiles and compare the extremes of a distribution. In addition, some key stakeholders may find that quantitative methods of prioritization fail to present a full picture, suggesting the need to use methods that combine quantitative and qualitative approaches.

Table 9.5. GENERIC WORKSHEET FOR PRIORITY SETTING

To Use	Sample Criteria (tailor to ensure criteria can be applied to all health issues being weighed)	Measure (cite-specific measure and data source if available)	Score (score data, assign points, or rank using identified method)	Weight[a] (assign value to criteria if desired)	Weighted Score (score multiplied by weight)	Priority Score (sum of weighted scores for each criterion used)
✓	Prevalence					
	Mortality rate					
	Community concern					
	Lost productivity (e.g., bed-disability days)					
	Premature mortality (e.g., years of potential life lost)					
	Medical costs to treat (or community economic costs)					
	Feasibility to prevent					
	Other:					

[a]A weight ensures that certain characteristics have a greater influence than others have in the final priority ranking. A sample formula might be: 2(Prevalence Score) + Community Concern Score + 3(Medical Cost Score) = Priority Score. In this example, the weight for prevalence is 2 and medical cost is 3. Users might enter data or assign scores (such as 1–5) for each criterion and use the formula to calculate a total score for the health event.

Source: Healthy People 2010 Toolkit.[40]

INNOVATION AND CREATIVITY IN PROGRAM
AND POLICY DEVELOPMENT

Another factor to consider in intervention development is innovation. Innovation has been defined as "a new method, idea, or product."[62] In many instances, there is a trade-off between the level to which a program is evidence based, through the scientific literature, and the degree to which it is innovative. Consider, for example, the evidence from a review of programs that promote seat belt use to prevent motor vehicle injuries. From these, there is strong evidence that enforcement programs are effective in promoting seat belt use and, hence, reducing motor vehicle injuries.[63] If you were planning to set up a program, would you follow what has already been done or try a new (and perhaps more innovative) approach? In practice, although it is crucial to search for programs that have worked in other places, there are several benefits to developing new program approaches. First, there is no guarantee that a program proven to work in one population or geographic area will yield the same results in another locality (see discussion of external validity in chapter 3). Second, because the evidence base in many areas of public health intervention is relatively weak, a continual discovery of new and innovative approaches is crucial. And third, the development of innovative programs can be motivating for the people carrying out programs and the community members with whom they work.

Creativity in Developing Priorities

Creativity and its role in effective decision making are not fully understood. Creativity is the process of developing original, imaginative, and innovative options. To understand the role of creativity in decision making, it is helpful to know about its nature and process and the techniques for nurturing it.

Researchers have sought to understand the characteristics of creative people. Above a threshold in the intelligence quotient, there does not appear to be a strong correlation between creativity and intelligence.[64] There also seem to be few differences in creativity between men and women.[65] Several other characteristics have been consistently associated with creativity. The typical period in the life cycle of greatest creativity appears to be between the ages of 30 and 40 years. It also seems that more creative people are less susceptible to social influences than those who are less creative.

The creative process has been described in four stages: preparation, incubation, insight, and verification.[66] The preparation phase is highly dependent on the education and training of the individual embarking on the creative process. Incubation usually involves a period of relaxation after a period of preparation. The human mind gathers and sorts data, and then needs time for ideas to jell. In the incubation period, it is often useful to direct energies toward some other pursuits before returning to the task at hand. In the insight phase, one gradually or rapidly becomes aware of a new idea or approach. And finally, in the verification phase, the individual verifies the appropriateness of the idea or solution. In the business setting, this would include consumer surveys or focus groups to test the acceptance of a new product.

Within an organizational setting, a number of processes can enhance creativity in decision making. It is important to identify ways to create a trusting work environment, to reward creativity within an organization, and to encourage the appropriate level of risk-taking among employees, ensuring that individual freedom and autonomy are not unduly constrained. The risks of creativity were summarized by a manager[67]:

> With creativity comes uncertainty. Whenever you have uncertainty people feel uncomfortable and insecure. If [a creative decision] is not successful, the negative things that can happen to you are ten times greater than the positive things. (pp. 723–724)

DEVELOPING AND USING ANALYTIC FRAMEWORKS

Analytic frameworks (also called *logic models* or *causal frameworks*) have benefited numerous areas of public health practice, particularly in developing and implementing clinical and community-based guidelines.[68-70] An analytic framework is a diagram that depicts the interrelationships between program resources, intervention activities, outputs, shorter term intervention outcomes, and longer term public health outcomes. The major purpose of an analytic framework is to map out the linkages on which to base conclusions about intervention effectiveness. An underlying assumption is that various linkages represent "causal pathways," some of which are mutable and can be intervened on. Numerous types of analytic frameworks are described in Battista and Fletcher.[71] Logic models and their role in action planning are discussed in chapter 10.

People designing public health interventions often have in mind an analytic framework that leads from program inputs to health outputs if the program works as intended. It is important for planning and evaluation purposes that what Lipsey has termed this "small theory" of the intervention be made explicit early, often in the form of a diagram.[72] In attempting to map inputs, mediators, and outputs, it important to determine whether mediators, or constructs, lie "upstream" or "downstream" from a particular intervention. As an analytic framework develops, the diagram also identifies key outcomes to be considered when formulating a data collection plan is formulated. These are then translated into public health indicators (i.e., measures of the extent to

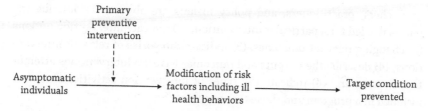

Figure 9.3: Generic analytic framework showing effects of primary prevention. *Source:* Battista & Fletcher.[71]

which targets in health programs are being reached). Besides helping to identify key information to be collected, an analytic framework can also be viewed as a set of hypotheses about program action, including the time sequence in which program-related changes should occur; these can later guide data analysis. If the program is subsequently successful in influencing outcomes at the end of this causal chain, having measures of the intermediate steps available aids interpretation by clarifying how those effects came about. Conversely, if little change in ultimate outcomes is observed, having measures of intermediate steps can help to diagnose where the causal chain was broken.

Analytic frameworks can be relatively simple or complicated, with every possible relationship between risk factors, interventions, and health outcomes. A generic analytic framework is shown in Figure 9.3.[71] A more comprehensive approach may describe potential relationships between sociopolitical context, social position, the health care system, and long-term health outcomes, as described in Figure 9.4.[73] By developing this and related diagrams,

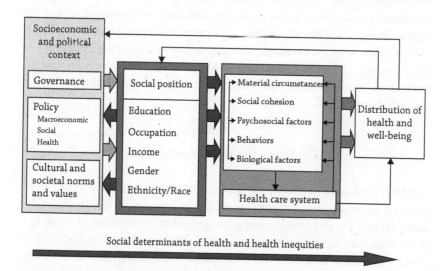

Figure 9.4: Analytic framework depicting the social determinants of health equity. *Source:* World Health Organization.[73]

researchers, practitioners, and policy makers are able to (1) describe the inputs needed for a particular intervention; (2) indicate intervention options for changing relevant outcomes; (3) indicate categories of relevant interventions; (4) describe the outputs and outcomes that the interventions attempt to influence; and (4) indicate the types of intervention activities that were included in a program and those that were not.[74, 75]

Constructing Analytic Frameworks

Several approaches and sources of information are beneficial as one begins to construct an analytic framework that will map intervention options related to a particular health issue. First, a comprehensive search of the scientific literature is essential. The methods outlined in chapter 8 form the basis for such a search. After this search, it is likely that the practitioner will find articles that show analytic frameworks, although these are likely to vary in completeness and sophistication. Another important part of developing a framework is the identification of mutable and immutable factors along the causal pathway. A mutable factor might relate to "exposure" to a mass media campaign on a particular health issue. Conversely, an immutable factor would be a person's gender.

It is helpful to construct analytic frameworks in a professional working group. The advantages to a group process are twofold: (1) after the literature is assembled, several members of the group can independently draft initial analytic frameworks on the same topic; and (2) when initial frameworks are available, review by a small group is likely to improve the modeling. It is important to note that the construction of an analytic framework should not be viewed as a static process. As more literature and the intervention process proceeds, the framework should be modified to fit advancing knowledge of determinants. If a work group finds it too difficult to construct an analytic framework, it may indicate that the program is too complex or that its basis is not well documented.

Considering the Broad Environment

One key component in developing analytic frameworks and subsequent interventions is consideration of the "upstream" causes of poor health status.[76,77] These factors are increasingly being recognized in the context of social epidemiology, that is, the socioenvironmental determinants of health, such as poverty and social isolation.[78] As shown in Table 9.6, the larger environment, including physical, social, legal, and cultural factors, needs to be fully considered as an intervention target.[79] Focus on environmental and policy factors

Table 9.6. CONTRASTING APPROACHES TO DISEASE PREVENTION

Health Area	Individual	Environmental and Policy[a]
Smoking	Smoking cessation classes	Cigarette taxation
	Hypnosis	Clean indoor air laws
	Nicotine patch	Regulation of cigarette advertising
Stress	Stress reduction classes	Reduced work demands
		Affordable child care
		Crime prevention programs
Diet and weight loss	Exercise programs	Public transportation
	Cooking classes	Affordable housing near workplace
	How-to-read food labels	Urban public recreation areas
		Food security programs
		Funding for farmers' markets

[a]Includes the physical, legal, social, and cultural environments.
Source: Adapted from Yen and Syme.[79]

is increasingly being recognized as an efficient and effective means for public health interventions.[79–81]

Even though the ultimate goal is individual behavior change, environmental programs can be designed at several different levels. Social support may be built for behavior change within a worksite, and community-wide policies may be enacted to support the same health-promoting behavior. These so-called ecological interventions are discussed in more detail in chapters 5 and 10.

SUMMARY

The public health practitioner has many tools at her or his fingertips for identifying and prioritizing program and policy options. This chapter has summarized several approaches that have proved useful for public health practitioners. As one proceeds through this process, several key points should be kept in mind.

KEY CHAPTER POINTS

- The public health practitioner has many tools at her or his fingertips for identifying and prioritizing program and policy options.
- In public health decision making, there is often not one "correct" answer.
- Although decisions are made in the context of uncertainty and risk, classical decision theory suggests that when managers have complete information, they behave rationally.

- Group decision making has advantages and disadvantages, but in most instances, the former outweigh the latter.
- Priorities should not be set on quantitative factors alone.
- It is often useful to apply a prioritization process on a smaller scale initially when stakes are lower.
- Analytic frameworks can enhance decision making, reviews of evidence, program planning, and program evaluation.

SUGGESTED READINGS AND SELECTED WEBSITES

Suggested Readings

Krueger RA, Casey MA. *Focus Groups: A Practical Guide for Applied Research.* 4th ed. Thousand Oaks, CA: Sage Publications, 2009.

Leider JP, Resnick B, Kass N, et al. Budget- and priority-setting criteria at state health agencies in times of austerity: a mixed-methods study. *Am J Public Health.* Jun 2014;104(6):1092–1099.

Maciosek MV, Coffield AB, Flottemesch TJ, Edwards NM, Solberg LI. Greater use of preventive services in U.S. health care could save lives at little or no cost. *Health Aff (Millwood).* Sep 2010;29(9):1656–1660.

Simoes EJ, Land G, Metzger R, Mokdad A. Prioritization MICA: a Web-based application to prioritize public health resources. *J Public Health Manag Pract.* Mar-Apr 2006;12(2):161–169.

Vilnius D, Dandoy S. A priority rating system for public health programs. *Public Health Reports* 1990;105(5):463–470.

Selected Websites

Centers for Disease Control and Prevention (CDC) Program Performance and Evaluation Office (PPEO) <http://www.cdc.gov/eval/resources/index.htm>. The CDC PPEO has developed a comprehensive list of evaluation documents, tools, and links to other websites. These materials include documents that describe principles and standards, organizations and foundations that support evaluation, a list of journals and online publications, and access to step-by-step manuals.

County Health Rankings and Roadmaps Action Center <http://www.countyhealthrankings.org/roadmaps/action-center/choose-effective-policies-programs>. The County Health Rankings and Roadmaps Action Center provides guidance on selecting evidence-informed policies and programs that target priority health issues. The Action Center also provides additional learning and resources relevant to selecting a program or policy for a community.

Disease Control Priorities Project (DCCP) <http://www.dcp2.org>. The DCPP is an ongoing effort to assess disease control priorities and produce evidence-based analysis and resource materials to inform health policymaking in developing countries. DCPP has produced eight volumes providing technical resources that can assist developing countries in improving their health systems and, ultimately, the health of their people.

Guide to Community Preventive Services (the *Community Guide*) <http://www.thecommunityguide.org/index.html>. The *Community Guide* provides guidance in choosing evidence-based programs and policies to improve health and prevent disease at the community level. The Task Force on Community Preventive Services—an independent, nonfederal, volunteer body of public health and prevention experts appointed by the Director of the CDC—has systematically reviewed more than 200 interventions to produce the recommendations and findings available at this site. The topics covered in the *Community Guide* currently include adolescent health, alcohol-excessive consumption, asthma, birth defects, cancer, cardiovascular disease, diabetes, emergency preparedness, health communication, health equity, HIV/AIDS, STIs and pregnancy, mental health, motor vehicle injury, nutrition, obesity, oral health, physical activity, social environment, tobacco, vaccination, violence, and worksite.

Healthy People <http://www.healthypeople.gov/>. Healthy People provides science-based, 10-year national objectives for promoting health and preventing disease in the United States. Since 1979, Healthy People has set and monitored national health objectives to meet a broad range of health needs, encourage collaborations across sectors, guide individuals toward making informed health decisions, and measure the impact of prevention activity.

Sustainable Development Goals (SDGs) <http://www.un.org/sustainabledevelopment/>. This site provides insight and resources on the SDGs developed by world leaders at a historic United Nations Summit in 2015. These 17 goals build on the success of the Millennium Development Goals and aim to transform our world through goals such as eliminating poverty.

Role of a Facilitator: Guiding an Event Through to a Successful Conclusion <https://www.mindtools.com/pages/article/RoleofAFacilitator.htm>. This site provides tips and resources on how to facilitate a successful and productive meeting.

Partners in Information Access for the Public Health Workforce <http://phpartners.org/>. Partners in Information Access for the Public Health Workforce is a collaboration of US government agencies, public health organizations, and health sciences libraries that provides timely, convenient access to selected public health resources on the Internet.

REFERENCES

1. Haire-Joshu D, McBride T, eds. *Transdisciplinary Public Health: Research, Education, and Practice*. San Francisco, CA: Jossey-Bass Publishers; 2013.
2. Maciosek MV, Coffield AB, Flottemesch TJ, Edwards NM, Solberg LI. Greater use of preventive services in U.S. health care could save lives at little or no cost. *Health Aff (Millwood)*. Sep 2010;29(9):1656–1660.
3. Maciosek MV, Coffield AB, Edwards NM, Flottemesch TJ, Solberg LI. Prioritizing clinical preventive services: a review and framework with implications for community preventive services. *Annu Rev Public Health*. Apr 29 2009;30:341–355.
4. Leider JP, Resnick B, Kass N. Tradeoffs in resource allocation at state health agencies. *J Public Health Manag Pract*. Nov-Dec 2014;20(6):566–579.
5. Leider JP, Resnick B, Kass N, et al. Budget- and priority-setting criteria at state health agencies in times of austerity: a mixed-methods study. *Am J Public Health*. Jun 2014;104(6):1092–1099.
6. Farrelly MC, Pechacek TF, Thomas KY, Nelson D. The impact of tobacco control programs on adult smoking. *Am J Public Health*. Feb 2008;98(2):304–309.
7. Brownson RC, Baker EA, Leet TL, Gillespie KN, True WR. *Evidence-Based Public Health*. 2nd ed. New York, NY: Oxford University Press; 2011.

8. Green LW. Health education's contribution to public health in the twentieth century: a glimpse through health promotion's rear-view mirror. *Annual Review of Public Health*. 1999;20:67–88.

9. World Health Organization. The Sustainable Development Goals 2015–2030. http://una-gp.org/the-sustainable-development-goals-2015-2030/.   Accessed October 8, 2016.

10. Simon HA. *Administrative Behavior: A Study of Decision-Making Processes in Administrative Organizations*. 4th ed. New York, NY: Free Press; 1997.

11. Gheaus A. Solidarity, justice and unconditional access to healthcare. *J Med Ethics*. Jun 28 2016.

12. Sogoric S, Dzakula A, Rukavina TV, et al. Evaluation of Croatian model of polycentric health planning and decision making. *Health Policy*. Mar 2009;89(3):271–278.

13. Eddy DM. Oregon's methods. Did cost-effectiveness analysis fail? *JAMA*. 1991;266(3):417–420.

14. Klevit HD, Bates AC, Castanares T, Kirk PE, Sipes-Metzler PR, Wopat R. Prioritization of health care services: a progress report by the Oregon health services commission. *Archives of Internal Medicine*. 1991;151:912–916.

15. Oregon Health Authority. Health Evidence Review Commission: Prioritization Methodology.   http://www.oregon.gov/oha/herc/Pages/Prioritization-Methodology.aspx. Accessed July 15, 2016.

16. Swinburn B, Egger G, Raza F. Dissecting obesogenic environments: the development and application of a framework for identifying and prioritizing environmental interventions for obesity. *Preventive Medicine*. 1999;29(6 Pt 1):563–570.

17. Simmons A, Mavoa HM, Bell AC, et al. Creating community action plans for obesity prevention using the ANGELO (Analysis Grid for Elements Linked to Obesity) Framework. *Health Promot Int*. Dec 2009;24(4):311–324.

18. Braun KL, Nigg CR, Fialkowski MK, et al. Using the ANGELO model to develop the children's healthy living program multilevel intervention to promote obesity preventing behaviors for young children in the U.S.-affiliated Pacific Region. *Child Obes*. Dec 2014;10(6):474–481.

19. Cauchi D, Rutter H, Knai C. An obesogenic island in the Mediterranean: mapping potential drivers of obesity in Malta. *Public Health Nutr*. Dec 2015;18(17):3211–3223.

20. Canadian Task Force on the Periodic Health Examination. The periodic health examination. Canadian Task Force on the Periodic Health Examination. *Can Med Assoc J*. Nov 3 1979;121(9):1193–1254.

21. US Preventive Services Task Force. *Guide to Clinical Preventive Services: An Assessment of the Effectiveness of 169 Interventions*. Baltimore: Williams & Wilkins; 1989.

22. Coffield AB, Maciosek MV, McGinnis JM, et al. Priorities among recommended clinical preventive services (1). *Am J Prev Med*. 2001;21(1):1–9.

23. Maciosek MV, Coffield AB, Edwards NM, Flottemesch TJ, Goodman MJ, Solberg LI. Priorities among effective clinical preventive services: results of a systematic review and analysis. *Am J Prev Med*. Jul 2006;31(1):52–61.

24. Partnership for Prevention. Rankings of Preventive Services for the US Population. https://www.prevent.org/National-Commission-on-Prevention-Priorities/Rankings-of-Preventive-Services-for-the-US-Population.aspx.   Accessed   July 15, 2016.

25. Maciosek MV, Coffield AB, McGinnis JM, et al. Methods for priority setting among clinical preventive services. *Am J Prev Med*. 2001;21(1):10–19.

26. Patrick DL, Wickizer TM. Community and health. In: Amick BCI, Levine S, Tarlov AR, Chapman Walsh D, eds. *Society and Health*. New York, NY: Oxford University Press; 1995:46–92.

27. Hahn RA, Teutsch SM, Rothenberg RB, Marks JS. Excess deaths from nine chronic diseases in the United States, 1986. *JAMA*. 1990;264(20):2654–2659.

28. Carvette ME, Hayes EB, Schwartz RH, Bogdan GF, Bartlett NW, Graham LB. Chronic disease mortality in Maine: assessing the targets for prevention. *J Public Health Manag Pract*. 1996;2(3):25–31.

29. Hoffarth S, Brownson RC, Gibson BB, Sharp DJ, Schramm W, Kivlaham C. Preventable mortality in Missouri: excess deaths from nine chronic diseases, 1979-1991. *Mo Med*. 1993;90(6):279–282.

30. Kindig D, Peppard P, Booske B. How healthy could a state be? *Public Health Rep*. Mar-Apr 2010;125(2):160–167.

31. Fukuda Y, Nakamura K, Takano T. Increased excess deaths in urban areas: quantification of geographical variation in mortality in Japan, 1973-1998. *Health Policy*. May 2004;68(2):233–244.

32. Regidor E, Inigo J, Sendra JM, Gutierrez-Fisac JL. [Evolution of mortality from principal chronic diseases in Spain 1975-1988]. *Med Clin (Barc)*. Dec 5 1992;99(19):725–728.

33. Garcia M, Bastian B, Rossen L, et al. Potentially Preventable Deaths Among the Five Leading Causes of Death—United States, 2010 and 2014. *MMWR*. 2016;65(45):1245–1255.

34. Hanlon J, Pickett G. *Public Health Administration and Practice*. Santa Clara, CA: Times Mirror/Mosby College Publishing; 1982.

35. Meltzer M, Teutsch SM. Setting priorities for health needs and managing resources. In: Stroup DF, Teutsch SM, eds. *Statistics in Public Health. Quantitative Approaches to Public Health Problems*. New York, NY: Oxford University Press; 1998:123–149.

36. Murray CJ, Frenk J. Health metrics and evaluation: strengthening the science. *Lancet*. Apr 5 2008;371(9619):1191–1199.

37. Simoes EJ, Land G, Metzger R, Mokdad A. Prioritization MICA: a Web-based application to prioritize public health resources. *J Public Health Manag Pract*. Mar-Apr 2006;12(2):161–169.

38. Simons-Morton BG, Greene WH, Gottlieb NH. *Introduction to Health Education and Health Promotion*. 2nd ed. Prospect Heights, IL: Waveland Press; 1995.

39. Sogoric S, Rukavina TV, Brborovic O, Vlahugic A, Zganec N, Oreskovic S. Counties selecting public health priorities—a "bottom-up" approach (Croatian experience). *Coll Antropol*. Jun 2005;29(1):111–119.

40. US Department of Health and Human Services. *Healthy People 2010 Toolkit*. Washington, DC: US Department of Health and Human Services; 2001.

41. Vilnius D, Dandoy S. A priority rating system for public health programs. *Public Health Reports*. 1990;105(5):463–470.

42. Griffin RW. *Management*. 7th ed. Boston, MA: Houghton Mifflin Company; 2001.

43. Von Bergen CW, Kirk R. Groupthink. When too many heads spoil the decision. *Management Review*. 1978;67(3):44–49.

44. Golembiewski R. *Handbook of Organizational Consultation*. 2nd ed. New York, NY: Marcel Dekker, Inc.; 2000.

45. Janis IL. *Groupthink*. Boston, MA: Houghton Mifflin; 1982.

46. Sunstein C, Hastie R. *Wiser: Getting Beyond Groupthink to Make Groups Smarter*. Boston, MA: Harvard Business Review Press; 2015.

47. Ramanadhan S, Viswanath K. Priority-setting for evidence-based health outreach in community-based organizations: A mixed-methods study in three Massachusetts communities. *Transl Behav Med.* Jun 1 2013;3(2):180–188.

48. Lu TH, Huang YT, Chiang TL. Using the diamond model to prioritize 30 causes of death by considering both the level of and inequality in mortality. *Health Policy.* Nov 2011;103(1):63–72.

49. Simoes EJ, Mariotti S, Rossi A, et al. The Italian health surveillance (SiVeAS) prioritization approach to reduce chronic disease risk factors. *Int J Public Health.* Aug 2012;57(4):719–733.

50. Missouri Department of Health and Senior Services. Priorities MICA. http://health.mo.gov/data/mica/PriorityMICA/index.html. Accessed October 28, 2016.

51. Green LW, Kreuter MW. Commentary on the emerging *Guide to Community Preventive Services* from a health promotion perspective. *American Journal of Preventive Medicine.* 2000;18(1S):7–9.

52. National Association of County and City Health Officials. First Things First: Prioritizing Health Problems. http://archived.naccho.org/topics/infrastructure/accreditation/upload/Prioritization-Summaries-and-Examples.pdf. Accessed July 23, 2016.

53. Last JM. *A Dictionary of Public Health.* New York, NY: Oxford University Press; 2007.

54. Crisp J, Pelletier D, Duffield C, Adams A, Nagy S. The Delphi Method? *Nursing Research.* 1997;46(2):116–118.

55. Dalkey N, Helmer O. An experimental application of the Delphi method to the use of experts. *Management Science.* 1963;9:458–467.

56. Rauch W. The decision Delphi. *Technological Forecasting and Social Change.* 1979;15:159–169.

57. Witkin BR, Altschuld JW. *Conducting and Planning Needs Assessments. A Practical Guide.* Thousand Oaks, CA: Sage Publications; 1995.

58. Krueger RA, Casey MA. *Focus Groups: A Practical Guide for Applied Research.* 4th ed. Thousand Oaks, CA: Sage Publications; 2009.

59. Delbecq AL, Van de Ven AH. *Group Techniques for Program Planning.* Glenview, IL: Scott, Foresman; 1975.

60. Association of State and Territorial Health Officials. *ASTHO Profile of State Public Health, Volume Three.* Arlington, VA: Association of State and Territorial Health Officials; 2014.

61. Turnock BJ. *Public Health: What it is and How it Works.* 6th ed. Sudbury, MA: Jones and Bartlett Publishers; 2016.

62. Stevenson A, Lindberg C, eds. *The New Oxford American Dictionary.* 3rd ed. New York, NY: Oxford University Press; 2010.

63. Centers for Disease Control and Prevention. Motor-vehicle occupant injury: Strategies for increasing use of child safety seats, increasing use of safety belts, and reducing alcohol-impaired driving. A report of the Task Force on Community Preventive Services. *MMWR.* 2001;50(RR-7):1–16.

64. Cicirelli V. Form of the relationship between creativity, IQ, and academic achievement. *J Educ Psych.* 1965;56(6):303–308.

65. Anastasi A, Schaefer CE. Note on the concepts of creativity and intelligence. *Journal of Creative Behavior.* 1971;5(2):113–116.

66. Busse TV, Mansfield RS. Theories of the creative process: a review and a perspective. *Journal of Creative Behavior.* 1980;4(2):91–103.

67. Ford C, Gioia D. Factors influencing creativity in the domain of managerial decision making. *J Manag.* 2000;26(4):705–732.

68. Woolf SH, DiGuiseppi CG, Atkins D, Kamerow DB. Developing evidence-based clinical practice guidelines: lessons learned by the US Preventive Services Task Force. *Annual Review of Public Health.* 1996;17:511–538.

69. McLaughlin JJ, GB. Logic models: A tool for telling your program's performance story. *Eval Program Planning.* 1999;22:65–72.

70. Task Force on Community Preventive Services. Guide to Community Preventive Services. www.thecommunityguide.org. Accessed June 5, 2016.

71. Battista RN, Fletcher SW. Making recommendations on preventive practices: methodological issues. *American Journal of Preventive Medicine.* 1988;4 Suppl:53–67.

72. Lipsey M. Theory as method: small theories of treatments. *New Directions for Evaluation.* 2007;114:30–62.

73. WHO. *Closing the gap in a generation: health equity through action on the social determinants of health. Final Report of the Commission on Social Determinants of Heal\th.* Geneva: WHO; 2008.

74. Briss PA, Brownson RC, Fielding JE, Zaza S. Developing and using the *Guide to Community Preventive Services:* lessons learned About evidence-based public health. *Annu Rev Public Health.* Jan 2004;25:281–302.

75. Briss PA, Zaza S, Pappaioanou M, et al. Developing an evidence-based *Guide to Community Preventive Services:* Methods. The Task Force on Community Preventive Services. *Am J Prev Med.* 2000;18(1 Suppl):35–43.

76. McKinlay JB. Paradigmatic obstacles to improving the health of populations— implications for health policy. *Salud Publica Mex.* Jul-Aug 1998;40(4):369–379.

77. McKinlay JB, Marceau LD. Upstream healthy public policy: lessons from the battle of tobacco. *Int J Health Serv.* 2000;30(1):49–69.

78. Berkman LF. Social epidemiology: social determinants of health in the United States: are we losing ground? *Annu Rev Public Health.* Apr 29 2009;30:27–41.

79. Yen IH, Syme SL. The social environment and health: a discussion of the epidemiologic literature. *Annual Review of Public Health.* 1999;20:287–308.

80. McKinlay JB. The promotion of health through planned sociopolitical change: Challenges for research and policy. *Social Science and Medicine.* 1993;36(2):109–117.

81. McKinlay JB, Marceau LD. To boldly go. *Am J Public Health.* 2000;90(1):25–33.

CHAPTER 10

✧

Developing an Action Plan and Implementing Interventions

Even if you're on the right track, you'll get run over if you just sit there.
Will Rogers

After a particular intervention—a program or policy—has been identified, sound planning techniques can ensure that the program is implemented effectively. It can be argued that planning is the most fundamental and most important administrative function.[1] Developing and implementing effective programs and policies requires sound management skills. Public health management is the process of constructing, implementing, and evaluating organized responses to a health problem or a series of interrelated health problems.[2] One of the goals of an evidence-based process is to make rational and well-grounded decisions—a key management function. Important decisions always carry some element of risk. Sound management and planning are iterative, generally do not lead to a single option, and do not eliminate the risk for making poor judgments.[2] In addition, complex public health problems are rarely resolved by implementing a single program or policy. Rather, change often requires a set of actions. The goal of action planning is, therefore, to maximize the chances of efficient use of resources and effective delivery of specific programs and policies that are part of an overall strategic plan. Previous chapters provide data to help guide the managerial decisions regarding *which* programs or policies to implement. This chapter deals with action planning—the process of putting a program or policy into effect. In implementation, one seeks to accomplish the setting up, management, and execution of the program.[1]

In the context of community change, sound action planning is one of the key factors predicting success.[3] The focus of this chapter is on *action planning*, that is, planning for a defined program, organizational, policy, or environmental change with specific, time-dependent outcomes, compared with ongoing planning that is a regular function within an organization.

Effective action plans have several key characteristics. First, they have clear goals and objectives. Second, the roles and responsibilities of important stakeholders are clarified and respected. Third, there are clear mechanisms for accountability. Fourth, the plans are comprehensive in that they describe specific steps, timelines, and roles and responsibilities. Although it is recognized that it is important to utilize multiple intervention tactics (communication, behavioral, policy, regulatory, environmental) to create change, each tactic should have a specific comprehensive action plan for its implementation. Such a plan includes a listing of all possible action steps and anticipated changes. This is an area in which a sound analytic framework (see chapter 9) can be especially useful in describing potential interventions and their effects. The plan must also have mechanisms for evaluation. Finally, the intervention tactics laid out within each plan need to be based on sound scientific evidence.

In simple terms, intervention (program or policy) development consists of planning, implementation, and evaluation (Figure 10.1). The earlier chapters in this book described the tools, strategies, and steps needed to determine which issues should be addressed by a public health intervention. In this chapter, our attention turns to the matter of implementation: "What specific actions can we take that are most likely to contribute to the changes in health or health behaviors we seek?"

To cover some essential issues for successful action planning, this chapter is organized in five main sections designed to highlight ecological frameworks, give examples of theories that can increase the likelihood of carrying out effective interventions, review key principles of planning, outline steps in action planning, and acknowledge important aspects of coalition-based interventions (which are covered in chapter 5).

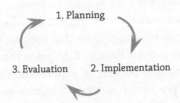

1. Planning

3. Evaluation   2. Implementation

Figure 10.1: A simple planning cycle for program development and implementation.

BACKGROUND

Effective action planning takes into account essentially all of the issues and approaches covered elsewhere in this book. For example, let's assume one is broadly concerned with the public health needs of a community. Early on, a partnership or coalition would have been established through which multiple stakeholders and community members are engaged in defining the main issues of concern and developing, implementing, and evaluating the intervention. The process would begin with a community assessment. This would start by examining epidemiologic data and prioritizing which health issues to address. After the quantitative data describing the main health issues have been established, additional community assessments (quantitative and qualitative) can be conducted to determine the specific needs and assets of the population of interest and the context (social, political, economic) within which the health problem exists. Through this process one would have identified the specific population and contextual issues using a wide range of local data sets.[4] Factors would be examined across the ecological framework (as described in chapter 5). In addition to a full community assessment, systematic reviews of the literature and cost-effectiveness studies would be reviewed to assist in determining possible intervention approaches, including a review of programmatic, organizational, policy, and environmental change interventions.

After a small set of possible interventions is identified one would then prioritize which intervention is best to implement (see chapter 9). Previous work has identified a number of issues to consider when prioritizing which intervention to conduct in a particular community or assessing readiness of a community to engage in a particular intervention (Box 10.1).[5-9] As described in chapter 5, information on issues to consider during prioritization can be collected as part of a complete community assessment. Consideration of these factors is needed to determine the levels of the ecological framework (individual behavior, organizational, environmental, or policy level change) that are most appropriate for intervention, the intervention strategy that is best for a specific community, and the content and processes that should be used for implementing the intervention.

ECOLOGIC FRAMEWORKS FOR ACTION PLANNING

Ecological frameworks emphasize the importance of individual, interpersonal, organizational, community (social and economic), and health policy factors because of the effect these variables have on individual behavior change and because of their direct effect on health.[10] In fact, the most effective

---

Box 10.1

QUESTIONS TO CONSIDER WHEN ASSESSING READINESS FOR INTERVENTION OPTIONS

- Is there a common understanding among community members and leaders regarding the nature of the problem and its determinants?
- Are community-based organizations capable of engaging in the desired intervention, or is it possible to build the capacity of these organizations (staff, resources, leadership support, knowledge of public health frameworks, cultural competence, and humility)?
- Does the intervention require that organizations work together? If so, what is the capacity of these organizations to work together (communication patterns, history, trust, group process skills, share data)?
- Is there a champion for the intervention approach?
- Are the skills needed to implement the intervention available?
- What has been done before in this community and other similar communities?
- Can the intervention be adapted or modified to fit the community of interest? In terms of culture, geography, educational level, other important factors?
- Do leaders (elected, appointed, and lay) support the intervention?
- Is the community supportive of the approach?
- Are there resources to implement the approach?
- Can the existing community infrastructures support the intervention? If not, can the infrastructures be enhanced or built?

Adapted Plested et al.,[5] Baker et al.,[6] and Robinson et al.[7]

---

interventions probably act at multiple levels because communities are made up of individuals who interact in a variety of social networks and within a particular context.[11] The assessment of needs and resources, literature review, and evaluation of available data sets should guide which level (or levels) of the ecological framework is the appropriate level for intervention.

An ecological framework is a useful way to organize objectives and intervention approaches (Table 10.1). Programs focused on changing *individual* behavior may provide information and teach skills to enable individuals to change their behaviors. These programs may focus on changing knowledge, attitudes, beliefs, and behaviors and may be conducted individually, in groups, or online.[12] Various theories can be useful in directing practitioners to specific strategies that are appropriate to use in changing individual behavior, organizational and environmental conditions, and policies that influence health and health behaviors (as described later in this chapter). Some theories, such as the stages-of-change theory, suggest that different approaches

Table 10.1 SUMMARY OF OBJECTIVES AND INTERVENTION APPROACHES
ACROSS LEVELS OF AN ECOLOGICAL FRAMEWORK

	Individual	Interpersonal	Organizational	Community	Health Policy
Objectives address	Knowledge	Programs	Programs	Programs	Ordinances
	Attitudes	Practices	Practices	Practices	Regulations
	Behavior	Social support	Policies	Policies	Laws
		Social networks	Agency environment	Built environment	
Approaches	Information	Develop new social ties	Organizational change	Social change	Political action
	Education	Lay health advisors	Networking	Media advocacy	Lobbying
	Training	Peer support groups	Organizational development	Coalition building	Media advocacy
	Counseling		Environmental changes	Community development	Policy advocacy
				Environmental changes	Coalition building

Source: Adapted from Simons-Morton, Green and Gottlieb[69]

are likely to be more or less useful, depending on the individual's readiness
for change.[11]

To address *interpersonal* factors, many programs include strategies to
strengthen social support.[13,14] As described by Israel,[15] these programs may
act in various ways. For example, programs may attempt to strengthen existing networks by working with families and friends. A program aimed at
strengthening existing social networks to enhance individual behavior change
might invite family members to join exercise facilities or take cooking classes
together. Alternatively, programs may develop new network ties through
social support groups or may enhance the capacity of natural helpers, such as
people in positions of respect in a community, to provide health-related information and assistance. Programs may also seek to provide Web-based support
using social media or online interactive games.[16,17] Programs may also seek to
enhance the total network through lay health advisors.[15] Lay health advisors
are lay people to whom others normally turn to for advice, emotional support,
and tangible aid.[18] Lay health advisors may provide information on specific
health risks or behaviors or on services available to address various health
needs. They may also assist clients in improving their communication skills
or establish linkages with health and human service agencies for efficient and

appropriate referral.[19] In some instances, building social ties may be a secondary aim of programs that primarily focus on other types of community-based activities.

Interventions at the organizational level may occur in two ways. The first is that organizations can support positive behavior change among their employees or those served by their organization through the implementation of individual behavior change programs, policy changes, or environmental changes. Organizations such as child care facilities, schools, and worksites are particularly important for enhancing public health because people spend one-third to one-half of their life in such settings. In this way, the organization is a setting for change. Alternately, public health and community-based organizations may create administrative changes that enhance diffusion of evidence-based interventions that have proved useful in other settings. These might include infrastructure development; workforce development and capacity building, including networking and multisectoral engagement, cultural capacity and humility, and leadership skills such as conflict management; and data management systems that can be shared.[20–23]

Public health interventions may also attempt to create changes in community and health policy or environmental factors. These efforts often focus on creating changes in community structures, processes, and policies. Changes in community structures or processes could include development of community parks, libraries, or educational facilities and may also involve changes in decision-making structures to incorporate points of view that were previously unheard. In terms of policy changes, these programs may, for example, focus on creating smoke-free public places to support changes in individual smoking behavior and attempt to alter community norms around smoking. Alternately, efforts may be focused on creating policy and environmental changes in other social, community, or economic factors such as housing, jobs, wages, education, and physical structures that influence health and health behaviors.[24] For example, an intervention may succeed at changing attitudes and intentions to increase consumption of fruits and vegetables, but there are no jobs—and therefore no funds—to purchase the produce; or the jobs that are available do not pay a wage that allows for purchase of produce or maintenance of utilities required for refrigeration and heating of food. Interventions aimed at encouraging economic development and living wages can alter capacity to change behavior.[25]

The use of ecological frameworks also emphasizes that individual, interpersonal, organizational, community, and health policy factors are interrelated, and programs that address one level are likely to enhance outcomes at the other levels.[26] For example, new health policy might be implemented in a worksite that employs a significant proportion of a town's population, and this might result in a change in social norms throughout a community. It is also important to note that ecological frameworks are important to consider whether the program is categorical (focused on a particular disease process) or a broadly defined community program like community development. Programs that focus on a disease category such as breast cancer and receive categorical funding to change individual behavior (e.g., getting mammograms) will enhance their ability to influence this behavior if they consider the impact of interpersonal and organizational factors and intervene accordingly.[26,27] This may entail providing low- or no-cost mammograms, changing the policy in the state so that more women are eligible for low- or no-cost mammograms, developing a lay health advisor approach to enhance breast cancer screening, or changing transportation systems to give women better access to screening and treatment services. Multilevel interventions (intervening at more than one level of the ecological framework) are increasingly recognized as important to address the complexity of factors influencing health behaviors and health outcomes (Box 10.2).[28-30] Although it is conceptually important to incorporate multiple levels, it remains difficult to tease apart the unique and synergistic contribution of intervention at each level.[31, 32]

Box 10.2

AN ECOLOGICAL APPROACH TO REDUCE DIABETES DISPARITIES

Within the United States there are significant disparities in diabetes: 15.9% of American Indians/Alaska Natives, 13.2% of non-Hispanic blacks, 12.8% of Hispanics, and 9% of Asian Americans have diagnosed diabetes compared with 7.6% of non-Hispanic whites.[28] To address these disparities the Alliance to Reduce Disparities in Diabetes implemented multicomponent interventions that addressed multiple levels of the ecological framework across five sites within the United States.[30] Individual level interventions focused on patient education and self-management. Provider interventions addressed cultural competency and communication. Systems level interventions focused on enhancing care coordination and community and organizational policy changes. While having this common framework, each of the five sites adapted and tailored the specific interventions to fit their community and cultural context. Evaluations were conducted for each level of the intervention and included clinical outcomes (e.g., changes in hemoglobin A1c, blood pressure, lipids, and weight), self-report scales (e.g., quality of life, perceived competence scale for diabetes, resources and supports for self-management), and tracking of systems changes (e.g., incorporating community health workers into the health care system).[29] The cross-site evaluation found improved quality of life and self-care behaviors and significant decreases in hemoglobin A1c level.

THE ROLE OF LOGIC MODELS AND THEORY
IN CREATING PROGRAMS AND POLICIES

The effectiveness of public health interventions can be enhanced by the use of systematic planning frameworks (described later), logic models, and theory (e.g., the transtheoretical model, social learning theory, policy development theories).[33]

When used in program planning, a logic model outlines specific activities and explains how they will lead to the accomplishment of objectives and how these objectives will enhance the likelihood of accomplishing program goals.[34] For example, a logic model lays out what the program participants will do (attend an educational session on breast cancer screening at their church) and what it will lead to (increased knowledge regarding risk factors for breast cancer and specific methods of breast cancer screening), which will in turn will have an impact (increase breast cancer screening rates), with the intention that this will produce a long-term outcome (decreased morbidity due to breast cancer). Logic models can be particularly helpful when interventions act on more "upstream" factors (such as education and employment) or "midstream" factors (such as organizational readiness to collaborate or share data) so that the intended influence on health behaviors and health outcomes is clearly articulated.[35] Several authors have conceptualized this process somewhat differently, yet the overall intent is that the intervention be laid out with specific activities intended to achieve certain objectives that in turn are expected to have an impact on clearly delineated outcomes, in both the near term and long term.

The specific intervention activities to be developed should be determined by their ability to meet the objectives outlined in the logic model and should be based on sound theories or models of behavioral, organizational, or community change. The specific activities should be developed with attention to the frameworks and planning tools described later. Whereas theory helps practitioners ask the right questions and understand why people are not living more health-promoting lifestyles or following medical advice, or understand the factors influencing implementation of organizational or community level policies that influence health, planning frameworks describe what needs to be done before developing and organizing a program or policy—and both help to identify what should be monitored or measured during evaluation.[11]

Theory

A theory is a set of interrelated concepts, definitions, and propositions that presents a systematic view of events or situations by specifying relations among variables in order to explain and predict events or situations.[11]

Theories and models explain behavior and suggest ways to achieve behavior change. As noted by Bandura, in advanced disciplines like mathematics, theories integrate laws; whereas in newer fields such as public health or behavioral science, theories describe or specify the determinants influencing the phenomena of interest.[36] As a result, in terms of action planning, theory can point to important intervention strategies. For example, individual level theories (e.g., health belief model, transtheoretical model of change, theory of planned behavior[11,33,36]) suggest that perceptions are important in maintaining behavior and that it is therefore important to include some strategies to alter perceptions; whereas if skills are considered important to change behavior (i.e., social learning theory[36]), then some strategy to alter skills must be included in the intervention. If laws and rules influence health and behavior, policies need to be enacted and enforced to support health. Policy theories and frameworks suggest that determinants of policy change include increasing knowledge of the problem and building support for change. Useful strategies such as developing policy briefs and engaging leadership can help to create the needed policy changes.[37,38] Organizational theories and frameworks point to policies, regulations, and structures that influence behaviors and health or characteristics within organizations that facilitate implementation of health-related interventions, including leadership support, funding, and collaborative relationships and networks.[9,39]

COMMON PRINCIPLES ACROSS PLANNING FRAMEWORKS

Numerous frameworks for planning have been proposed over the past few decades. Among the earliest approaches was a simple program evaluation and review technique (PERT) chart. As described by Breckon and colleagues,[40] this was a graphically displayed timeline for the tasks necessary in the development and implementation of a public health program. Subsequent approaches have divided program development into various phases, including needs assessment, goal setting, problem definition, plan design, implementation, and evaluation. There are numerous other planning frameworks that have proved useful for various intervention settings and approaches. Among them are the following:

- Predisposing, Reinforcing and Enabling Constructs in Educational/environmental Diagnosis and Evaluation, with its implementation phase: Policy, Regulatory, and Organizational Constructs in Educational and Environmental Development (PRECEDE-PROCEED)[41]
- Intervention Mapping[42]
- Developing a state health improvement plan (SHIP)[43]

Each of these frameworks has been used to plan and implement successful programs. The PRECEDE-PROCEED model alone has generated thousands of documented health promotion applications in a variety of settings and across multiple health problems. Others, such as the SHIP process, are explicitly linked to accreditation standards and measures.[43] Rather than providing a review of each of these planning frameworks, key planning principles have been abstracted that appear to be crucial to the success of interventions in community settings and are common to each framework. Those principles include the following:

1. Data should guide the development of programs. Elsewhere in this book, many types and sources of data are described that are useful in summarizing a community's health status, needs, and assets in the community to make changes.
2. Community members should participate in the process. As discussed in chapter 5, active participation by a range of community members in setting priorities, planning interventions, and making decisions enhances the viability and staying power of many public health programs.
3. Participants should develop an intervention strategy that addresses more than one level of the ecological framework. Based on a participatory process, community members are encouraged to develop intervention strategies across multiple sectors, including community, schools, and health care facilities.
4. The community capacity for health promotion should be increased. A systematic planning process can be repeated to address various health priorities. Such an approach aims to increase capacity to improve public health by enhancing the community's skills in health planning and health promotion.
5. Evaluation should emphasize feedback and program improvement. Sound evaluation improves program delivery, and timely feedback to the community is essential.

A STEPWISE APPROACH TO SUCCESSFUL ACTION PLANNING

The preceding frameworks and keys to intervention success suggest a series of steps for successful action planning (Box 10.3).[44,45] Previous chapters have dealt with a number of these steps, and chapter 11 addresses evaluation issues. This section will highlight several key issues involved in some of these steps, including adaptation, staff training and capacity building, developing action plans, assessing resource needs, and identifying and training staff.

Box 10.3
STEPS IN DESIGNING A SUCCESSFUL PUBLIC HEALTH INTERVENTION

---

1. Develop partnership with appropriate organizations, agencies, and community members
2. Review health data; determine contributing factors
3. Conduct full community assessment
4. Undertake systematic reviews of the literature and cost-effectiveness studies to identify existing programs and policies
5. Assess feasibility and potential for adaptation with organizational partners and those affected by the intervention . . . determine potential barriers and solutions
6. Select and adapt specific intervention program, environmental change, or policy
7. Develop logic model specifying specific goal, objectives, and action steps for the intervention selected
8. Develop the evaluation plan for activities, objectives, and goal
9. Obtain support in the setting for intervention (e.g., community, health care, schools)
10. Develop work plan and timetables
11. Assess resource needs
12. Identify, train, and supervise workers
13. Pilot-test intervention and evaluation
14. Monitor and evaluate program or policy
15. Use evaluation results to modify intervention as appropriate

Adapted from The Planned Approach to Community Health (PATCH)[44] and Davis et al.[45]

Adaptation

After an intervention approach has been determined, it is important to consider how to adapt the intervention to the population, culture, and context of interest.[46,47] This requires that community members and existing community-based organizations have an active role in the initial assessments and the development, implementation, and evaluation of interventions. This type of approach is consistent with community-based participatory research (CBPR). Israel and colleagues define CBPR as a collaborative approach to research that equitably involves, for example, community members, organizational representatives, and researchers in all aspects of the research process.[48] The partners contribute unique strengths and shared responsibilities to enhance understanding of a given phenomenon and the social and cultural dynamics of the community. This can improve the ability to integrate the knowledge gained with action to improve the health and well-being of community members.[48] Driven by values of social or environmental justice,[49] CBPR creates the structures needed for all partners to engage in improving community health. These structures are co-created by all partners and provide the opportunity for all partners to learn from each other (co-learning).[50, 51]

One of the challenges that a program often encounters when adapting an intervention is the tension between fidelity, or keeping the key ingredients of an intervention that made it successful, and adaptation to fit the community of interest.[52] Adapting interventions from one location to another requires considerations regarding the determinants of the health issue, the population, culture and context, and political and health care systems.[47,53–56] Lee and colleagues have developed a useful approach for planned adaptation that includes four steps: (1) examining the evidence-based theory of change, (2) identifying population differences, (3) adapting the program content, and (4) adapting evaluation strategies.[57]

There are several issues to consider in adapting an intervention that has been effective in one setting and with one population into another setting and population. Among these are attributes of applicability (whether the intervention process can be implemented in the local setting) such as the political environment, public acceptance of the intervention, cultural norms regarding the issue and the intervention proposed, history of the relationship between the community and the organization implementing the intervention including the history of trust, engagement of the community in the intervention development and implementation, and resources available for program.[47] Other factors relate to transferability (whether the intervention effectiveness is similar in the local setting and the original study), baseline risk factors, population characteristics, and the capacity to implement the intervention.[56,58] There are some aspects of an intervention that are relatively benign to change (e.g., the name of the intervention or the graphics used), whereas changing other aspects of the intervention may be somewhat concerning (e.g., the sector of the community where the intervention is implemented) or advised against (e.g., eliminating training modules).[59]

Work conducted with the National Community Committee of the Prevention Research Centers identified 10 considerations to take into account when adapting evidence-based physical activity programs with and within racial and ethnic minority communities (Box 10.4).[60] Although these were developed for physical activity, some may also be important to consider in developing programs for other interventions aimed at reducing health disparities.[60]

Box 10.4
THING TO CONSIDER WHEN ADAPTING EVIDENCED-BASED PROGRAMS WITH AND WITHIN RACIAL/ETHNIC COMMUNITIES (EXAMPLE IS FOR PHYSICAL ACTIVITY PROMOTION)

1. **Attend to culture**
   - Require ongoing cultural competency training for all staff (e.g., those who have experienced racial or ethnic discrimination, those who have been subjected to racial or ethnic discrimination, and those who have benefited from racial or ethnic discrimination)
   - Recognize a history of mistrust or mistreatment by social and medical professionals and services
   - Recognize diversity within and among groups regarding cultural norms
   - Recognize the complexity and differences within and across racial and ethnic minority populations
   - Recognize differences in the meaning of physical activity across communities
   - Consider the location of programs and resources in communities
   - Recognize the variety of responses that may occur with weight loss related to physical activity (e.g., concern regarding sickness, gaining weight to be attractive)
   - Recognize that it is considered acceptable, and sometimes preferable, in some racial and ethnic minority communities for individuals to be heavier
2. **Build on previous studies and work in the community**
   - Review recommendations from the *Guide to Community Preventive Services (Community Guide)*, learning from what others have done, including essential elements for a specific intervention but adapting for local racial and ethnic minority communities, based on conversations and previous experiences within the intended community
3. **Tailor the intervention (e.g., media messages, programs, policies, environmental changes) to the population and community you intend to serve in terms of the following:**
   - Reading level
   - Education level and the quality of the education
   - Available resources and infrastructures (e.g., parks, recreation centers, trails)
   - Individual and family characteristics (e.g., age and age-related norms, work, complex family structures, health conditions)
   - Availability of jobs and the unemployment rate
   - Incarceration and crime rate

- Knowledge and attitudes of your targeted community regarding physical activity and disease
- Readiness to engage in physical activity
- Physical activity that is most frequently practiced in the specific community
- The challenges that occur when information and support provided by health professionals, family, friends, and public health officials differs with regard to the importance and benefit of physical activity

4. **Engage the community in the planning, implementation and evaluation of the intervention**
   - Educate community partners about the research process overall, not just the intervention including community members and organizations from the beginning and continuing to engage them throughout the process
   - Hire lay health advisors and providing training and certification
   - Consider including individuals from nontraditional places

5. **Use existing or create new community infrastructures within the racial and ethnic minority community to support the intervention**
   - Provide transportation offering child care options
   - Involve local businesses
   - Consider the availability and number of recreational facilities
   - Create linkages between existing structures and new initiatives
   - Create linkages between existing structures within and outside of racial and ethnic minority communities

6. **Ensure appropriate intervention resources, including the following:**
   - Money
   - In-kind support
   - Incentives for participants
   - Liability insurance
   - Long-term and bridge funding to ensure sustainability
   - Funding restrictions
   - Full-time, gainful employment for community members
   - Resources that build community capacity for developing and managing resources
   - Resources that allow flexibility in responding to community needs beyond the specific intervention and in ways that facilitate the building of relationships within and among community members
   - Building on existing strengths in the community considering the use and enhancement of settings where the community frequents and has had a positive experience with (e.g., pharmacy, barber shops, child care)

7. **Assess and ensure actual and perceived personal and environmental safety**
   - Provide street lights and sidewalks

- Creating initiatives that recognize concern regarding interpersonal crime and gangs
- Create and enforce safe dog policies
- Ensure safe stairs and doors in buildings where activities are held
- Recognize and address the fear and perceptions created when individuals loiter (i.e., hang out) (individuals engaging in these actions may be inappropriately perceived as intimidating)
- Recognize and understand that some individuals may feel a greater sense of safety, and decreased vulnerability, with a larger body size

8. **Create community support**
   - Assess, build, and evaluate the trust among and within the groups who will implement the intervention
   - Assess, build, and evaluate trust and buy-in from racial and ethnic minority and broader community leaders and stakeholders

9. **Conduct a full community assessment, including the following:**
   - Physical activity rates
   - Community resources
   - Density of the community (e.g., number of people in the area and the size of the area)
   - Partnership capacity
   - Level and types of partnership collaboration
   - Relationships of racial and ethnic minority community with broader community
   - Socioeconomic indicators of the community

10. **Recognize the importance of gender issues, including the following:**
    - Traditional role expectations and personal expectations
    - The way men and women interact when developing intervention strategies
    - Gender issues that may be different across the lifespan
    - The positive and negative impacts on relationships when partners are, or are not, physically active

Adapted from Baker et al.[60]

Developing Action Plans

After general adaptation considerations have been discussed, it is time to develop action plans. Developing action plans requires developing program objectives and specific activities to achieve these objectives. To develop program objectives, it is essential to understand the components of sound program objectives.[1,2] This is of paramount importance because planning and evaluation are based on a series of objectives. A rigorous commitment to setting and monitoring objectives builds quality control into a program or policy and allows for midcourse corrections through process evaluation (see chapter 11). An intervention objective should include a clear identification of the health issue or risk factor being addressed, the at-risk population being addressed, the current status of the health issue or risk factor in the at-risk population, and the desired outcome of the intervention. A clearly defined objective can guide both the development of intervention content and the selection of appropriate communication channels. It also facilitates the development of quantitative evaluation measures that can be used to monitor the success of the intervention and to identify opportunities for improvement. Importantly, a clearly defined objective will improve the coordination of activities among the various partners participating in the intervention. Many have suggested that objectives need to be SMART—specific, measurable, achievable, realistic, and time bound.[61] More generally, several aspects of sound objective-setting have been described[1]:

- There should be sound scientific evidence to support the objectives.
- The result to be achieved should be important and understandable to a broad audience.
- Objectives should be prevention oriented and should address health improvements that can be achieved through population-based or health-service interventions.
- Objectives should drive action and suggest a set of interim steps (intermediate indicators) that will achieve the proposed targets within the specified time frame.
- The language of objectives should be precise, avoiding use of general or vague verbs.
- Objectives should be measurable and may include a range of measures— health outcomes, behavioral risk factors, health service indicators, or assessments of community capacity. They should count assets and achievements and look to the positive.
- Specific timetables for completion of objectives should be described.

Table 10.2 presents examples of sound objectives from national and state governmental sectors. These are drawn from the strategic plans and other planning materials of the programs noted. Some have found it helpful to start with more simple objectives to ensure that they link to both goals and activities, and then work from there to make the objectives "SMART."

Developing the Work Plan and Timetables

A detailed action plan that includes the development of a work plan and a specific timeline for completion will enhance the chances of a successful

Table 10.2. EXAMPLES OF OBJECTIVES AND THEIR LINKAGES
TO ACTION STRATEGIES

Level/Organization	Objective	Action Strategies
National/ US Department of Health and Human Services	Increase the proportion of children and adolescents aged 2 years through 12th grade who view television, videos, or play video games for no more than 2 hours a day.	Provide family-based support, in combination with electronic monitoring devices, to decrease screen time.
National/ US Department of Health and Human Services	Reduce the proportion of persons in the population with hypertension	Engage community health workers in health education and outreach interventions to improve blood pressure.

Source: https://www.healthypeople.gov/2020/topics-objectives/topic/heart-disease-and-stroke/objectives #4555
http://www.thecommunityguide.org/index.html.

program. Defining lines of authority and communication is crucial for a community-based intervention in which numerous activities may occur simultaneously. In conjunction, the time frame for the program or policy should be carefully mapped in the form of a timeline. For externally funded projects like grants and contracts, this timeline corresponds to the funding period. A timeline is a graphic presentation of information, including a list of all activities (or milestones) and designating when they are to be accomplished. Basic timeline construction includes the following[1]:

1. A complete listing of activities, grouped by major categories
2. Ascertaining which activities need to be done first
3. Determining how long each activity will take
4. Determining when each and every activity is to begin and finish
5. Establishing the time units that are most appropriate (weeks, months, years)

A sample timeline is shown in Table 10.3. Although there are many ways to organize a timeline, this example groups activities into four main categories: (1) administration; (2) intervention development and implementation; (3) data collection and evaluation; and (4) analysis and dissemination. For internal purposes it is useful to add another component to this timeline—that of the personnel intended to carry out each task. Doing this in conjunction with the timeline will allow for assessment of workload and personnel needs at various times throughout the proposed project. Another important component of program delivery is the assessment of program implementation: "How

Table 10.3. [a]EXAMPLE TIME LINE FOR IMPLEMENTATION OF A PUBLIC HEALTH INTERVENTION.

Activity	Month											
	1	2	3	4	5	6	7	8	9	10	11	12
Administration												
• Hire and train staff	x	x										
• Assemble research team	x	x										
• Conduct staff meetings	x	x	x	x	x	x	x	x	x	x	x	x
• Oversee and manage budget	x	x	x	x	x	x	x	x	x	x	x	x
Intervention development and implementation												
• Conduct focus groups to refine interventions			x	x								
• Pilot-test interventions					x	x						
• Finalize interventions and begin delivery							x	x	x			
Data collection and evaluation												
• Test and finalize questionnaires					x	x						
• Review pilot data and refine data collection approaches							x	x				
• Conduct process evaluation									x	x	x	x
• Conduct impact evaluation									x	x	x	x
Analysis and dissemination (all year 2 or year 3 activities)												
• Edit data and conduct data entry												
• Refine and conduct analyses												
• Write rough draft and final project report												
• Present findings at regional and national meetings												

[a]Only year 1 is displayed as an example.

well was the program delivered?" These issues are covered in more detail in chapter 11 within the context of process evaluation.

Assessing Resource Needs

Another step in action planning is determining the resources required to implement a particular program or policy. Resources can be grouped into five general areas:

1. *Available funds:* How many direct funds are available? What are the sources? Are there limitations on how and when funds can be spent? Are funds internal or external to a program or agency? Are there "in-kind" funds?
2. *Personnel:* How many and what types of personnel are needed? What type of training will be needed for program staff? What personnel do collaborating organizations bring to the project?
3. *Equipment and Materials:* What types of equipment and supplies are needed for the program? Are there certain pieces of equipment that can be obtained "in-kind" from participating partners?
4. *Facilities:* For some types of interventions, is significant infrastructure needed (such as clinics, hospitals, or mobile vans)?
5. *Travel:* Is there travel directly related to carrying out the project? Are there related travel expenses for other meetings or presentations in professional settings?

A generic budget planning worksheet is provided in Table 4.3.

Staff Training and Capacity Building

As an intervention develops, adequate staff and volunteer training is essential for smooth implementation of interventions. In the early phases, it is important to ensure that all members of a partnership (academic, practice, and community) have the level of information and skills needed to take part in the evidence-based planning and decision-making process. Other types of training may focus on leadership development or strategic planning. Additional training may then take place to provide the specific information and skills required for the chosen intervention. Formal training should be provided for staff members who have a limited background in specific intervention areas such as policy advocacy, health behavior change, evaluation, media communications, or coalition building. Special attention should also be given to basic skills such as planning, budgeting, personnel management, written and verbal communication, and cultural appropriateness. It is also important to consider

Table 10.4.   GENERIC BUDGET PLANNING WORKSHEET

Line Item	Internal Resources (new budget allocation)	Internal In-Kind (reallocation of existing resources)	External Resources (grants, contracts, other public or private sources)	External In-Kind (donated services or nonfinancial resources)
Personnel (staff or contractors)				
Examples:				
Coordinator				
Data manager				
Health educator				
Evaluator				
Administrative support staff				
Technical support/ consultants				
Subject matter experts				
Meeting facilitators				
Graphic designer				
Marketing/public relations specialist				
Copy writer/editor				
Website designer				
Fringe benefits				
Equipment and materials				
Examples:				
Office supplies				
Meeting supplies				
Computer supplies				
Graphic design software				
Data software				
Audio equipment				
Presentation equipment				
Other equipment purchase				
Computer/copier				
Maintenance				
Facilities				
Examples:				
Clinical space				
Space for group meetings				
Conference and meeting rooms				

Table 10.4 CONTINUED

Line Item	Internal Resources (new budget allocation)	Internal In-Kind (reallocation of existing resources)	External Resources (grants, contracts, other public or private sources)	External In-Kind (donated services or nonfinancial resources)
Travel				
Examples:				
Staff meeting travel, lodging, and per diem				
Steering group travel and lodging				
Mileage associated with program implementation				
Other nonpersonnel service costs				
Examples:				
Conference call services				
Long-distance services				
Website service				
Transcription costs for focus group tapes				
Indirect/overhead costs				
Total costs				

the utilization of local community members, or what some have called lay health advisors, community health workers, or promotoras.[62-65] Community members may have expertise in many areas that make their engagement important, and they can be trained to implement the specific intervention and can be given ongoing support as needed.[66] The training of all staff, community health workers, and others should be included as a necessary first step in the work plan, and the persons responsible for training should be listed in the work plan.

When addressing training needs, several key questions come to mind:

- In which areas does each staff member need training?
- Who should conduct the training?

- Do some people have unused skills that could be useful to an intervention?
- How best should community members be oriented and trained regarding an intervention?
- How can training be time efficient?
- How can training bring in principles of adult learning?

Pilot-Testing the Intervention and Framing the Evaluation

Pilot testing is an important part of intervention development. A pilot test is a "mini-study" carried out with a small number of individuals (often 20 or fewer) to detect any problems with intervention and evaluation strategies. Carefully examining the results of a pilot test can obviate problems before a large scale intervention—where the stakes are higher—is undertaken. A pilot test allows one to accomplish the following:

1. Refine the original hypotheses or research questions.
2. Produce information that will help improve evaluation approaches.
3. Improve curriculum materials or evaluation instruments.
4. Test approaches for data imputation and analysis.
5. Uncover politically sensitive issues, allowing program planners to better anticipate difficulties.
6. Estimate costs for people, equipment, materials, and time.
7. Ascertain the cultural appropriateness of interventions in diverse populations by inclusion in program development.
8. Enhance the marketability of an intervention with senior agency administrators when a pilot test is successful.

To the extent possible, a pilot test should be conducted in the same manner as that intended for the full program. In some cases, a pilot study may use qualitative methods, such as focus groups or individual interviews, which are not part of the main project. However, pilot tests can also provide an opportunity to examine the utility and appropriateness of quantitative instruments. Pilot test participants should be similar to those who will be in the actual project. Generally, pilot test participants should not be enrolled in the main project; therefore it is sometimes useful to recruit pilot participants from a separate geographic region.[67] Complete notes should be taken during the pilot test so that the project team can debrief with all needed information.

SUMMARY

This chapter provides an overview of various approaches to action planning along with several related issues. An important caveat should be kept in mind when planning an intervention. It has been suggested that sometimes a disproportionate amount of effort and resources go into the planning process compared with the actual intervention.[68] The diagnostic phases are often resource intensive to avoid action planning that leads to weak interventions. The key is to expend enough resources during the assessment and planning processes to be sure that the intervention focuses on a problem that is defined in a way that is potentially solvable and that the right intervention is chosen, while ensuring that adequate resources are available for actual implementation. It is also crucial that well-trained practitioners are available for intervention delivery.

KEY CHAPTER POINTS

- Ecological frameworks encourage the use of comprehensive, multilevel interventions that emphasize the importance of individual, interpersonal, organizational, community (social and economic), and health policy factors.
- The assessment of needs and resources, literature review, and evaluation of available data sets should guide which level of the ecological framework is the appropriate level for intervention
- A stepwise and systematic approach to action planning can enhance the chances of intervention success.
- The use of a logic model and theory will increase the likelihood for success in designing, implementing, and evaluating public health interventions.
- It is critical to adapt programs and policies to the population, culture, and context of interest.

SUGGESTED READINGS AND SELECTED WEBSITES
Suggested Readings

Bartholomew Eldredge LK, Markham CM, Ruiter RAC, Kok G, Fernandez ME, Parcel GS. *Planning Health Promotion Programs: An Intervention Mapping approach.* 4th ed. San Francisco, CA: Jossey-Bass Publishers; 2016.

Glanz K, Rimer B, Viswanath K, eds. *Health Behavior and Health Education.* 5th ed. San Francisco, CA: Jossey-Bass Publishers; 2015.

Green LW, Kreuter MW. *Health Promotion Planning: An Educational and Ecological Approach.* 4th ed. New York, NY: McGraw-Hill; 2005.

McLeroy KR, Bibeau D, Sleekier A, Glanz K. An ecological perspective on health promotion programs. *Health Education Quarterly* 1988;15:351–377.

Timmreck TC. *Planning, Program Development, and Evaluation. A Handbook for Health Promotion, Aging and Health Services.* 2nd ed. Boston, MA: Jones and Bartlett Publishers; 2003.

Selected Websites
Centers for Disease Control and Prevention—Assessment & Planning Models, Frameworks & Tools <https://www.cdc.gov/stltpublichealth/cha/assessment.

html>. This site provides information on key elements of, as well as differences between, assessment and planning frameworks. It also provides tools and resources for commonly used planning models and frameworks.

Community Tool Box <http://ctb.ku.edu/en/>. The Community Tool Box is a global resource for free information on essential skills for building healthy communities. It offers more than 7,000 pages of practical guidance on topics such as leadership, strategic planning, community assessment, advocacy, grant writing, and evaluation. Sections include descriptions of the task, step-by-step guidelines, examples, and training materials.

Developing and Sustaining Community-Based Participatory Research Partnerships: A Skill-Building Curriculum <http://www.cbprcurriculum. info/>. This evidence-based curriculum is intended as a tool for community-institutional partnerships that are using or planning to use a community based-participatory research (CBPR) approach to improve health. It is intended for use by staff of community-based organizations, staff of public health agencies, and faculty, researchers, and students at all skill levels. Units provide a step-by-step approach, from the development of the CBPR partnership through the dissemination of results and planning for sustainability. The material and information presented in this curriculum are based on the work of the Community-Institutional Partnerships for Prevention Research Group that emerged from the Examining Community-Institutional Partnerships for Prevention Research Project.

Health Education Resource Exchange (HERE) in Washington <http://here.doh.wa.gov/>. This clearinghouse of public health education and health promotion projects, materials, and resources in the State of Washington is designed to help community health professionals share their experience with colleagues. The website includes sections on community projects, educational materials, health education tools, and best practices.

Knowledge for Health (K4Health) <https://www.k4health.org>. Funded by USAID and implemented by The Johns Hopkins Bloomberg School of Public Health, the mission of the K4Health project is to increase the use and dissemination of evidence-based, accurate, and up-to-date information to improve health service delivery and health outcomes worldwide. The site offers eLearning opportunities, results of needs assessment activities, and toolkits for family planning and reproductive health, HIV/AIDS, and other health topics.

Management Sciences for Health <http://erc.msh.org/>. Since 1971, Management Sciences for Health (MSH), a nonprofit organization, has worked in more than 140 countries and with hundreds of organizations. MSH resources communicate effective management practices to health professionals around the world. This site, the Manager's Electronic Resource Center, covers topics such as conducting local rapid assessments, working with community members, and developing leaders. The site links to case studies and toolkits from around the world.

National Cancer Institute, Health Behavior Constructs <http://cancercontrol.cancer.gov/brp/research/constructs/index.html>. This site provides definitions of major theoretical constructs employed in health behavior research, and information about the best measures of these constructs. The National Cancer Institute has also published a concise summary of health behavior theories in *Theory at a Glance, Second Edition*. http://www.sbccimplementationkits.org/demandrmnch/wp-content/uploads/2014/02/Theory-at-a-Glance-A-Guide-For-Health-Promotion-Practice.pdf.

Planned Approach to Community Health <http://wonder.cdc.gov/wonder/prevguid/ p0000064/P0000064.asp>. The Planned Approach to Community Health (PATCH), developed by the Centers for Disease Control and Prevention and their partners, is widely recognized as an effective model for planning, conducting, and evaluating community health promotion and disease prevention programs. It is used by diverse communities in the United States and several nations to address a variety of health concerns such as cardiovascular disease, HIV, injuries, teenage pregnancy, and access to health care. The PATCH Guide is designed to be used by the local coordinator and contains "how to" information on the process, things to consider when adapting the process to a community, and sample over-heads and handout materials.

REFERENCES

1. Timmreck TC. *Planning, Program Development, and Evaluation. A Handbook for Health Promotion, Aging and Health Services.* 2nd ed. Boston, MA: Jones and Bartlett Publishers; 2003.
2. Dyal WW. *Program Management. A Guide for Improving Program Decisions.* Atlanta, GA: Centers for Disease Control and Prevention; 1990.
3. Fawcett SB, Francisco VT, Paine-Andrews A, Schultz JA. A model memorandum of collaboration: a proposal. *Public Health Rep.* 2000;115(2–3):174–179.
4. Brownson RC, Baker EA, Leet TL, Gillespie KN, True WR. *Evidence-Based Public Health.* 2nd ed. New York, NY: Oxford University Press; 2011.
5. Plested BA, Edwards RW, Jumper Thurman P. *Community readiness: a handbook for successful change.* Fort Collins, CO: Triethnic Center for Prevention Research; 2005.
6. Baker EA, Brennan Ramirez LK, Claus JM, Land G. Translating and disseminating research- and practice-based criteria to support evidence-based intervention planning. *J Public Health Manag Pract.* Mar-Apr 2008;14(2):124–130.
7. Robinson K, Farmer T, Riley B, Elliott SJ, Eyles J, Team CI. Realistic expectations: Investing in organizational capacity building for chronic disease prevention. *American Journal of Health Promotion.* May-Jun 2007;21(5):430–438.
8. Bay Area Regional Health Inequities Initiative. Local Health Department Organizational Self-Assessment for Achieving Health Equity: Toolkit and Guide to Implementation. http://barhii.org/download/toolkit/self_assessment_toolkit. pdf. Accessed September 5, 2016.
9. Cohen BE, Schultz A, McGibbon E, et al. A Conceptual Framework of Organizational Capacity for Public Health Equity Action (OC-PHEA). *Can J Public Health.* May-Jun 2013;104(3):e262–e266.
10. Baker EA, Brownson CA. Defining characteristics of community-based health promotion programs. *J Public Health Manag Pract.* 1998;4(2):1–9.
11. Glanz K, Rimer B, Viswanath K, eds. *Health Behavior and Health Education.* 5th ed. San Francisco, CA: Jossey-Bass Publishers; 2015.
12. Wantland DJ, Portillo CJ, Holzemer WL, Slaughter R, McGhee EM. The effectiveness of Web-based vs. non-Web-based interventions: a meta-analysis of behavioral change outcomes. *J Med Internet Res.* Nov 10 2004;6(4):e40.
13. O'Malley AJ, Christakis NA. Longitudinal analysis of large social networks: estimating the effect of health traits on changes in friendship ties. *Stat Med.* Apr 30 2011;30(9):950–964.

14. Umberson D, Crosnoe R, Reczek C. Social relationships and health behavior across life course. *Annu Rev Sociol*. Aug 1 2011;36:139–157.

15. Israel BA. Social networks and health status: linking theory, research, and practice. *Patient Couns Health Educ*. 1982;4(2):65–79.

16. Edwards M, Wood F, Davies M, Edwards A. "Distributed health literacy": longitudinal qualitative analysis of the roles of health literacy mediators and social networks of people living with a long-term health condition. *Health Expect*. Oct 2013;18(5):1180–1193.

17. Eysenbach G, Powell J, Englesakis M, Rizo C, Stern A. Health related virtual communities and electronic support groups: systematic review of the effects of online peer to peer interactions. *BMJ*. May 15 2004;328(7449):1166.

18. Israel BA. Social networks and social support: implications for natural helper and community level interventions. *Health Educ Q*. 1985;12(1):65–80.

19. Eng E, Young R. Lay health advisors as community change agents. *Family and Community Health*. 1992;151:24–40.

20. Aarons GA, Ehrhart MG, Farahnak LR, Sklar M. Aligning leadership across systems and organizations to develop a strategic climate for evidence-based practice implementation. *Annu Rev Public Health*. 2014;35:255–274.

21. Allen P, Brownson R, Duggan K, Stamatakis K, Erwin P. The makings of an evidence-based local health department: identifying administrative and management practices. *Frontiers in Public Health Services & Systems Research*. 2012;1(2).

22. Kelly CM, Baker EA, Williams D, Nanney MS, Haire-Joshu D. Organizational capacity's effects on the delivery and outcomes of health education programs. *J Public Health Manag Pract*. Mar-Apr 2004;10(2):164–170.

23. Ward M, Mowat D. Creating an organizational culture for evidence-informed decision making. *Healthc Manage Forum*. Autumn 2012;25(3):146–150.

24. World Health Organization. *Closing the Gap in a Generation: Health Equity Through Action on the Social Determinants of Health. Final Report of the Commission on Social Determinants of Health*. Geneva: WHO; 2008.

25. Morris JN, Donkin AJ, Wonderling D, Wilkinson P, Dowler EA. A minimum income for healthy living. *J Epidemiol Community Health*. Dec 2000;54(12):885–889.

26. Sallis J, Owen N. Ecological models of health behavior. In: Glanz K, Rimer B, Vishwanath K, eds. *Health Behavior: Theory, Research, and Practice*. 2nd ed. San Francisco, CA: Jossey-Bass Publishers; 2015:43–64.

27. McLeroy KR, Bibeau D, Steckler A, Glanz K. An ecological perspective on health promotion programs. *Health Education Quarterly*. 1988;15:351–377.

28. Centers for Disease Control and Prevention. National Diabetes Statistics Report, 2014. http://www.cdc.gov/diabetes/pdfs/data/2014-report-estimates-of-diabetes-and-its-burden-in-the-united-states.pdf. Accessed October 20, 2016.

29. Collinsworth A, Vulimiri M, Snead C, Walton J. Community health workers in primary care practice: redesigning health care delivery systems to extend and improve diabetes care in underserved populations. *Health Promot Pract*. Nov 2014;15(2 Suppl):51S–61S.

30. Lewis MA, Bann CM, Karns SA, et al. Cross-site evaluation of the Alliance to Reduce Disparities in Diabetes: clinical and patient-reported outcomes. *Health Promot Pract*. Nov 2014;15(2 Suppl):92S–102S.

31. Clauser SB, Taplin SH, Foster MK, Fagan P, Kaluzny AD. Multilevel intervention research: lessons learned and pathways forward. *J Natl Cancer Inst Monogr*. May 2012;2012(44):127–133.

32. Cleary PD, Gross CP, Zaslavsky AM, Taplin SH. Multilevel interventions: study design and analysis issues. *J Natl Cancer Inst Monogr*. May 2012;2012(44):49–55.

33. Glanz K, Bishop DB. The role of behavioral science theory in development and implementation of public health interventions. *Annu Rev Public Health*. Apr 21 2010;31:399–418.

34. Knowlton L, Phillips C. *The Logic Model Guidebook: Better Strategies for Great Results*. 2nd ed. Thousand Oaks, CA: Sage Publications; 2012.

35. Institute of Medicine. *Speaking of Health: Assessing health communications strategies for diverse populations*. Washington, DC: National Academies Press; 2002.

36. Bandura A. *Social Foundations of Thought and Action: A Social Cognitive Theory*. Englewood Cliffs, NJ: Prentice Hall; 1986.

37. Dodson EA, Eyler AA, Chalifour S, Wintrode CG. A review of obesity-themed policy briefs. *Am J Prev Med*. Sep 2012;43(3 Suppl 2):S143–S148.

38. Uneke CJ, Ezeoha AE, Uro-Chukwu H, et al. Enhancing the capacity of policymakers to develop evidence-informed policy brief on infectious diseases of poverty in Nigeria. *Int J Health Policy Manag*. Sep 2015;4(9):599–610.

39. Brownson RC, Allen P, Duggan K, Stamatakis KA, Erwin PC. Fostering more-effective public health by identifying administrative evidence-based practices: a review of the literature. *Am J Prev Med*. Sep 2012;43(3):309–319.

40. Breckon DJ, Harvey JR, Lancaster RB. *Community Health Education: Settings, Roles, and Skills for the 21st Century*. 4th ed. Rockville, MD: Aspen Publishers; 1998.

41. Green LW, Kreuter MW. *Health Promotion Planning: An Educational and Ecological Approach*. 4th ed. New York, NY: McGraw Hill; 2005.

42. Bartholomew L, Parcel G, Kok G, Gottlieb N, Fernandez M. *Planning Health Promotion Programs: An Intervention Mapping Approach*. 3rd ed. San Francisco, CA: Jossey-Bass Publishers; 2011.

43. Association of State and Territorial Health Officials. Developing a state health improvement plan: Guidance and resources. http://www.astho.org/WorkArea/DownloadAsset.aspx?id=6597. Accessed September 10, 2016.

44. (Entire issue devoted to descriptions of the Planned Approach to Community Health [PATCH]). *Journal of Health Education*. 1992;23(3):131–192.

45. Davis JR, Schwartz R, Wheeler F, Lancaster R. Intervention methods for chronic disease control. In: Brownson RC, Remington PL, Davis JR, eds. *Chronic Disease Epidemiology and Control*. 2nd ed. Washington, DC: American Public Health Association; 1998:77–116.

46. Stirman SW, Miller CJ, Toder K, Calloway A. Development of a framework and coding system for modifications and adaptations of evidence-based interventions. *Implement Sci*. 2013;8:65.

47. Wallerstein N, Duran B. Community-based participatory research contributions to intervention research: the intersection of science and practice to improve health equity. *Am J Public Health*. Apr 1 2010;100(Suppl 1):S40–S46.

48. Israel BA, Schulz AJ, Parker EA, Becker AB. Review of community-based research: assessing partnership approaches to improve public health. *Annual Review of Public Health*. 1998;19:173–202.

49. Cargo M, Mercer SL. The value and challenges of participatory research: strengthening its practice. *Annu Rev Public Health*. Apr 21 2008;29:325–350.

50. Israel B, Eng E, Schultz A, Parker E, eds. *Methods in community-based participatory research for health*. 2nd ed. San Francisco, CA: Jossey-Bass Publishers; 2013.

51. Viswanathan M, Ammerman A, Eng E, et al. *Community-based participatory research: assessing the evidence*. Rockville, MD: Agency for Healthcare Research and

Quality Publication: Evidence Report/Technology Assessment No. 99 (Prepared by RTI—University of North Carolina Evidence-based Practice Center under Contract No. 290-02-0016). AHRQ Publication 04-E022- 2; July 2004 2004. 04-E022-2.

52. Allen J, Linnan L, Emmons K. Fidelity and its relationship to implementation effectiveness, adaptation and dissemination. In: Brownson R, Colditz G, Proctor E, eds. *Dissemination and Implementation Research in Health: Translating Science to Practice.* New York, NY: Oxford University Press; 2012:281–304.

53. Barrera M, Jr., Castro FG, Strycker LA, Toobert DJ. Cultural adaptations of behavioral health interventions: a progress report. *J Consult Clin Psychol.* Apr 2012;81(2):196–205.

54. Castro FG, Barrera M, Jr., Holleran Steiker LK. Issues and challenges in the design of culturally adapted evidence-based interventions. *Annu Rev Clin Psychol.* 2010;6:213–239.

55. Cuijpers P, de Graaf I, Bohlmeijer E. Adapting and disseminating effective public health interventions in another country: towards a systematic approach. *Eur J Public Health.* Apr 2005;15(2):166–169.

56. Wang S, Moss JR, Hiller JE. Applicability and transferability of interventions in evidence-based public health. *Health Promotion International.* Mar 2006;21(1):76–83.

57. Lee SJ, Altschul I, Mowbray CT. Using planned adaptation to implement evidence-based programs with new populations. *Am J Community Psychol.* Jun 2008;41(3-4):290–303.

58. Castro FG, Barrera M, Jr., Martinez CR, Jr. The cultural adaptation of prevention interventions: resolving tensions between fidelity and fit. *Prev Sci.* Mar 2004;5(1):41–45.

59. Lezin N, Rolleri A, Wilson M, Fuller T, Firpo-Triplett R, Barth R. *Reducing the Risk Adaptation Kit.* Santa Cruz, CA: ETR Associates; 2011.

60. Baker E, Motton F, Lewis E. Issues to consider when adapting evidence-based physical activity interventions with and within racial/ethnic minority communities. *International Public Health Journal.* 2012;4(3):285–294.

61. Rogers T, Chappelle E, Wall H, Barron-Simpson R. *Using DHDSP Outcome Indicators for Policy and Systems Change for Program Planning and Evaluation.* Atlanta, GA: Centers for Disease Control and Prevention; 2011.

62. Ayala GX, Vaz L, Earp JA, Elder JP, Cherrington A. Outcome effectiveness of the lay health advisor model among Latinos in the United States: an examination by role. *Health Educ Res.* Oct 2010;25(5):815–840.

63. Braun R, Catalani C, Wimbush J, Israelski D. Community health workers and mobile technology: a systematic review of the literature. *PLoS One.* 2013;8(6):e65772.

64. Lehmann U, Sanders D. *Community Health Workers: What Do We Know About Them? The State of the Evidence on Programmes, Activities, Costs and Impact on Health Outcomes of Using Community Health Workers.* Geneva: World Health Organization; 2007.

65. Viswanathan M, Kraschnewski J, Nishikawa B, et al. Outcomes of community health worker interventions. *Evid Rep Technol Assess (Full Rep).* Jun 2009(181):1–144, A141-142, B141-114, passim.

66. Fleury J, Keller C, Perez A, Lee SM. The role of lay health advisors in cardiovascular risk reduction: a review. *Am J Community Psychol.* Sep 2009;44(1-2):28–42.

67. McDermott RJ, Sarvela PD. *Health Education Evaluation and Measurement. A Practitioner's Perspective*. 2nd ed. New York, NY: WCB/McGraw-Hill; 1999.
68. Sleekier A, Orville K, Eng E, Dawson L. Summary of a formative evaluation of PATCH. *Journal of Health Education*. 1992;23(3):174–178.
69. Simons-Morton BG, Greene WH, Gottlieb NH. *Introduction to Health Education and Health Promotion*. 2nd ed. Prospect Heights, IL: Waveland Press; 1995.

CHAPTER 11

ᴄᴧᴐ

Evaluating the Program or Policy

One of the great mistakes is to judge policies and programs by their intentions rather than their results.

Milton Friedman

Evaluation is an essential part of the evidence-based public health process, answering questions about program needs, the process of implementation, and tracking of outcomes. It can (1) help to plan programs in a way to enhance the likelihood that they will be effective, (2) allow for midcourse corrections and changes, (3) help determine whether the program or policy has been effective, and (4) provide information for planning the next program or policy. This chapter reviews some of the key issues to consider in conducting an evaluation and provides linkages to a diverse literature (within and outside public health) for those wishing to go beyond these basics.

BACKGROUND

What Is Evaluation?

Evaluation is the process of analyzing programs and policies and the context within which they occur to determine whether changes need to be made in implementation and to assess the intended and unintended consequences of programs and policies; this includes, but is not limited to, determining whether they are meeting their goals and objectives. Evaluation is "a process that attempts to determine as systematically and objectively as possible the relevance, effectiveness, and impact of activities in light of their objectives."[1] There is variation in the methods used to evaluate programs and perhaps even more variation in the language used to describe each of the various evaluation techniques. There are both quantitative and qualitative evaluation methods and techniques, with the strongest approaches generally including a blending of these (i.e., mixed methods).[2,3] A comprehensive review of evaluation is beyond the scope of any single chapter and is the focus of numerous other textbooks.[4-7] This chapter reviews some of the critical issues to consider in conducting an evaluation, such as representation of stakeholders in all aspects of the evaluation, types of evaluation, how to decide on the appropriate evaluation methods (e.g., exploratory evaluation, program vs. policy evaluation), and considerations when disseminating evaluation findings.

There has been considerable discourse in the literature about the various paradigmatic approaches to evaluation and scientific inquiry. A paradigm is a set of beliefs or a model that helps to guide scientific inquiry. Many of the differences in the paradigms used to guide inquiry within public health are epistemological (i.e., they reflect different perspectives on the relationship between the inquirer and what can be known) and ontological (i.e., they reflect different perspectives on the nature of reality and what can be known about it). These paradigms are discussed in detail elsewhere.[8-11] Although a complete discussion of these issues is beyond the intent of this chapter, it is essential to recognize that the choices one makes in this regard influence the data collected, the interpretation of the data, and the utilization of evaluation results.[12,13] For example, although most individuals in the field would agree that evaluation in the absence of some stakeholder involvement is generally less useful, there are instances when evaluation is conducted after the program has been completed and data have already been collected. As will be discussed in more depth later in the chapter, this limits the potential for stakeholder involvement in deciding on the types of questions to ask (i.e., what is important to them), the data to be collected, and the way data are collected. In these instances, the evaluation decisions are influenced by program planning factors such as timing, expertise, available resources, and available data. Alternately, there are instances when the focus of the evaluation and the type of data collected are decided by the program implementers without the input of a wider group of stakeholders because of the belief that involvement of stakeholders would somehow "contaminate" the evaluation results.

Why Evaluate?

There are many reasons for public health practitioners to evaluate programs and policies. First, practitioners in the public sector must be accountable to national leaders, state policy makers, local governing officials, and citizens for the use of resources.[14] Similarly, those working in the private and nonprofit sectors must be accountable to their constituencies, including those providing the funds for programs and policy initiatives. Evaluation also forms the basis for making choices when resources are limited (as they always are), in part by helping to determine the costs and benefits of the various options (for more about this, see chapter 4). Finally, evaluation is also a source of information for making midcourse corrections, improving programs and policies, and serving as the basis for deciding on future programs and policies. It is closely related to the program planning issues and steps described in chapter 10 (Table 11.1).

In the early stages of planning and evaluation, it is useful to consider a set of factors (so-called utility standards) that help to frame the reasons for and uses of an evaluation (Table 11.2).[15-17] In part, these standards frame a set of questions, such as the following:

- Who needs to be involved in providing data for the evaluation?
- Who should conduct the evaluation?
- How should data be collected??

Table 11.1. LINKAGES BETWEEN PROGRAM PLANNING AND EVALUATION

Program Planning Activity	Evaluation Data/Sources
Goal	• Outcome data: Assess changes in morbidity, mortality, disability, quality of life
	—Social indicator data
	—Census data
	—National, state, or local survey data
Objectives	• Impact data: Track knowledge, attitude, and behavioral/skill changes
	—Programmatic surveys
	—National, state, or local survey data
	—Qualitative data (observations, interviews, diaries, content analysis)
Action Steps	• Process data: Assess how well a program is being delivered
	—Records of program attendance
	—Survey of participant satisfaction
	—Observational data of environment
Program Planning	• Formative data: Determine whether a program is feasible and appropriate
	—Individual or group interviews
	—Surveys of knowledge or attitudes

Table 11.2. UTILITY STANDARDS FOR EVALUATION

Standard	Description
Stakeholder identification	Persons involved in or affected by the evaluation should be identified so that their needs can be addressed
Evaluator credibility	The persons conducting the evaluation should be trustworthy and competent in performing the evaluation for findings to achieve maximal credibility and acceptance
Information scope and selection	Information collected should address pertinent questions regarding the program and be responsive to the needs and interests of clients and other specified stakeholders
Values identification	The perspectives, procedures, and rationale used to interpret the findings should be carefully described so that the bases for value judgments are clear
Report clarity	Evaluation reports should clearly describe the program being evaluated, including its context and the purposes, procedures, and findings of the evaluation so that essential information is provided and easily understood
Report timeliness and dissemination	Substantial interim findings and evaluation reports should be disseminated to intended users so that they can be used in a timely fashion
Evaluation impact	Evaluations should be planned, conducted, and reported in ways that encourage follow-through by stakeholders to increase the likelihood of the evaluation being used

Source: Joint Committee on Standards for Educational Evaluation.[15,16]

- How do we construct measures to learn what we need to know?
- What should be included in an evaluation report?
- How might evaluation of a policy differ than an evaluation of a program?

The Role of Stakeholders

As discussed in chapter 6, a stakeholder is anyone who is involved in the program or policy operations, is served by the program or policy, is affected by it, or will use the evaluation results.[18] It is important to include representatives of all of these groups in the design of the program or policy as well as in the design, implementation, and interpretation of evaluation results. The inclusion of these lay and professional perspectives will ensure that all voices are considered in the evaluation and that all will benefit from the evaluation. For staff, inclusion in the evaluation process can provide opportunities to develop skills and abilities in evaluation design and interpretation and can ensure that changes suggested in program implementation are consistent with their work experiences. (It is critical to ensure staff that program evaluation is not evaluation of *personnel*.[18]) In terms of affected audiences, inclusion in the evaluation process can increase their investment in the program and ensure that their interests and desires are considered when changes are made in programs and policies. Administrators and program funders need to be included to ensure that evaluation activities are conducted with an understanding of where the program or policy fits within the broader organizational or agency mission and to answer questions most urgent to these groups.[18] Regardless of who is included, it is essential that the relationships among these stakeholders be based on mutual trust, respect, and open communication.

Before the evaluation begins, all key stakeholders need to agree on the program goals and objectives, along with the purpose of the evaluation. Each stakeholder may harbor a different opinion about the program goals and objectives and the purpose of the evaluation, and these differences should be discussed and resolved before the evaluation plan is developed and implemented. There are several group process techniques that can be helpful in this regard. For example, the nominal group technique and the multivoting method (chapter 9) all offer opportunities for individual voices to be heard while, at the same time, providing a process for prioritization.

After the purpose of the evaluation has been agreed on, the next step is to turn stakeholder questions into an evaluation design. The specific roles and responsibilities of each group of stakeholders in creating the questions that guide the evaluation and in developing the methods to collect data may vary. In some evaluation designs, the stakeholders may be notified as decisions are made or have minimal input into evaluation decisions.[12] There are also other evaluation approaches (participatory, collaborative, or empowerment evaluation), in which stakeholders are seen as coequal partners in all evaluation decisions, including which questions are to be answered, which data are collected, how data are collected and analyzed, and how results are interpreted.[19] Some of these designs emphasize stakeholder participation as a means of ensuring that the evaluation is responsive to stakeholder needs, whereas other designs involve stakeholders to increase the control and ownership.[10,12] The role of the stakeholders will depend in part on the desires of the stakeholders and the paradigm guiding the evaluation. In all cases, everyone involved should have a clear understanding of their role in the evaluation process.

Before data collection, all stakeholders should also agree on the extent to which the data collected will be kept confidential, not only in terms of protecting the confidentiality of participants in data collection (a nonnegotiable condition for protecting evaluation participants), but also in terms of how information will be shared within the group of stakeholders (all at once or some notified before others). The group should also reach consensus on how and when information will be communicated outside the immediate group of stakeholders, what will be shared, and by whom.[12]

TYPES OF EVALUATION

There are several types of evaluation, including those related to program formation, context, process, impact, and outcome. Each type has a different purpose and is thus appropriate at different stages in the development of the program or policy. Initial evaluation efforts should focus on population needs and the implementation of program activities, commonly called formative or process evaluation. Impact evaluations and outcome evaluations are only appropriate after the program has been functioning for a sufficient amount of time to see potential changes. The exact timing will depend on the nature of the program and the changes expected or anticipated. Further, each type of evaluation involves different evaluation designs and data collection methods. Choices of which evaluation types to employ are based in part on the interests of the various stakeholders and the resources available.

Formative Evaluation

The goal of formative evaluation is to determine whether an element of a program or policy (e.g., materials, messages, strategy) is feasible, appropriate, and meaningful for the target population.[20] It should be conducted when intervention approaches are being determined, before program or policy initiation. Formative evaluation data can be collected through quantitative (questionnaires) or qualitative (individual or group interviews) methods. Information that is useful at this stage is documentation of the context, or setting, within which the health concern is occurring, including an assessment of the social, economic, and physical environment factors.[10,11,18,20] To fully assess context, it is important to document the current knowledge and attitudes of the intended audience about various behaviors and their perspectives on proposed programs and policies. For example, suppose a new program for healthy eating is proposed for school children. Formative evaluation questions might include the following:

- What are the attitudes among school officials toward the proposed healthy eating program?
- What are current barriers for policies for healthy eating?
- Are there certain schools that have healthier food environments than others?
- What are the attitudes among schoolchildren toward healthier food choices?
- What, if anything, has been tried in the past, and what were the results?

After these data are collected and analyzed by the relevant stakeholders, a action plan should be developed. (Chapter 10 describes this process in detail.) The action plan is essential to evaluation. A key component of the action plan is the development of a logic model (an analytic framework) (described in chapter 9). A logic model lists specific activities that are designed (based on evidence) to lead to the accomplishment of objectives, which, in turn, will enhance the likelihood of accomplishing program goals. A logic model lays out what outputs or activities will occur (an educational session on breast cancer screening at a church) and what they will lead to (increased knowledge among participants regarding risk factors for breast cancer and specific methods of breast cancer screening), which will in turn have an impact (increased breast cancer screening rates), with the intention that this will therefore produce a long-term outcome (decreased morbidity due to breast cancer). As discussed in chapter 10, intervention activities and objectives should be based on the best evidence available.

Several authors have conceptualized this process somewhat differently[6,12,21]; however, the overall intent is that the program or policy should be laid out in such a way that it specifies the activities and the program objectives that are expected to affect clearly delineated proximal and distal outcomes. Although any logic model is obviously limited in its ability to predict the often important unintended consequences of programs and policies, many argue that, even with this limitation, a logic model is mandatory to evaluate a program effectively. Rossi and colleagues have stated that evaluation in the absence of a logic model results in a "black box" effect in that the evaluation may provide information with regard to the effects but not the processes that produced the effects.[12] Moreover, because so many of the distal outcomes in public health are not evident until long after a program is implemented (e.g., decreases in morbidity due to lung cancer as a result of a tobacco control program), it is essential to ascertain whether more proximal outcomes (e.g., decreases in current smoking rates) are being achieved.

Process Evaluation

Process evaluation assesses the way an intervention (program or policy) is implemented, rather than its effectiveness.[20] It can function as a form of quality control by assessing what occurs during implementation compared with what is intended. Process evaluation addresses the following questions:

- To what extent is the program or policy being implemented as planned?
- Are materials and content appropriate for the population of focus?
- For program interventions:

- How many are attending educational sessions? Who is attending? Who is not attending?
- Are all potential participants participating equally? Is the program reaching the intended audience?
- Does the program have sufficient resources?
- What percentage of the program are participants receiving?
- For policy interventions:
  - How many people are covered by the policy?
  - Are the intended audiences aware of the policy?
  - Is the policy being consistently enforced?
  - Does the policy reach all people equitably?

These data are important to document changes that have been, and need to be, made to the program or policy to enable it to be implemented more effectively. Information for process evaluation can be collected through quantitative and qualitative methods, including observations, field notes, interviews, questionnaires, program records, environmental audits, and local newspapers and publications.

Impact Evaluation

Impact evaluation assesses the extent to which program objectives are being met. Some also refer to this as an assessment of intermediate or proximal outcomes, to acknowledge both the importance of short-term effects and that impact evaluation can assess intended as well as unintended consequences.[10] Impact evaluation is probably the most commonly reported type of evaluation in the public health literature.

Impact evaluation requires that all program objectives be clearly specified. A challenge in conducting an impact evaluation is the presence of many program objectives and their variable importance among stakeholders. There are also instances when a national program is implemented at many sites. The national program is likely to require each site to track the attainment of certain objectives and goals. Each site, however, may also have different specific program objectives and activities that they enact to accomplish local and national objectives and achieve the desired changes in outcomes. They may, therefore, be interested in tracking these local program activities and objectives in addition to the national requirements for reporting on program outcomes. Because no evaluation can evaluate all program components, stakeholders should come to an agreement before collecting data as to which objectives will be measured at what times.

It may be appropriate to alternate the types of data collected over months or years of a program to meet multiple programmatic and stakeholder needs. For example, suppose one was evaluating the changes in physical activity in a community over a 5-year period. In the initial phases of a program, it may be important to collect baseline data to understand the effects of the environment on physical activity. At each time point, it may be important to collect data on a set of core items (e.g., rates of physical activity) but alternate the data collected for some domains of questions (time 2: data on the role of social support; time 3: data on attitudes toward policies). Moreover, impact evaluation should not occur until participants have completed the program as planned or until policies have been established and implemented for some time. For example, if a program is planned to include five educational sessions, it is not useful to assess impact on objectives after the participants have attended only two sessions. It is also important to include assessments after the program has been completed to determine whether the changes made as a result of the program have been sustained over time.

Program objectives assessed by impact evaluation may include changes in knowledge, attitudes, or behavior. For example, changes in knowledge about risk factors associated with breast cancer or the benefits of early detection might be tracked through the use of a questionnaire administered before and after an educational campaign or program. Similarly, changes in attitude might be ascertained by assessing a participant's intention to obtain a mammogram both before and after an intervention through the use of a questionnaire. In the case of policy interventions (e.g., a policy enacted to make mammography a covered benefit for all women), objectives assessed by impact evaluation might track the rate of mammography screening before and after enactment of the policy.

The Importance of Reliability and Validity

As described in more depth in chapter 3, validity is the extent to which a measure accurately captures what it is intended to capture and reliability is the likelihood that the instrument will get the same result time after time.[1] Changes associated with public health programs can be tracked through the use of preintervention to postintervention questionnaires. It is often useful to use items from questionnaires that have already been used to evaluate other programs. Many instruments are available in peer-reviewed articles on the subject of interest (see chapter 8 on reviewing the scientific literature). If the items are not included in a scientific article, it is possible to contact the researcher and obtain the items or questionnaire directly from them.

For individual-level interventions, practitioners should consider using measures that have been tested in various surveillance systems such as the Behavioral Risk Factor Surveillance System (BRFSS). Begun in 1984, the BRFSS is the largest telephone health survey in the world.[22,23] Reviews of the reliability and validity of BRFSS data show risk factor prevalence rates comparable to other national surveys that rely on self-reports.[24] Among the survey questions used in the BRFSS, measures determined to be of high reliability and high validity were current smoker, blood pressure screening, height, weight, and several demographic characteristics.[25] Measures of both moderate reliability and validity included when last mammography was received, clinical breast exam, sedentary lifestyle, intense leisure-time physical activity, and fruit and vegetable consumption.

Even if the instruments under consideration have been shown to be valid and reliable in one population (e.g., residents of an urban area), it may be important to assess the reliability and validity of measures in the particular population being served by the program (e.g., a rural population). For example, it may be necessary to translate the items from English into other languages in a way that ensures that participants understand the meaning of the questions. This may require more than a simple word-for-word translation. (Some words or phrases may be culturally defined and may not have a direct translation.). In addition, the multicultural nature of public health necessitates that the methods used to collect data and the analysis and reporting of the data reflect the needs, customs, and preferences of diverse populations. It is important to determine that the measures are appropriate for the population that is to be surveyed in terms of content (meeting program objectives), format (including readability and validity), and method of administering the questionnaire (e.g., self-administered versus telephone).[23,24] Changes in technologies may affect the reliability, validity, and feasibility of various data collection methods. For example, data are often collected by telephone, an effective method during the time when land lines were the norm. The greater use of cell phones, answering machines, voice mail, and caller ID has contributed to declines in response rates and has increased costs of conducting telephone surveys.[26]

Issues of validity and reliability are somewhat different, but no less important, in the collection of qualitative data. The concept outlined by Lincoln and colleagues[11] and Shenton[27] is "trustworthiness" of qualitative data. Trustworthiness involves establishing credibility (confidence in the findings), transferability (applicable in other contexts), dependability (repeatable), and confirmability (shaped by the respondent and not the interviewer).

Design and Analysis Considerations

It is also important to consider the evaluation design that is most appropriate to assess the impact of a program or policy. Although this is described in chapter 7, there are a few additional considerations, particularly when conducting community-based programs. One particularly important issue to consider is the unit of assignment to intervention or control versus unit of analysis. Several authors have suggested ways to address these concerns.[28-30] For example, by using the individual as the unit of analysis, it is possible to use relatively fewer communities and collect more data, adjusting for the correlation among individuals within the same unit of assignment (e.g., within communities or within schools) through statistical means.[29,31,32] Alternately, one can collect fewer data across more communities or separate the communities into tracks, with some receiving the interventions and others being assigned to a control or delayed-treatment group. Others have suggested that the use of control groups may not necessarily be the best approach. Rather, the use of naturalistic inquiry and case studies, which provide in-depth descriptions of single or multiple cases, may be more useful in some evaluations.[33]

As described in chapter 5, qualitative data collection (e.g., individual or group interviews) can also be used to evaluate program impact by documenting changes, exploring the factors related to these changes, and determining the extent to which the intervention, as opposed to other factors, has influenced these changes. Moreover, qualitative data can be particularly helpful in assessing the unintended consequences of programs and policies.[10] Qualitative data must also adhere to standards and criteria of excellence, but these criteria are different than those used for quantitative measures.[34]

Outcome Evaluation

Outcome evaluation provides long-term feedback on changes in health status, morbidity, mortality, and quality of life that can be attributed to the intervention. These more distal outcomes are difficult to attribute to a particular program or policy because it takes so long for the effects to be seen and because changes in these outcomes are influenced by factors outside the scope of the program or policy itself. Assessment of an intervention's influence on these outcomes, therefore, is often thought to require certain types of evaluation designs (experimental and quasi-experimental rather than observational) and long-term follow-up (described in chapter 7). Some programs and policies, however, may rely on the published literature to extrapolate from proximal to distal outcomes. For example, the link between smoking and lung cancer is well established. Thus it may be possible to extrapolate from a decrease in smoking rates to the number of lung cancer cases prevented (the concept of population attributable risk described in chapter 3).

Data that are collected for purposes of outcome evaluation are more likely to be quantitative than qualitative and include social indicator data collected by the Centers for Disease Control and Prevention (CDC), the World Health Organization (WHO), state or provincial health departments, and local surveillance systems such as those sponsored by hospitals or health care systems. An evaluation that has included both impact and outcome data is shown in Box 11.1.[35-37] Qualitative data, however, can be useful in outcome evaluations to enhance understanding of the meaning and interpretation of quantitative findings and increase credibility of the results for many stakeholders.

Some kinds of data will enhance the quality of outcome evaluation. For example, it is helpful to have predata and postdata available on the outcomes of interest. Comparison or control groups can assist in determining whether the changes in desired outcomes are due to the intervention or to other factors. It is also important to have complete data; data collected as part of the program should not be systematically missing from a site or from some segment of the population of interest. In addition, secondary data, or data collected as part of surveillance systems, are most useful if they adequately and completely cover the subgroups of the population that the program or policy is intended to influence. For example, it may be important to have sufficient data to determine whether there are differences in effect by race, age, or gender. The data, regardless of their source, should be collected using reliable and valid measures and be analyzed using techniques that are appropriate for the questions asked and the types of data being used.

Box 11.1
EVALUATING A COMMUNITY-LEVEL INITIATIVE TO REDUCE OBESITY

Shape Up Somerville is a long-term community health initiative in Somerville, Massachusetts.[35] Starting in 1998, Shape Up Somerville aimed to reduce obesity by increasing active living and healthy eating through a variety of community-based (school, community, municipal) programmatic and policy interventions. Progress was tracked through process, impact, and outcome evaluation. In terms of process evaluation, indicators included changes in school curriculum, participation in community forums, and the number of medical professionals trained on obesity guidelines and screening practices. In terms of impact evaluation, indicators included partnership and community capacity; the development, approval, and implementation of a variety of policies (e.g., school wellness policies, bike lane policies, and vending machine policies); and behavioral changes (e.g., consumption of fruits and vegetables, physical activity and sports, and TV watching behaviors).[36] In terms of outcome evaluation, the team assessed changes in body mass index (BMI).[37] Evaluation methods included surveys, interviews and focus groups, BMI measurement, and environmental audits.

Metrics for Impact and Outcome Evaluation

Quantitative metrics for evaluation can be grouped in broad categories, including health outcomes, determinants, and correlates. The CDC conducted a systematic review to identify a total of 42 widely used metrics for community health (Table 11.3). Many of these are widely available at the state, county, and city levels throughout the United States and in other countries.

Although adequate indicators have been developed for mortality endpoints and for many behavioral risk factors like cigarette smoking or lack of leisure-time activity, shorter term (intermediate) markers are needed. The rationale for intermediate indicators is founded in the need for evaluators to assess program change in periods of months or years, rather than over longer periods of time. Environmental and policy indicators (unobtrusive measures) may also be useful as an intermediate measure for documenting behavioral changes. Examples of these indicators include the number of state laws banning smoking, the number of private worksites banning smoking, the miles of trails in a community, or the availability of low-fat foods in local restaurants (see chapter 5 for more description of metrics).

DECIDING ON THE APPROPRIATE EVALUATION METHODS

There are many issues to consider in deciding the appropriate methods to use for a particular evaluation, including the type of data to collect (e.g., qualitative vs. quantitative data). Qualitative data may include individual and group interviews; diaries of daily or weekly activities; records, newspapers, and other forms of mass media; and photographs, photovoice, and other visual and creative arts (e.g., music, poems). Quantitative data include surveys or questionnaires, surveillance data, and other records. Either form of data may be collected as primary data (designed for purposes of the evaluation at hand) or secondary data (existing data collected for a purpose other than the evaluation at hand, but still capable of answering the current evaluation questions to some extent).

These different types of data are often associated with different paradigmatic approaches (i.e., differences regarding what is known and how knowledge is generated) (Table 11.4). Quantitative data are generally collected using a positivist paradigm, or what is often called the "dominant" paradigm. As discussed earlier in this chapter, a paradigm offers guidance because it provides a set of understandings about the nature of reality and the relationship between the knower and what can be known. Within a positivist paradigm, what is known is constant, separate from the method

Table 11.3. [a]FREQUENTLY RECOMMENDED HEALTH METRICS

Health Outcomes		Health Determinants and Correlates			
Mortality	Morbidity	Health Care (access and quality)	Health Behaviors	Demographics and Social Environment	Physical Environment
Mortality— leading causes of death (9)	Obesity (6)	Health insurance coverage (6)	Tobacco use/ smoking (8)	Age (9)	Air quality (4)
Infant mortality (6)	Low birth weight (3)	Provider rates (primary care physicians, dentists) (5)	Physical activity (5)	Sex (6)	Water quality (3)
Injury-related mortality (3)	Hospital utilization (4)	Asthma-related hospitalization (4)	Nutrition (4)	Race/ethnicity (9)	Housing (5)
Motor vehicle injury mortality (3)	Cancer rates (4)		Unsafe sex (3)	Income (9)	
Suicide (4)	Motor vehicle injury (4)		Alcohol use (4)	Poverty level (6)	
Homicide (4)	Overall health status (4)		Seat belt use (3)	Educational attainment (6)	
	Sexually transmitted infections (chlamydia, gonorrhea, syphilis) (4)		Immunizations and screenings (5)	Employment status (6)	
	AIDS (3)			Foreign born (3)	
	Tuberculosis (4)			Homelessness (3)	
				Language spoken at home (3)	
				Marital status (3)	
				Domestic violence and child abuse (3)	
				Violence and crime (4)	
				Social capital/social support (4)	

[a]Numbers in parenthesis indicate the number of 10 Guidance Documents that recommended that specific outcome or determinant/correlate.

Adapted from Centers for Disease Control and Prevention. *Community Health Assessment for Population Health Improvement: Resource of Most Frequently Recommended Health Outcomes and Determinants.* Atlanta, GA: CDC; 2013.

Table 11.4 COMPARISON OF QUANTITATIVE AND QUALITATIVE
EVALUATION APPROACHES

Type of Evaluation	Type of Data	Method of Collection/Analysis
Quantitative	• Survey questionnaire	• Phone, in-person, online, mail
	• Social indicator data	• National (CDC WONDER, Census, BRFSS, WHO)
	• Geographic Information Systems	• Secondary review of archival data
	• Environmental assessments	• Primary data collection or secondary review of data
Qualitative	• Open-ended questions	• Phone, in-person, mail questionnaire
	• Individual interviews	• Phone, in-person
	• Diaries	• Self-administered
	• Group interviews and focus groups	• In-person, telephone conference calls
	• Newspapers, newsletters, and printed materials	• Primary collection or secondary review of archival data (content analysis)
	• Photography	• Primary data collection
	• Observation and environmental assessments	• Single or multiple observation, structured and unstructured

of generating knowledge, the person conducting the inquiry, and the context within which the inquiry is conducted. On the other end of the spectrum, qualitative data are often collected within alternative paradigms that include critical theory and constructionism. Although these alternative paradigms vary, they generally suggest that knowledge is dependent on the context and the interaction between the researcher and the participant in a study. It is important to note, however, that quantitative and qualitative data may be collected and analyzed using any paradigm as the guiding framework for the design of the study. For example, community-based evaluations are often conducted within an alternative paradigm but may utilize either qualitative or quantitative data, or may include both types (i.e., mixed methods).

Data Triangulation

Triangulation involves using both quantitative and qualitative data in the data collection and analysis process. Such mixed-methods approaches often result in greater validity of inferences, more comprehensive findings, and more insightful understanding.[3,38] Although beyond the scope of this chapter, detailed descriptions are available on mixed-methods designs, data collection methods, and analytic approaches.[2] Triangulation generally involves the use of multiple methods of data collection or analysis to determine points of commonality or disagreement.[39] Triangulation is often beneficial because of the complementary nature of the data. Though quantitative data provide an excellent opportunity to determine *how* variables are related to other variables for large numbers of people, they provide little in the way of understanding *why* these relationships exist (so-called contextual evidence[40,41]). Qualitative data, on the other hand, can help provide information to explain quantitative findings, or what has been called "illuminating meaning."[39] The triangulation of qualitative and quantitative data can provide powerful evidence of effectiveness and can also provide insight into the processes of change in organizations and populations.[42] There are many examples of the use of triangulation of qualitative and quantitative data to evaluate health-related programs and policies (see Box 11.2 for an example from HIV prevention).[43]

Other methods of triangulation have been described. These include "investigator triangulation," in which more than one investigator collects or analyzes raw data.[44] When consensus emerges, the results may have higher validity. In "theory triangulation," study findings are corroborated with existing social or behavioral science theories.[45]

The Role for Exploratory Evaluation

Exploratory evaluation (also known as evaluability assessment) is a pre-evaluation activity designed to maximize the chances that any subsequent evaluation will result in useful information.[5] It can be a precursor to either quantitative or qualitative evaluation and is often cost-effective because it can prevent costly evaluation of programs and policies whose logic model is not plausible or whose activities and resources are not sufficient or relevant (evidence based?) to achieve the objectives.[46]

Although the concept of exploratory evaluation has been around since the mid-1970s when it was first used by the US Department of Health, Education, and Welfare,[47] the method has been underutilized in public health.[46] The use of exploratory evaluation for public health topics has been relatively narrow; examples include promotion of physical activity,[48] healthy eating,[49] and rape prevention.[50]

As summarized by Trevisan[51] and Leviton and colleagues,[46] exploratory evaluation was designed to remedy several common problems in evaluation. First, there have been complaints from policy makers that evaluations are not always useful. Second, an exploratory evaluation can shed light on

Box 11.2
MIXED-METHODS EVALUATION OF AN HIV PREVENTION PROGRAM

Health care providers (e.g., physicians, nurses, physician assistants) play an important role in motivating and supporting HIV-infected patients in making behavior changes. To reduce HIV risk, the Partnership for Health (PfH) intervention is an evidence-based program that is clinician delivered and designed to reduce risky sexual behaviors through provider-patient discussions on safer sex and disclosure of HIV status.[43] Over a 6-year period, the program was disseminated to 776 individuals from 104 different organizations across 21 states or territories. A cross-sectional, mixed-method (qualitative and quantitative) evaluation was performed to assess the dissemination, implementation, and sustainability of the PfH program. There were three central evaluation questions: (1) How effective is the PfH program in reaching the target audience? (2) Did the PfH training lead to changed provider-patient practices? (3) What barriers and successes were experienced during implementation? An online survey was administered to all people trained in PfH from 2007 to 2013. Most respondents (79%) reported using PfH, but only 32% used the program with every patient. Open-ended questions identified the challenges in PfH implementation, which included a lack of buy-in from organizations, lack of leadership involvement, and staffing changes. Three keys to success were noted: a strong clinic coordinator, a champion for the program, and support from leadership. Using a relatively simple and inexpensive evaluation design, the team was able to assess the reach of PfH, challenges, and facilitators for improved dissemination, implementation, and sustainability of the program.

stakeholder disagreements (about the program goals, logic, how to measure success), which may suggest that a program is not ready for evaluation. Third, the underlying logic for a program may not be clear or realistic (i.e., it is not clear how particular interventions will achieve desired results). Fourth, the cost of an evaluation may be prohibitive. And finally, the relevant decision makers may be unwilling to make changes on the basis of evaluation.

The steps of an exploratory evaluation can be summarized by eight questions that have been adapted from the early work of Strosberg and Wholey[47]:

1. What resources, activities, objectives, and causal assumptions make up the program or policy?

2. Do those above the program managers at the higher levels of the organization agree with the program manager's description of the intervention?
3. To what extent does the program or policy have agreed-on measures and data sources?
4. Does the description of the intervention correspond to what is actually found in the field?
5. Are planned activities and resources likely to achieve objectives?
6. Does the intervention have well-defined uses for information on progress toward its measurable objectives?
7. What portion of the program or policy is ready for evaluation of progress toward agreed-on objectives?
8. What evaluation and management options should organizational leaders consider?

For public health practitioners, exploratory evaluation has many benefits and can lead to more effective and efficient evaluations.[46] For those seeking to learn more about exploratory evaluation, several sources are useful.[5, 46, 47]

Evaluation of Dissemination and Implementation Projects

There is growing emphasis on dissemination and implementation (D&I) research, which seeks to accelerate the adoption of evidence-based interventions in particular populations and settings.[52] Research on D&I has now taught us several important lessons about how evidence-based programs are spread: (1) D&I does not occur spontaneously, (2) passive approaches to D&I are largely ineffective, and (3) single-source prevention messages are generally less effective than comprehensive approaches.[53]

When evaluating the D&I of an evidence-based practice, it is generally not necessary to re-prove the effectiveness of the intervention (e.g., whether smoking bans decrease nonsmokers' exposure to secondhand smoke). Rather, one is more interested in understanding the fidelity of intervention implementation, process measures, or indicators of sustainability.[54] When addressing these D&I issues, a modified evaluation framework is needed. There are more than 60 models for D&I research, many of which have a practice-oriented focus.[55] A useful model for D&I evaluation is the RE-AIM framework, which takes a staged approach to measure Reach, Efficacy/Effectiveness, Adoption, Implementation, and Maintenance.[56] In RE-AIM, reach refers to the participation rate within the target population and the characteristics of participants versus nonparticipants. Efficacy/effectiveness relates to the impact of an intervention on specified outcome criteria. Adoption applies at the system level and concerns the percentage and representativeness of organizations that will adopt a given program or policy. Implementation refers to intervention integrity, or the quality and consistency of delivery when the intervention is replicated in real-world settings. And finally, maintenance (or sustainability) describes the long-term change at both individual and system/organizational levels. Practitioner-friendly tools (e.g., https://sustaintool.org/) can be useful in assessing program sustainability.[57] RE-AIM has been applied across numerous risk factors, diseases, and settings.[58] Its usefulness in evaluating the impact of public health policies has also been documented.[59] So-called hybrid evaluation designs answer both effectiveness and D&I questions in the same evaluation.[60]

Using Evaluation to Create Change

Another important consideration in the design and implementation of the evaluation is the intent of the evaluation with regard to the creation of knowledge versus the creation of change. Many traditional forms of evaluation act to assess the extent to which a program has met its objectives. Newer methods of evaluation include participants in the evaluation process with the intent of creating changes in the social structure and increasing the capacity of participants to self-evaluate.[61] These later forms of evaluation are often called empowerment evaluation, participatory action research, or community-based participatory research.[10,19,61–63] Such evaluation methods assess program goals and objectives as they relate to individuals, as well as the context within which individuals live (including economic conditions, education, community capacity, social support, and control).

Change can also come in the form of public health policy (described later). To improve public health outcomes, evidence-based public health policy is developed through a continuous process that uses the best available quantitative and qualitative evidence.[64] Persuasive use of results of policy evaluations can be critical in the shaping of successful legislative and organizational change.[17]

Policy Evaluation Versus Program Evaluation

Although there are many similarities in using evaluation to assess the implementation and effectiveness of programs and health policy, there are some significant differences that should be noted. Just as with program planning, there are several stages in a policy cycle, including agenda setting, formulation, decision making, implementation, and maintenance or termination.[65] In considering evaluation within the context of the policy cycle, the first decision is the utilization of data in the agenda setting or policy formation stage and the policy design or formulation stage. This is similar to a community assessment but is likely to differ in terms of consideration of whether or not the issue warrants a public or government intervention. If there is evidence that policy change is warranted, the question becomes whether current policies adequately address the concern or there is a need to modify existing legislation, create new policy, or enforce existing policy. Issues of cost-effectiveness and public opinion are as likely to have a significant impact on the answers to these questions as are other data collected.

The next phase of the policy cycle is policy implementation. Process data are useful at this stage, with a focus on the extent to which the policy is being implemented according to expectations of the various stakeholders. The last stage in the policy cycle is policy maintenance or termination. In this stage, longer term data are appropriate, with a focus on the extent to which the policy has achieved its objectives and goals.

Policy evaluations are critical to understanding the impact of policies on community- and individual-level behavior changes. They should include "upstream" (e.g., presence of zoning policies supportive of physical activity), "midstream" (e.g., the enrollment in walking clubs), and "downstream" (e.g., the rate of physical activity) factors.[66–68] By far, the most quantitative measures are routinely available from long-standing data systems for downstream outcomes.

Benchmarks include programmatic as well as structural, social, and institutional objectives and goals. For example, 5 years after implementation of a state law requiring insurance coverage of cancer screenings, several questions might be addressed:

- Do health care providers know about the law?
- Do persons at risk for cancer know about the law?
- Have cancer screening rates changed?
- Are all relevant segments of the population being affected by the law?

There are several challenges in evaluating health policies. One is that the acceptable timing of the evaluation is likely to be determined more by legislative sessions than programmatic needs.[69] Because of the wide variety of objectives and goals, it is important to acknowledge from the outset that evaluation results provide but one piece of data that is used in decision making regarding maintaining or terminating a health policy. This is in part because the evaluation of public health policy must be considered part of the political process. The results of evaluations of public policy inevitably influence the distribution of power and resources. Therefore, although it is essential to conduct rigorous evaluations, it must be acknowledged that no evaluation is completely objective, value-free, or neutral.

Resource Considerations

Resources are also important to consider in determining the appropriate evaluation methods. Resources to consider may include time, money, personnel, access to information, and staff. It is important to assess stakeholder needs in determining the type of evaluation to conduct. It may be that stakeholders require information to maintain program funding or to justify the program or policy to constituents. Alternately, participants may feel that previous interventions have not met their needs and may request certain types of data to alleviate these concerns. Similarly, program administrators in a collaborative program may require information about the benefit of the collaboration or information on how to improve the evaluation in order to fix managerial problems that are occurring before other process, impact, or outcome measures can be assessed.

The methods of evaluation used should not, however, be constrained by the skill and comfort level of the evaluator. Because there are a broad range of evaluation skills that can be utilized, and few evaluators have all of these skills, there is a temptation to see needs through the evaluator's lens of ability. It is far more useful to define the method of evaluation by the other factors mentioned earlier and the questions asked, and then bring together a group of evaluators who have the various skills necessary to conduct the evaluation.[10] In doing so, it is important to consider the ability of the evaluators to work with others who have different technical skills as well as the availability of resources to bring together these multiple types of expertise.

DISSEMINATION: MEMBER VALIDATION, REPORTING, AND USING DATA

After the data are collected and analyzed, it is important to provide the various stakeholders with a full reporting of the information collected and the recommendations for program or policy improvements. A formal report should include background information on the evaluation, such as the purpose of the evaluation (including the focus on process, impact, or outcome questions), the various stakeholders involved, a description of the program, including program goals and objectives, a description of the methodology used, and the evaluation results and recommendations.[4,5,18] Some important questions to consider when reporting evaluation data are shown in Table 11.5.[70-72] Perhaps

Table 11.5. QUESTIONS TO CONSIDER WHEN REPORTING
EVALUATION INFORMATION

Question	Considerations
Who are the different *audiences* (potential consumers) that should be informed?	Key stakeholders (people and agencies)
	Participants in the program
	Public health practitioners
	Policy makers
	Public health researchers
	The general public
What is your *message*?	Focus on what you want people to remember
	Keep it concise and actionable
	Think of a core message and one or two related messages
	Make it understandable
How will you inform the community about the results of your intervention (the *medium*)?	Town meetings
	Meetings of local organizations (civic groups)
	Newspapers articles, feature stories
	Online articles
	Journal articles
	Social media
Who will assume responsibility for presenting the results?	Public health practitioners
	Public health researchers
	Community members
What are the implications for program improvement?	Need for new or different personnel or training of existing staff
	Need for new resources
	Refinement of intervention options
	Changes in time lines or action steps

Adapted from The Planned Approach to Community Health (PATCH)[70,72] and Grob.[71]

most important, the report should tell readers something they do not already know, in a concise format.[71] The "Mom Test" is also important for any evaluation report—where months or years of evaluation effort needs to be boiled down to a few key sentences that are easily understood by a broad audience and that are specific, are inspiring, and will elicit a response.[71] For example: "Our reading improvement program that started last year in our schools is working. Reading levels are up significantly in every classroom where it was tried."

The development and dissemination of evaluation findings have changed dramatically over the past 20 years. A few decades ago, the typical evaluation report would be a hard-copy volume that might also be reduced to an executive summary. Newer approaches take advantage of electronic information technology by using websites, videos, electronic newsletters, and infographics. The newer approaches to data visualization (e.g., infographics) help in presenting data in an accessible and appealing way to stakeholders who are often inundated with information.[73,74] An example of an info-graphic is shown in Figure 11.1.[75] Real-time visualizations of data can also be powerful tools for presenting quantitative data (http://www.healthdata.org/gbd/data-visualizations).

Utilization of the report and the specific recommendations may depend on the extent to which stakeholders have been involved in the process to this point and the extent to which the various stakeholders have been involved in

305 DEATHS
DUE TO POVERTY

263 DEATHS
DUE TO LESS THAN HIGH SCHOOL EDUCATION

COMBINED THE NUMBER OF DEATHS COULD FILL OVER
7 METROLINK CARS

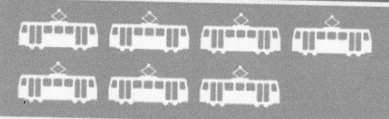

THE ESTIMATED COST OF THIS LOSS OF LIFE IS APPROXIMATELY
$4.0 BILLION

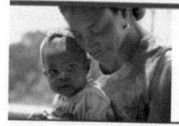

To Find Out More Click Below

Explore how many lives could be saved in our community if we improved education.

Figure 11.1: Infographic showing the effects of poverty on mortality in St. Louis, Missouri.
Source: For the Sake of All, 2014.[75]

the data analysis and interpretation. One useful method is to conduct some sort of member validation of the findings before presenting a final report. This is particularly important if the participants have not had other involvement in data analysis and interpretation. Member validation is a process by which the preliminary results and interpretations are presented back to those who provided the evaluation data. These participants are asked to comment on the results and interpretations, and this feedback is used to modify the initial interpretations.

Utilization of the evaluation report is also influenced by its timeliness and the match between stakeholder needs and the method of reporting the evaluation results.[6,18,71] Often, evaluation results are reported back to the funders and program administrators and published in academic journals, but not provided to community-based organizations or community members themselves. The ideal method of reporting the findings to each of these groups is likely to differ. For some stakeholders, formal written reports are helpful, whereas for others, an oral presentation of results or information placed in newsletters or on websites might be more appropriate. It is, therefore, essential that the evaluator considers the needs of all the stakeholders and provides the evaluation results back to the various interest groups in appropriate ways. This includes, but is not limited to, ensuring that the report enables the various stakeholders to utilize the data for future program or policy initiatives.

SUMMARY

Evaluation is a critical step in an evidence-based process of encouraging and creating health-promoting changes among individuals and within communities. As with planning, it is important to provide resources for the evaluation efforts that are appropriate to the scope of the program or policy.

KEY CHAPTER POINTS

- Because evaluation can influence the distribution of power and resources in communities, it is essential that evaluators strive to include key stakeholders early in the process.
- Information gathered should be shared with all stakeholders in ways that are understandable and useful.
- The types of data used (qualitative, quantitative) should be appropriate to the questions asked. Practitioners are encouraged to seek out other experts from multiple disciplines to assist them with venturing into new data collection approaches.

- It is important to conduct evaluation across the life of a program (formative, process, impact, and outcome) to ensure proper implementation and monitoring.
- Newer techniques, such as exploratory evaluation, can be a precursor to either quantitative or qualitative evaluation and are often cost-effective.
- Practitioners are encouraged to publish results of their program and policy evaluations and to disseminate their findings widely. This process creates new and generalizable knowledge that can be highly beneficial to public health professionals and, ultimately, to the communities they serve.

SUGGESTED READINGS AND SELECTED WEBSITES
Suggested Readings

Fink A. *Evaluation Fundamentals: Insights Into Program Effectiveness, Quality, and Value.* 3rd ed. Thousand Oaks, CA: Sage Publications; 2014.

Israel BA, Cummings KM, Dignan MB, et al. Evaluation of health education programs: current assessment and future directions. *Health Education Quarterly.* 1995;22(3):364–389.

Leviton L, Kettel Khan L, Rog D, Dawkins N, Cotton D. Evaluability assessment to improve public health policies, programs and practices. *Annu Rev Public Health.* 2010;31:213–233.

Patton MQ. *Qualitative Evaluation and Research Methods.* 3rd ed. Thousand Oaks, CA: Sage Publications; 2002.

Posavac EJ. *Program Evaluation. Methods and Case Studies.* 8th ed. New York, NY: Routledge; 2016.

Shadish W, Cook T, Campbell D. *Experimental and Quasi-Experimental Designs for Generalized Causal Inference.* Boston, MA: Houghton Mifflin; 2002.

Timmreck TC. *Planning, Program Development, and Evaluation. A Handbook for Health Promotion, Aging and Health Services.* 2nd ed. Boston, MA: Jones and Bartlett Publishers; 2003.

Wholey J, Hatry H, Newcomer K, eds. *Handbook of Practical Program Evaluation.* 4th ed. San Francisco, CA: Jossey-Bass Publishers; 2015.

Selected Websites
American Evaluation Association <http://www.eval.org/p/cm/ld/fid=51>. The American Evaluation Association is an international professional association of evaluators devoted to the application and exploration of program evaluation, personnel evaluation, technology, and many other forms of evaluation.

Centers for Disease Control and Prevention (CDC) Program Performance and Evaluation Office (PPEO) <http://www.cdc.gov/eval/resources/index.htm>. The CDC PPEO has developed a comprehensive list of evaluation documents, tools, and links to other websites. These materials include documents that describe principles and standards, organizations and foundations that support evaluation, a list of journals and online publications, and access to step-by-step manuals.

Community Health Status Indicators (CHSI) Project <http://wwwn.cdc.gov/communityhealth >. The Community Health Status Indicators (CHSI) Project includes 3,141 county health status profiles representing each county in the United States excluding territories. Each CHSI report includes data on access and utilization of health care services, birth and death measures, Healthy People 2020 targets and US birth and death rates, vulnerable populations, risk factors for premature deaths, communicable diseases, and environmental health. The goal of CHSI is to give local public health agencies another tool for improving their community's health by identifying resources and setting priorities.

Community Tool Box <http://ctb.ku.edu/en/>. The Community Tool Box is a global resource for free information on essential skills for building healthy communities. It offers more than 7,000 pages of practical guidance on topics such as leadership, strategic planning, community assessment, advocacy, grant writing, and evaluation. Sections include descriptions of the task, step-by-step guidelines, examples, and training materials.

RE-AIM.org <http://www.re-aim.org/>. With an overall goal of enhancing the quality, speed, and public health impact of efforts to translate research into practice, this site provides an explanation of and resources (e.g., planning tools, measures, self-assessment quizzes, FAQs, comprehensive bibliography) for those wanting to apply the RE-AIM framework.

Research Methods Knowledge Base <http://www.socialresearchmethods.net/kb/>. The Research Methods Knowledge Base is a comprehensive Web-based textbook that covers the entire research process, including formulating research questions; sampling; measurement (surveys, scaling, qualitative, unobtrusive); research design (experimental and quasi-experimental); data analysis; and writing the research paper. It uses an informal, conversational style to engage both the newcomer and the more experienced student of research.

United Nations (UN) Development Programme's Evaluation Office <http://erc.undp.org/index.html>. The UN Development Programme is the UN's global development network, an organization advocating for change and connecting countries to knowledge, experience, and resources to help people build a better life. This site on evaluation includes training tools and a link to their *Handbook on Planning, Monitoring and Evaluating for Development Results*, available in English, Spanish and French. The Evaluation Resource Center allows users to search for evaluations by agency, type of evaluation, region, country, year, and focus area.

W. K. Kellogg Foundation Evaluation Handbook <http://www.wkkf.org/resource-directory/resource/2010/w-k-kellogg-foundation-evaluation-handbook>. The W. K. Kellogg Foundation Evaluation Handbook provides a framework for thinking about evaluation as a relevant and useful program tool. It includes a guide to logic model development, a template for strategic communications, and an overall framework designed for project directors who have evaluation responsibilities.

REFERENCES

1. Porta M, ed. *A Dictionary of Epidemiology*. 6th ed. New York, NY: Oxford University Press; 2014.
2. Creswell J, Plano Clark V. *Designing and Conducting Mixed Methods Research*. 2nd ed. Thousand Oaks, CA: Sage Publications; 2011.
3. Greene J, Benjamin L, Goodyear L. The merits of mixing methods in evaluation. *Evaluation*. 2001;7(1):25–44.

4. Fink A. *Evaluation Fundamentals: Insights Into Program Effectiveness, Quality, and Value.* 2nd ed. Thousand Oaks, CA: Sage Publications; 2015.

5. Newcomer K, Hatry H, Wholey J, eds. *Handbook of Practical Program Evaluation.* 4th ed. San Francisco, CA: Jossey-Bass Publishers; 2015.

6. Patton M. *Qualitative Evaluation and Research Methods.* 4th ed. Thousand Oaks, CA: Sage Publications; 2014.

7. Timmreck TC. *Planning, Program Development, and Evaluation. A Handbook for Health Promotion, Aging and Health Services.* 2nd ed. Boston, MA: Jones and Bartlett Publishers; 2003.

8. Committee on Evaluating Progress of Obesity Prevention Efforts. *Evaluating Obesity Prevention Efforts: A Plan for Measuring Progress.* Washington, DC: Institute of Medicine of The National Academies; 2013.

9. Fetterman DM, Kaftarian SJ, Wandersman A. *Empowerment Evaluation: Knowledge and Tools for Self-Assessment & Accountability.* Thousand Oaks, CA: Sage Publications; 1996.

10. Israel BA, Cummings KM, Dignan MB, et al. Evaluation of health education programs: current assessment and future directions. *Health Education Quarterly.* 1995;22(3):364–389.

11. Lincoln Y, Lynham S, Guba E. Paradigmatic controversies, contradictions, and emerging confluences, revisited. In: Denzin N, Lincoln Y, eds. *Handbook of Qualitative Research.* 4th ed. Thousand Oaks, CA: Sage Publications; 2011:163–188.

12. Rossi PH, Lipsey MW, Freeman HE. *Evaluation: A Systematic Approach.* 7th ed. Thousand Oaks, CA: Sage Publications; 2004.

13. Shadish W, Cook T, Campbell D. *Experimental and Quasi-Experimental Designs for Generalized Causal Inference.* Boston, MA: Houghton Mifflin; 2002.

14. Jack L Jr., Mukhtar Q, Martin M, et al. Program evaluation and chronic diseases: methods, approaches, and implications for public health. *Prev Chronic Dis.* Jan 2006;3(1):A02.

15. Joint Committee on Standards for Educational Evaluation. *Program Evaluation Standards: How to Assess Evaluations of Educational Programs.* 2nd ed. Thousand Oaks, CA: Sage Publications; 1994.

16. Yarbrough D, Shulha L, Hopson R, Caruthers F. *The Program Evaluation Standards: A Guide for Evaluators and Evaluation Users.* 3rd ed. Thousand Oaks, CA: Sage Publications; 2011.

17. Shadish WR. The common threads in program evaluation. *Prev Chronic Dis.* Jan 2006;3(1):A03.

18. Centers for Disease Control and Prevention. Framework for program evaluation in public health. *MMWR.* 1999;48(RR-11):1–40.

19. Arora PG, Krumholz LS, Guerra T, Leff SS. Measuring community-based participatory research partnerships: the initial development of an assessment instrument. *Prog Community Health Partnersh.* Winter 2015;9(4):549–560.

20. Thompson N, Kegler M, Holtgrave D. Program evaluation. In: Crosby R, DiClemente R, Salazar L, eds. *Research Methods in Health Promotion.* San Francisco, CA: Jossey-Bass Publishers; 2006:199–225.

21. Bartholomew L, Parcel G, Kok G, Gottlieb N, Fernandez M. *Planning Health Promotion Programs: An Intervention Mapping Approach.* 3rd ed. San Francisco, CA: Jossey-Bass Publishers; 2011.

22. Centers for Disease Control and Prevention. Behavioral Risk Factor Surveillance System. http://www.cdc.gov/brfss/. Accessed August 30, 2016.

23. Mokdad AH. The Behavioral Risk Factors Surveillance System: past, present, and future. *Annu Rev Public Health*. Apr 29 2009;30:43–54.
24. Pierannunzi C, Hu SS, Balluz L. A systematic review of publications assessing reliability and validity of the Behavioral Risk Factor Surveillance System (BRFSS), 2004-2011. *BMC Med Res Methodol*. 2013;13:49.
25. Nelson DE, Holtzman D, Bolen J, Stanwyck CA, Mack KA. Reliability and validity of measures from the Behavioral Risk Factor Surveillance System (BRFSS). *Soz Praventivmed*. 2001;46(Suppl 1):S3–S42.
26. Kempf AM, Remington PL. New challenges for telephone survey research in the twenty-first century. *Annu Rev Public Health*. 2007;28:113–126.
27. Shenton A. Strategies for ensuring trustworthiness in qualitative research projects. *Education for Information*. 2994;22:63–75.
28. Koepsell TD, Wagner EH, Cheadle AC, et al. Selected methodological issues in evaluating community-based health promotion and disease prevention programs. *Annual Review of Public Health*. 1992;13:31–57.
29. Murray DM, Varnell SP, Blitstein JL. Design and analysis of group-randomized trials: a review of recent methodological developments. *Am J Public Health*. Mar 2004;94(3):423–432.
30. Thompson B, Coronado G, Snipes SA, Puschel K. Methodologic advances and ongoing challenges in designing community-based health promotion programs. *Annu Rev Public Health*. 2003;24:315–340.
31. Murray DM. *Design and Analysis of Group-Randomized Trials*. New York, NY: Oxford University Press; 1998.
32. Murray DM, Pals SL, Blitstein JL, Alfano CM, Lehman J. Design and analysis of group-randomized trials in cancer: a review of current practices. *J Natl Cancer Inst*. Apr 2 2008;100(7):483–491.
33. Yin RK. *Case Study Research: Design and Methods*. 5th ed. Thousand Oaks, CA: Sage Publications; 2014.
34. Noble H, Smith J. Issues of validity and reliability in qualitative research. *Evid Based Nurs*. Apr 2015;18(2):34–35.
35. Economos CD, Curtatone JA. Shaping up Somerville: a community initiative in Massachusetts. *Prev Med*. Jan 2009;50(Suppl 1):S97–S98.
36. Folta SC, Kuder JF, Goldberg JP, et al. Changes in diet and physical activity resulting from the Shape Up Somerville community intervention. *BMC Pediatr*. 2013;13:157.
37. Coffield E, Nihiser AJ, Sherry B, Economos CD. Shape Up Somerville: change in parent body mass indexes during a child-targeted, community-based environmental change intervention. *Am J Public Health*. Feb 2014;105(2):e83–e89.
38. Casey D, Murphy K. Issues in using methodological triangulation in research. *Nurse Res*. 2009;16(4):40–55.
39. Steckler A, McLeroy KR, Goodman RM, Bird ST, McCormick L. Toward integrating qualitative and quantitative methods: an introduction. *Health Education Quarterly*. 1992;19(1):1–8.
40. Brownson RC, Baker EA, Leet TL, Gillespie KN, True WR. *Evidence-Based Public Health*. 2nd ed. New York, NY: Oxford University Press; 2011.
41. Rychetnik L, Hawe P, Waters E, Barratt A, Frommer M. A glossary for evidence based public health. *J Epidemiol Community Health*. Jul 2004;58(7):538–545.
42. Tarquinio C, Kivits J, Minary L, Coste J, Alla F. Evaluating complex interventions: perspectives and issues for health behaviour change interventions. *Psychol Health*. Jan 2015;30(1):35–51.
43. August EM, Hayek S, Casillas D, Wortley P, Collins CB, Jr. Evaluation of the dissemination, implementation, and sustainability of the "Partnership for Health" intervention. *J Public Health Manag Pract*. Oct 19 2015.

44. Guyatt G, Rennie D, Meade M, Cook D, eds. *Users' Guides to the Medical Literature. A Manual for Evidence-Based Clinical Practice.* 3rd ed. Chicago, IL: American Medical Association Press; 2015.

45. Carter N, Bryant-Lukosius D, DiCenso A, Blythe J, Neville AJ. The use of triangulation in qualitative research. *Oncol Nurs Forum.* Sep 2014;41(5):545–547.

46. Leviton LC, Khan LK, Rog D, Dawkins N, Cotton D. Evaluability assessment to improve public health policies, programs, and practices. *Annu Rev Public Health.* Apr 21 2010;31:213–233.

47. Strosberg MA, Wholey JS. Evaluability assessment: from theory to practice in the Department of Health and Human Services. *Public Adm Rev.* Jan-Feb 1983;43(1):66–71.

48. Dwyer JJ, Hansen B, Barrera M, et al. Maximizing children's physical activity: an evaluability assessment to plan a community-based, multi-strategy approach in an ethno-racially and socio-economically diverse city. *Health Promot Int.* Sep 2003;18(3):199–208.

49. Durham J, Gillieatt S, Ellies P. An evaluability assessment of a nutrition promotion project for newly arrived refugees. *Health Promot J Austr.* Apr 2007;18(1):43–49.

50. Basile KC, Lang KS, Bartenfeld TA, Clinton-Sherrod M. Report from the CDC: Evaluability assessment of the rape prevention and education program: summary of findings and recommendations. *J Womens Health (Larchmt).* Apr 2005;14(3):201–207.

51. Trevisan M. Evaluability assessment from 1986 to 2006. *Am J Evaluation.* 2007;28:209–303.

52. Rabin B, Brownson R. Developing the terminology for dissemination and implementation research. In: Brownson R, Colditz G, Proctor E, eds. *Dissemination and Implementation Research in Health: Translating Science to Practice.* New York, NY: Oxford University Press; 2012:23–51.

53. Brownson RC, Jones E. Bridging the gap: translating research into policy and practice. *Prev Med.* Oct 2009;49(4):313–315.

54. Brownson R, Colditz G, Proctor E, eds. *Dissemination and Implementation Research in Health: Translating Science to Practice.* New York, NY: Oxford University Press; 2012.

55. Tabak RG, Khoong EC, Chambers DA, Brownson RC. Bridging research and practice: models for dissemination and implementation research. *Am J Prev Med.* Sep 2012;43(3):337–350.

56. Glasgow RE, Vogt TM, Boles SM. Evaluating the public health impact of health promotion interventions: the RE-AIM framework. *Am J Public Health.* Sep 1999;89(9):1322–1327.

57. Luke DA, Calhoun A, Robichaux CB, Elliott MB, Moreland-Russell S. The Program Sustainability Assessment Tool: a new instrument for public health programs. *Prev Chronic Dis.* 2014;11:130184.

58. Dzewaltowski DA, Estabrooks PA, Klesges LM, Bull S, Glasgow RE. Behavior change intervention research in community settings: how generalizable are the results? *Health Promot Int.* Jun 2004;19(2):235–245.

59. Jilcott S, Ammerman A, Sommers J, Glasgow RE. Applying the RE-AIM framework to assess the public health impact of policy change. *Ann Behav Med.* Sep-Oct 2007;34(2):105–114.

60. Curran GM, Bauer M, Mittman B, Pyne JM, Stetler C. Effectiveness-implementation hybrid designs: combining elements of clinical effectiveness and implementation research to enhance public health impact. *Med Care.* Mar 2012;50(3):217–226.

61. Nitsch M, Waldherr K, Denk E, Griebler U, Marent B, Forster R. Participation by different stakeholders in participatory evaluation of health promotion: a literature review. *Eval Program Plann*. Oct 2013;40:42–54.

62. Cargo M, Mercer SL. The value and challenges of participatory research: strengthening its practice. *Annu Rev Public Health*. Apr 21 2008;29:325–350.

63. Israel BA, Schulz AJ, Parker EA, Becker AB. Review of community-based research: assessing partnership approaches to improve public health. *Annual Review of Public Health*. 1998;19:173–202.

64. Brownson RC, Chriqui JF, Stamatakis KA. Understanding evidence-based public health policy. *Am J Public Health*. Sep 2009;99(9):1576–1583.

65. Howlett M, Ramesh M, Perl A. *Studying Public Policy: Policy Cycles and Policy Subsystems*. 3rd ed. New York, NY: Oxford University Press; 2009.

66. McKinlay JB. Paradigmatic obstacles to improving the health of populations: implications for health policy. *Salud Publica Mex*. Jul-Aug 1998;40(4):369–379.

67. Krieger N. Proximal, distal, and the politics of causation: what's level got to do with it? *Am J Public Health*. Feb 2008;98(2):221–230.

68. Braveman P, Egerter S, Williams DR. The social determinants of health: coming of age. *Annu Rev Public Health*. 2011;32:381–398.

69. Brownson RC, Royer C, Ewing R, McBride TD. Researchers and policymakers: travelers in parallel universes. *Am J Prev Med*. Feb 2006;30(2):164–172.

70. Cockerill R, Myers T, Allman D. Planning for community-based evaluation. *Am J Evaluation*. 2000;21(3):351–357.

71. Grob G. Writing for impact. In: Newcomer K, Hatry H, Wholey J, eds. *Handbook of Practical Program Evaluation*. 4th ed. San Francisco, CA: Jossey-Bass Publishers; 2015:739–764.

72. US Department of Health and Human Services. *Planned Approach to Community Health: Guide for the Local Coordinator*. Atlanta, GA: Centers for Disease Control and Prevention; 1996.

73. Otten JJ, Cheng K, Drewnowski A. Infographics and public policy: using data visualization to convey complex information. *Health Aff (Millwood)*. Nov 2015;34(11):1901–1907.

74. Spiegelhalter D, Pearson M, Short I. Visualizing uncertainty about the future. *Science*. Sep 9 2011;333(6048):1393–1400.

75. Washington University in St. Louis. Creating economic opportunity for low-to-moderate income families in St. Louis. https://forthesakeofall.files.wordpress.com/2014/10/discussion-guide-community-1.pdf. Accessed September 30, 2016.

CHAPTER 12

༝

Opportunities for Advancing Evidence-Based Public Health

Luck is what happens when preparation meets opportunity.
Seneca

Modern society faces a myriad of complex and interrelated public health issues. To take these on in the most effective and efficient manner, we benefit from an evidence-based decision-making process. Although there is a great deal that remains to be learned, the evidence base on effective public health interventions has grown considerably in the past few decades, as has our understanding of how best to implement these initiatives.

Because many public health services are delivered by public health organizations (governmental and nongovernmental), there is growing knowledge on what needs to be in place for health departments to implement evidence-based intiatives.[1] The research base for effectiveness of public health agencies stems largely from practice-based research designed to understand how evidence is (or is not) disseminated and from systems research.[2,3] This work has led to the development of a set of agency (health department) level structures and activities that are positively associated with performance measures (e.g., achieving core public health functions, carrying out evidence-based interventions).[4] Five domains appear to be essential: workforce development, leadership, organizational climate and culture, relationships and partnerships, and financial processes.[4]

It is also essential to keep in mind that as the scientific evidence base grows and new health threats are identified, the process of evidence-based public health (EBPH) needs to take into account broad macro-level forces (so-called forces of change) that affect the physical, economic, policy, and sociocultural environments. Several important forces of change that are currently affecting public health include: the Patient Protection and Affordable Care Act, public health agency accreditation, climate change, Health in All policies initiatives, social media and informatics, demographic transitions, and globalized travel.[5,6] There are numerous ways in which these broad societal changes can be addressed in an EBPH framework (Table 12.1).

This chapter briefly describes an array of opportunities in public health that take into account these broader forces of change, as well as current priorities in public health, the body of available evidence, how the evidence is applied across various settings, and broader forces of change. Although these examples are not exhaustive, they are meant to illustrate the vast array of challenges and opportunities faced by public health practitioners in the coming years.

SHOW ME THE EVIDENCE

Expand the Evidence Base on Intervention Effectiveness

The growing literature on the effectiveness of preventive interventions in clinical and community settings[7,8] does not provide equal coverage of health problems. For example, the evidence base on how to increase immunization levels is much stronger than that for how to prevent poor health outcomes from a natural or human-made disaster. Even when we have interventions of proven effectiveness, the populations in which the interventions have been tested often do not include subpopulations with the greatest disease and injury burden. A greater investment of resources to expand the evidence base is therefore essential. Expanding the base of evidence also requires reliance on well-tested conceptual frameworks, especially those that pay close attention to translation of research to practice.[9,10] For example, RE-AIM helps program planners and evaluators to pay explicit attention to Reach, Efficacy/ Effectiveness, Adoption, Implementation, and Maintenance.[11] Building this evidence base is likely to benefit from greater use of natural experiments, particularly for addressing social and policy determinants of health.[12]

Build the Evidence on External Validity

As described in chapter 1, there are various forms of evidence. Some forms of evidence inform our knowledge about the etiology and prevention of disease.[13] Other data show the relative effectiveness of specific interventions to address a particular health condition. However, what is often missing is a body of evidence that can help to determine the generalizability of effectiveness of an intervention from one population and setting to another[14,15]—that

Table 12.1. FORCES OF CHANGE, THE USE OF EVIDENCE-BASED PUBLIC HEALTH, AND PRACTICE-BASED RESEARCH QUESTIONS[a]

Forces of Change	Example Issues	Using Evidence-Based Public Health (EBPH) or Administrative-Evidence Based Practices (A-EBP) to address Forces of Change	Sample Practice-Based Research Questions
Patient Protection and Affordable Care Act	The requirement of insurance carriers to provide first dollar coverage for primary and secondary preventive services	EBPH: Primary and secondary screening as recommended (level A and B) by the US Preventive Services Task Force	How do funding formulas, payment methods, policy decisions, and community health needs and risks influence the levels of investment made in public health strategies at local, state, and national levels?
Accreditation	The internal focus on quality improvement and performance management	A-EBP: In-service training for quality improvement or evidence-based decision making[4]	How do public health agency accreditation programs influence the effectiveness, efficiency, and outcomes of public health strategies delivered at local, state, and national levels?
Climate change	Emergency risk communication strategies with a special focus on outreach to vulnerable populations	EBPH: Health communication and social marketing: health communication campaigns that include mass media and health-related product distribution; community-based interventions implemented in combination to increase vaccinations in targeted population[8]	How do the content, quality, and timeliness of public health surveillance systems and informatics capabilities influence the effectiveness, efficiency, and outcomes of public health strategies delivered at local, state, and national levels?
Health in All policies	Policy decisions made outside the health sector affect the determinants of health	EBPH: Smoke-free policies in the workplace; promoting health equity in housing programs and policies[8] A-EBP: Build and/or enhance partnerships with schools, hospitals, community organizations, social services, private businesses, universities, law enforcement; a learning orientation with the presence of multidisciplinary, diverse management teams[4]	What conditions and strategies facilitate productive interorganizational relationships and patterns of interaction among organizations that contribute to public health strategies at local, state, and national levels?

(continued)

Table 12.1. CONTINUED

Forces of Change	Example Issues	Using Evidence-Based Public Health (EBPH) or Administrative-Evidence Based Practices (A-EBP) to address Forces of Change	Sample Practice-Based Research Questions
Social media and informatics	The use of social media for health behavior change	EBPH: Social marketing for reducing tobacco use and secondhand smoke exposure; promoting physical activity[8] A-EBP: Access to and free flow of information[4]	How do health information and communication technologies influence the effectiveness, efficiency, and outcomes of public health strategies delivered at local, state, and national levels (e.g., electronic health records, mobile health technologies, social media, electronic surveillance systems, geographic information systems, network analysis, predictive modeling)?
Demographic transitions	Screening and counseling for chronic diseases	EBPH: Interventions utilizing community health workers[8] Healthful diet and physical activity for cardiovascular disease prevention	How do supply-side and demand-side factors affect the racial, ethnic, socioeconomic, and cultural diversity of persons eating a healthy diet?
Globalized travel	Sexual transmission of new or emerging diseases	EBPH: Interventions to reduce sexual risk behaviors or increase protective behaviors[8]	How do the legal powers and duties of governmental public health agencies influence the effectiveness, efficiency, and outcomes of public health strategies delivered at local and state levels?

[a]Adapted from Erwin and Brownson.[6]

is, the core concepts of external validity, as described in chapter 3. The issues in external validity often relate to context for an intervention—for example, "What factors need to be taken into account when an internally valid program or policy is implemented in a different setting or with a different population subgroup?" "How does one balance the concepts of fidelity and reinvention?" If the adaptation process changes the original intervention to such an extent that the original efficacy data may no longer apply, then the program may be viewed as a new intervention under very different contextual conditions. Green has recommended that the implementation of evidence-based approaches requires careful consideration of the "best processes" needed when generalizing evidence to alternate populations, places, and times (e.g., what makes evidence useful).[16]

Consider Evidence Typologies

In reflecting on what works and what is ineffective it becomes apparent that trying to put interventions into these two broad categories (effective vs. ineffective) minimizes the ability of practitioners to discern what is most likely to be effective in their population and context. In addressing this concern several groups have begun to describe different categories of intervention evidence (Type 2), rather than simply indicating that an intervention is or is not "evidence based" (Table 12.2).[17,18] A similar type of typology is applied in the *Using What Works for Health* portal, providing practitioners with a range of evidence-based interventions across levels of evidence.[19] These categories of intervention build on work from Canada, the United Kingdom, Australia, the Netherlands, and the United States on how to recast the strength of evidence, emphasizing the "weight of evidence" and a wider range of considerations beyond efficacy. Although this continuum provides more variability in categorizing interventions, it has been noted that the criteria for assigning an intervention to one category or another often include research design, with randomized designs being weighted as most beneficial. However, adherence to a strict hierarchy of study designs may reinforce an "inverse evidence law" by which interventions most likely to influence whole populations (e.g., policy change) are least valued in an evidence matrix emphasizing randomized designs.[20-22]

Address Mis-Implementation in Public Health Practice

Mis-implementation is a process whereby effective interventions are ended or ineffective interventions are continued in public health settings (i.e., evidence-based decision making is not occurring).[23,24] Various other terms can be used in describing programs ending prematurely, such as de-adoption, termination, and discontinuation.[24] Most of the current literature focuses on overuse and underuse of clinical interventions and the cultural shift needed toward the acceptance of de-adoption within medicine.[25] More than 150 medical practices are deemed ineffective or unsafe.[26] There is sparse literature on mis-implementation in public health practice.

Table 12.2. TYPOLOGY FOR CLASSIFYING INTERVENTIONS BY LEVEL
OF SCIENTIFIC EVIDENCE[a]

Category	How Established	Considerations for Level of Scientific Evidence	Data Source Examples
Effective: 1st tier	Peer review via systematic review	Based on study design and execution External validity Potential side benefits or harms Costs and cost-effectiveness	*Community Guide* Cochrane reviews
Effective: 2nd tier	Peer review	Based on study design and execution External validity Potential side benefits or harms Costs and cost-effectiveness	Articles in the scientific literature Research-Tested Intervention Programs Technical reports with peer review
Promising	Intervention evaluation without formal peer review	Summative evidence of effectiveness Formative evaluation data Theory-consistent, plausible, potentially high-reach, low-cost, replicable	State or federal government reports (without peer review) Conference presentations Case studies
Emerging	Ongoing work, practice-based summaries, or evaluation of works in progress	Formative evaluation data Theory-consistent, plausible, potentially high-reach, low-cost, replicable Face validity	Evaluability assessments[b] Pilot studies NIH RePORTER data base Projects funded by health foundations

NIH = National Institutes of Health.
[a]Adapted from Brennan et al.[17] and Brownson et al.[18]
[b]A "pre-evaluation" activity that involves an assessment is an assessment before commencing an evaluation to establish whether a program or policy can be evaluated and what might be the barriers to its evaluation (also known as exploratory evaluation).

A richer understanding of mis-implementation will help us better allocate already limited resources to be used more efficiently. This knowledge will also allow researchers and practitioners to prevent the continuation of ineffective programs or discontinuation of effective programs. Previous studies have suggested that between 58% and 62% of public health programs are evidence based.[27,28] Even among programs that are evidence based, 37% of programs within state health departments are discontinued when they should continue.[23]

EXTEND THE REACH AND RELEVANCE OF EVIDENCE
Better Address Health Equity

To what degree do specific evidence-based approaches achieve health equity? For many interventions there is not a clear answer to this question. Despite the national goals aimed at eliminating health disparities, there are many areas in which we have not yet met these goals, or even moved in the right direction. For example, in both developed and developing countries, poverty is strongly correlated with poor health outcomes.[29] Yet, data show large and growing differences in disease burden and health outcomes between high- and low-income groups.[30,31] Most of the existing intervention research has been conducted among higher income populations, and programs focusing on elimination of health disparities have often been short-lived.[32] Policy, systems, and environmental interventions hold the potential to influence health determinants more broadly and could significantly reduce the growing disparities across a wide range of health problems.[33] When enough evidence exists, systematic reviews should focus specifically on interventions that show promise in improving health equity.[34-36]

As public health agencies address health equity more fully, numerous challenges exist in setting priorities and measuring progress. To overcome these challenges, innovative approaches are needed, including augmentation of existing population surveys, the use of combined data sets, and the generation of small-area estimates.[37]

Make Evidence More Accessible for Policy Audiences

Evidence becomes more relevant to policymakers when it involves a local example and when the effects are framed in terms of its direct impact on one's local community, family, or constituents.[38] In the policy arena, decision makers indicate that relevance to current debates is a critical factor in determining which research will be used and which proposals will be considered. Research on contextual issues and the importance of narrative communication that presents data in the form of story and helps to personalize issues is beginning to emerge.[39] Policy audiences are also more likely to respond to brief and creative ways for presenting data. For example, approaches to data visualization (e.g., infographics) make complex data more accessible and appealing to stakeholders who are often inundated with information.[40, 41]

Learn from Global Efforts

Nearly every public health issue has a global footprint because diseases do not know borders and shared solutions are needed. This can readily be seen if one lines up goals of the World Health Organization with national health plans. Although it is important to acknowledge that public health challenges in less developed countries are compounded by poverty and hunger, diminished public infrastructure, and the epidemiologic transition to behaviors that pose risks more typically found in higher income countries, EBPH decision making still has applicability. There are, however, few data available on the reach of EBPH across developed and less developed regions of the world. Early findings from a four-country study (Australia, Brazil, China, and the United States) show wide variations in knowledge of EBPH approaches, how that knowledge is developed, and how EBPH-related decisions are made.[42]

As this work develops there are many areas that are likely to lead to advances in EBPH. These could include (1) adapting methods of public health surveillance from one country to another[43]; (2) understanding how to adapt an effective intervention in one geographic region to the context of another geographic region[44,45]; (3) implementing innovative methods for building capacity in EBPH[46]; and (4) identifying effective methods for delivery of health care services in one country that could be applied to another.

WHAT GETS MEASURED GETS DONE
Set Priorities and Measure Progress

Establishing public health and health care priorities in an era of limited resources is a demanding task. The use of the analytic tools discussed in this book can make important contributions to priority setting. Measuring progress toward explicit goals has become an essential feature of goal setting. Global health priorities are set by initiatives such as the Sustainable Development Goals,[47] whereas national benchmarks are offered in strategic plans such as Healthy People 2020.[48] Progress toward both types of objectives can be tracked in periodic reports as long as (1) the resources required to collect these data are available and (2) data needs are aligned with the interventions being implemented at provincial, state, and local levels. Increasingly, these health priorities are focusing on social determinants of health or changes to the physical environment, which often are not tracked in public health surveillance systems.

Improve Surveillance of Policy-Related Variables

Public health surveillance, that is, the ongoing systematic collection, analysis, and interpretation of outcome-specific health data, is a cornerstone of public health.[49] In the United States we now have excellent epidemiologic data for estimating which population groups and which regions of the country are affected by a specific condition and how patterns are changing over time with respect to both acute and chronic conditions. To supplement these data, we need better information on a broad array of environmental and policy factors that determine these patterns. When implemented properly, policy surveillance systems can be an enormous asset for policy development and evaluation. These data allow us to compare progress among states, determine the types of bills that are being introduced and passed (e.g., school nutrition standards, safe routes to school programs), and begin to track progress over time.

BREAK DOWN THE HEALTH SILOS
Address the Tension Between Participatory Decision Making and Evidence-Based Public Health

Participatory approaches are designed to actively involve community-based organizations, governmental agencies, and community members in research and intervention projects.[50-53] These collaborative approaches are promising because they move beyond the "parachute" approach to public health practice and research (whereby community members are simply the objects of study) to one in which a wide variety of partners are actively involved in the process. Yet, there is a potential for tension between participatory approaches and evidence-based decision making. For example, a well-conducted community assessment might lead to a specific set of health-related priorities and intervention approaches (e.g., diabetes, arthritis, suicide, sexually transmitted infections). There may be community support for addressing some of these issues but not others. Moreover, although several of these may have common determinants (e.g., physical activity), there may be funding available for a particular disease (e.g., diabetes) and not others. It is important to develop structures for discussing these issues and weighing the best ways to move forward. Some communities may decide to apply for funds with one group and have another group continue to seek funding for other priority areas. Alternately, the group might support funding in one area, recognizing that addressing common determinants will assist in the prevention of a variety of health issues. Lastly, the assessment might find that there are underlying root causes of these issues, for example, inadequate transportation to resources and support services in a rural community. The community might incorporate policy development or environmental changes in order to develop these infrastructures in a way that they remain in the community beyond the grant funding.

Enhance Transdisciplinary Work Across Sectors and Systems

As illustrated at numerous points in this book, effective approaches to prevention will require attention from many sectors, including government, private industry, and academia.[54] This relates to the growing scholarly work on team science, which is often accomplished through transdisciplinary research. Transdisciplinary research provides valuable opportunities for practice-research collaboration to improve the health and well-being of both individuals and communities.[55-57] For example, tobacco control efforts have been successful in facilitating cooperation among disciplines such as advertising, policy, business, medical science, and behavioral science. Activities within these transdisciplinary tobacco networks try to fill the gaps between scientific discovery and research translation by engaging a wide range of partners. A transdisciplinary approach has also shown some evidence of effectiveness in obesity prevention in Canada.[58,59] As networks to promote public health develop, it will be important to engage new disciplines and organizations. It is particularly important to engage "nontraditional" partners (i.e., those whose mission is not directly focused on health) such as business and industry, local and state departments of transportation, city planners, and local and state media.

DEVELOP MORE EFFECTIVE LEADERS
Engage Leadership

As noted elsewhere in this book, leadership is essential to promote adoption of evidence-based decision making as a core part of public health practice.[60,61] This includes an expectation that decisions will be made on the basis of the best science, needs of the target population, and what will work locally. In some cases additional funding may be required, but in many circumstances not having the will to change (rather than dollars) is the major impediment. Recent practice-based research shows a number of actions from leaders in public health agencies that may increase the use of scientific information in decision making.[62] These actions include direct supervisor expectations for EBPH use and performance evaluation based partially on EBPH principles.[62]

Expand Training Opportunities

In the United States, the core public health workforce is employed in governmental settings, including 59 state and territorial public health agencies, nearly 3,000 local health departments, and many federal agencies (e.g., the Centers for Disease Control and Prevention, Environmental Protection Agency). In developing countries, a significant proportion of the public health workforce is supported by nongovernmental organizations (e.g., the World Health Organization, the United Nations Children's Fund, the World Bank).[63] A large percentage of this workforce has no formal education in public health. Therefore, more practitioner-focused training is needed on the rationale for EBPH, how to select interventions, how to adapt them to particular circumstances, and how to monitor their implementation.[64] As outlined in chapter 1, we would supplement this recommendation by inclusion of EBPH-related competencies.[13] Some training programs show evidence of effectiveness.[27,28,65] The most common format uses didactic sessions, computer labs, and scenario-based exercises, taught by a faculty team with expertise in EBPH. The reach of these training programs can be increased by emphasizing a train-the-trainer approach.[66] Other formats have been used, including Internet-based self-study,[67,68] CD-ROMs,[69] distance and distributed learning networks, and targeted technical assistance. Training programs may have greater impact when delivered by "change agents" who are perceived as experts yet share common characteristics and goals with trainees.[70] A commitment from leadership and staff to lifelong learning is also an essential ingredient for success.[71,72] Because many of the health issues needing urgent attention in local communities will require the involvement of other organizations (e.g., nonprofit groups, hospitals, employers), their participation in EBPH-related training efforts is essential.

Strengthen Academic-Practice Linkages

Another way to enhance capacity and leadership in EBPH and public health more broadly for the public health workforce is through academic-practice partnerships such as the Academic Health Department (AHD). A recent study of Council on Education for Public Health–accredited schools and programs of public health found that of 156 institutions surveyed, 117 completed the survey and 64 (55%) indicated that they had an AHD partnership.[73] The partnerships varied regarding their structure (formal vs. informal; written Memorandum of Understanding vs. not) and types of engagement, and the strongest benefits of such partnerships were clearly for the students involved by improving competencies of students, enhancing career opportunities of public health graduates, and improving public health graduates' preparation to enter the workforce. In addition, these kinds of academic-practice partnerships may address limitations in how evidence is generated for public health practice[74] and enhance the competencies of practitioners in EBPH particularly in the area of community health assessment.

Enhance Effectiveness and Efficiency Through Accreditation

A national voluntary accreditation program for public health agencies was established through the Public Health Accreditation Board (PHAB) in 2007.[75] As an effort to improve both the quality and performance of public health agencies at all levels, the accreditation process is structured around 12 domains. The accreditation process intersects with EBPH on at least three levels. First, the entire process is based on the predication that if a public health agency meets certain standards and measures, quality and performance will be enhanced. The evidence for such a predication, however, is incomplete and often relies on the type of best evidence available that can only be described as sound judgment, based on experience in practice. Second, domain 10 of the PHAB process is "Contribute to and Apply the Evidence Base of Public Health." Third, the prerequisites for accreditation—a community health assessment, a community health improvement plan, and an agency strategic plan—are key elements of EBPH (see chapter 6). As of November 2016, a total of 133 public health departments (141 local health departments, 20 state health departments, and one tribal health agency) had achieved accreditation through PHAB, covering 56% of the US population.[76]

Accreditation appears to confer numerous benefits, including increased transparency, strengthened management processes, and improved ability to identify organizational weaknesses.[77] The accreditation process also provides many opportunities for enhancing EBPH: the actual use of standards and measures presents opportunities to strengthen the evidence-base for accreditation, and, as EBPH evolves, new findings will help inform the refinement of standards and measures over time.

SUMMARY

Prevention was the major contributor to the health gains of the past century, yet it is vastly undervalued.[78] Public health history teaches us that a long "latency period" often exists between the scientific understanding of a viable disease prevention method and its widespread application on a population basis.[79] For example, it has been estimated that it takes 17 years for research to reach practice.[80-82] Many of the approaches to reduce this research-to-practice gap are outlined in this book—these remedies will allow us to expand the evidence base for public health, apply the evidence already in hand, address health equity, and therefore more fully achieve the promise of public health.

KEY CHAPTER POINTS

- The process of evidence-based public health should take into account broad macro-level forces of change that affect the physical, economic, policy, and sociocultural environments.
- New intervention evidence is constantly emerging and there is a need to collect more data on external validity.
- The reach and relevance of evidence is needed to better address health equity, gather more policy-relevant evidence, and learn from global efforts.
- There is need to continue to set priorities, measure progress and expand policy-related surveillance.
- Continued efforts are needed to break downs silos in public health and enhance contributions of disciplines that cross sectors.
- Emphasis is needed on leadership development to enhance EBPH that can be aided via practice-academic linkages and accreditation.

SUGGESTED READINGS AND SELECTED WEBSITES
Suggested Readings

Brownson RC, Allen P, Jacob RR, et al. Understanding mis-implementation in public health practice. *Am J Prev Med.* May 2015;48(5):543–551.

Burchett HE, Mayhew SH, Lavis JN, Dobrow MJ. When can research from one setting be useful in another? Understanding perceptions of the applicability and transferability of research. *Health Promot Int.* Sep 2012;28(3):418–430.

Erwin P, Brownson R. Macro trends and the future of public health practice. *Annu Rev Public Health.* 2016; Dec 15. [Epub ahead of print]

Fielding J, Kumanyika S. Recommendations for the concepts and form of Healthy People 2020. *Am J Prev Med.* Sep 2009;37(3):255–257.

Freudenberg N, Franzosa E, Chisholm J, Libman K. New approaches for moving upstream: how state and local health departments can transform practice to reduce health inequalities. *Health Educ Behav.* Apr 2015;42(1 Suppl):46S–56S.

Green LW. From research to "best practices" in other settings and populations. *Am J Health Behav.* 2001;25(3):165–178.

McGinnis JM. Does proof matter? Why strong evidence sometimes yields weak action. *Am J Health Promot.* May-Jun 2001;15(5):391–396.

Otten JJ, Cheng K, Drewnowski A. Infographics and public policy: using data visualization to convey complex information. *Health Aff (Millwood).* Nov 2015;34(11):1901–1907.

Selected Websites
Global Health Council <http://www.globalhealth.org/>. The Global Health Council is the world's largest membership alliance dedicated to saving lives by improving health throughout the world. Its diverse membership comprises health care

professionals and organizations that include nongovernmental organizations, foundations, corporations, government agencies, and academic institutions. This website provides policy briefs, research briefs, fact sheets, and roundtable discussions on many topics.

Kaiser Family Foundation <http://www.kff.org/>. The Kaiser Family Foundation (not associated with Kaiser Permanente or Kaiser Industries) is a nonprofit, private foundation that focuses on the major health care issues facing the United States and on the US role in global health policy. It compiles and presents public data and also develops its own research. Intended audiences are policymakers, the media, and the general public, and data are easily accessible. Links provide comparable data for American states (www.statehealthfacts.org) and for countries (www.globalhealthfacts.org).

National Conference of State Legislatures (NCSL) <http://www.ncsl.org/>. The NCSL is a bipartisan organization that serves the legislators and staffs of the nation's 50 states, its commonwealths, and its territories. NCSL provides research, technical assistance, and opportunities for policymakers to exchange ideas on the most pressing state issues. The NCSL site provides information about each state's governing bodies as well as bill summaries, reports, and databases on numerous public health policy topics.

Public Health Accreditation Board (PHAB) < http://www.phaboard.org/>. The PHAB is a nonprofit organization that handles the voluntary accreditation process for public health agencies (i.e., state and territorial health departments, centralized states, local health departments, multijurisdictional departments, and tribal health departments). The goal of this accreditation is to improve and protect the health of the public by assuring practice-focused and evidence-based standards.

RE-AIM.org <http://www.re-aim.org/>. With an overall goal of enhancing the quality, speed, and public health impact of efforts to translate research into practice, this site provides an explanation of and resources (e.g., planning tools, measures, self-assessment quizzes, FAQs, comprehensive bibliography) for those wanting to apply the RE-AIM framework.

Research-Tested Intervention Programs (RTIPS) <http://rtips.cancer.gov/rtips/index.do>. At this site, the National Cancer Institute translates research-tested intervention programs. Program materials are available to order or download, and the site provides details of an intervention such as the time required, suitable settings, and the required resources.

Using What Works: Adapting Evidence-Based Programs to Fit Your Needs <http://cancercontrol.cancer.gov/use_what_works/start.htm>. The National Cancer Institute provides a train-the-trainer course designed to teach health promoters how to adapt evidence-based programs to their local communities. Materials describe how to conduct a needs assessment and how to find, adapt, and evaluate evidence-based programs.

What Works for Health
<http://www.countyhealthrankings.org/roadmaps/what-works-for-health>. What Works for Health is a component of the Robert Wood Johnson Foundation's County Health Rankings and Roadmaps. This site provides information on choosing evidence-informed policies, programs, and system changes known to improve factors related to health. These factors come from four general categories: Health Behaviors, Clinical Care, Social and Economic Factors, and Physical Environment.

World Health Organization <http://www.who.int/en/>. The World Health Organization (WHO) is the directing and coordinating authority for health within the United

Nations system. It is responsible for providing leadership on global health matters, shaping the health research agenda, setting norms and standards, articulating evidence-based policy options, providing technical support to countries, and monitoring and assessing health trends. From this site, one can access *The World Health Report*, WHO's leading publication that provides an expert assessment on global health with a focus on a specific subject each year.

REFERENCES

1. Allen P, Brownson R, Duggan K, Stamatakis K, Erwin P. The makings of an evidence-based local health department: identifying administrative and management practices. *Frontiers in Public Health Services & Systems Research.* 2012;1(2).
2. Brownson R, Colditz G, Proctor E, eds. *Dissemination and Implementation Research in Health: Translating Science to Practice.* New York, NY: Oxford University Press; 2012.
3. Mays GP, Scutchfield FD. Advancing the science of delivery: public health services and systems research. *J Public Health Manag Pract.* Nov 2012;18(6):481–484.
4. Brownson RC, Allen P, Duggan K, Stamatakis KA, Erwin PC. Fostering more-effective public health by identifying administrative evidence-based practices: a review of the literature. *Am J Prev Med.* Sep 2012;43(3):309–319.
5. Erwin PC, Harris JK, Smith C, Leep CJ, Duggan K, Brownson RC. Evidence-based public health practice among program managers in local public health departments. *J Public Health Manag Pract.* Sep-Oct 2014;20(5):472–480.
6. Erwin P, Brownson R. Macro trends and the future of public health practice. *Annu Rev Public Health.* 2016; Dec 15. [Epub ahead of print].
7. Agency for Healthcare Research and Quality. Guide to Clinical Preventive Services, 2014. 3rd. http://www.ahrq.gov/professionals/clinicians-providers/guidelines-recommendations/guide/index.html. Accessed October 12, 2016.
8. Task Force on Community Preventive Services. Guide to Community Preventive Services. www.thecommunityguide.org. Accessed June 5, 2016.
9. Nilsen P. Making sense of implementation theories, models and frameworks. *Implement Sci.* 2015;10(1):53.
10. Tabak RG, Khoong EC, Chambers DA, Brownson RC. Bridging research and practice: models for dissemination and implementation research. *Am J Prev Med.* Sep 2012;43(3):337–350.
11. Glasgow RE, Vogt TM, Boles SM. Evaluating the public health impact of health promotion interventions: the RE-AIM framework. *Am J Public Health.* Sep 1999;89(9):1322–1327.
12. Petticrew M, Cummins S, Ferrell C, et al. Natural experiments: an underused tool for public health? *Public Health.* Sep 2005;119(9):751–757.
13. Brownson RC, Baker EA, Leet TL, Gillespie KN, True WR. *Evidence-Based Public Health.* 2nd ed. New York, NY: Oxford University Press; 2011.
14. Burchett H, Umoquit M, Dobrow M. How do we know when research from one setting can be useful in another? A review of external validity, applicability and transferability frameworks. *J Health Serv Res Policy.* Oct 2011;16(4):238–244.
15. Burchett HE, Mayhew SH, Lavis JN, Dobrow MJ. When can research from one setting be useful in another? Understanding perceptions of the applicability and transferability of research. *Health Promot Int.* Sep 2012;28(3):418–430.

16. Green LW. From research to "best practices" in other settings and populations. *Am J Health Behav*. 2001;25(3):165–178.

17. Brennan L, Castro S, Brownson RC, Claus J, Orleans CT. Accelerating evidence reviews and broadening evidence standards to identify effective, promising, and emerging policy and environmental strategies for prevention of childhood obesity. *Annu Rev Public Health*. Apr 21 2011;32:199–223.

18. Brownson RC, Fielding JE, Maylahn CM. Evidence-based public health: a fundamental concept for public health practice. *Annu Rev Public Health*. Apr 21 2009;30:175–201.

19. University of Wisconsin Population Health Institute. Using What Works for Health. http://www.countyhealthrankings.org/roadmaps/what-works-for-health/using-what-works-health. Accessed July 28, 2016.

20. Nutbeam D. How does evidence influence public health policy? Tackling health inequalities in England. *Health Promot J Aust*. 2003;14:154–158.

21. Ogilvie D, Egan M, Hamilton V, Petticrew M. Systematic reviews of health effects of social interventions: 2. Best available evidence: how low should you go? *J Epidemiol Community Health*. Oct 2005;59(10):886–892.

22. Kessler R, Glasgow RE. A proposal to speed translation of healthcare research into practice: dramatic change is needed. *Am J Prev Med*. Jun 2011;40(6):637–644.

23. Brownson RC, Allen P, Jacob RR, et al. Understanding mis-implementation in public health practice. *Am J Prev Med*. May 2015;48(5):543–551.

24. Gnjidic D, Elshaug AG. De-adoption and its 43 related terms: harmonizing low-value care terminology. *BMC Med*. 2015;13:273.

25. Gunderman RB, Seidenwurm DJ. De-adoption and un-diffusion. *J Am Coll Radiol*. Nov 2015;12(11):1162–1163.

26. Prasad V, Ioannidis JP. Evidence-based de-implementation for contradicted, unproven, and aspiring healthcare practices. *Implement Sci*. 2014;9:1.

27. Dreisinger M, Leet TL, Baker EA, Gillespie KN, Haas B, Brownson RC. Improving the public health workforce: evaluation of a training course to enhance evidence-based decision making. *J Public Health Manag Pract*. Mar-Apr 2008;14(2):138–143.

28. Gibbert WS, Keating SM, Jacobs JA, et al. Training the workforce in evidence-based public health: an evaluation of impact among US and international practitioners. *Prev Chronic Dis*. 2013;10:E148.

29. Subramanian SV, Belli P, Kawachi I. The macroeconomic determinants of health. *Annu Rev Public Health*. 2002;23:287–302.

30. Ezzati M, Friedman AB, Kulkarni SC, Murray CJ. The reversal of fortunes: trends in county mortality and cross-county mortality disparities in the United States. *PLoS Med*. Apr 22 2008;5(4):e66.

31. Kulkarni SC, Levin-Rector A, Ezzati M, Murray CJ. Falling behind: life expectancy in US counties from 2000 to 2007 in an international context. *Popul Health Metr*. Jun 15 2011;9(1):16.

32. Shaya FT, Gu A, Saunders E. Addressing cardiovascular disparities through community interventions. *Ethn Dis*. Winter 2006;16(1):138–144.

33. Freudenberg N, Franzosa E, Chisholm J, Libman K. New approaches for moving upstream: how state and local health departments can transform practice to reduce health inequalities. *Health Educ Behav*. Apr 2015;42(1 Suppl):46S–56S.

34. Masi CM, Blackman DJ, Peek ME. Interventions to enhance breast cancer screening, diagnosis, and treatment among racial and ethnic minority women. *Med Care Res Rev*. Oct 2007;64(5 Suppl):195S–242S.

35. Peek ME, Cargill A, Huang ES. Diabetes health disparities: a systematic review of health care interventions. *Med Care Res Rev.* Oct 2007;64(5 Suppl):101S–156S.

36. Petticrew M, Roberts H. Systematic reviews: do they "work" in informing decision-making around health inequalities? *Health Econ Policy Law.* Apr 2008;3(Pt 2):197–211.

37. Shah SN, Russo ET, Earl TR, Kuo T. Measuring and monitoring progress toward health equity: local challenges for public health. *Prev Chronic Dis.* 2014;11:E159.

38. Jones E, Kreuter M, Pritchett S, Matulionis RM, Hann N. State health policy makers: what's the message and who's listening? *Health Promot Pract.* Jul 2006;7(3):280–286.

39. Stamatakis K, McBride T, Brownson R. Communicating prevention messages to policy makers: the role of stories in promoting physical activity. *J Phys Act Health.* 2010;7(Suppl 1):S00–S107.

40. Otten JJ, Cheng K, Drewnowski A. Infographics and public policy: using data visualization to convey complex information. *Health Aff (Millwood).* Nov 2015;34(11):1901–1907.

41. Spiegelhalter D, Pearson M, Short I. Visualizing uncertainty about the future. *Science.* Sep 9 2011;333(6048):1393–1400.

42. deRuyter A, Ying X, Budd E, et al. Implementing evidence-based practices to prevent chronic disease: knowledge, knowledge acquisition, and decision-making across four countries. *9th Annual Conference on the Science of Dissemination and Implementation.* Washington, DC: NIH; 2016.

43. Schmid T, Zabina H, McQueen D, Glasunov I, Potemkina R. The first telephone-based health survey in Moscow: building a model for behavioral risk factor surveillance in Russia. *Soz Praventivmed.* 2005;50(1):60–62.

44. Cuijpers P, de Graaf I, Bohlmeijer E. Adapting and disseminating effective public health interventions in another country: towards a systematic approach. *Eur J Public Health.* Apr 2005;15(2):166–169.

45. Cambon L, Minary L, Ridde V, Alla F. Transferability of interventions in health education: a review. *BMC Public Health.* Jul 02 2012;12:497.

46. Diem G, Brownson RC, Grabauskas V, Shatchkute A, Stachenko S. Prevention and control of noncommunicable diseases through evidence-based public health: implementing the NCD 2020 action plan. *Glob Health Promot.* Sep 2016;23(3):5–13.

47. World Health Organization. The Sustainable Development Goals 2015–2030. http://una-gp.org/the-sustainable-development-goals-2015-2030/. Accessed October 8, 2016.

48. Fielding J, Kumanyika S. Recommendations for the concepts and form of Healthy People 2020. *Am J Prev Med.* Sep 2009;37(3):255–257.

49. Thacker SB, Berkelman RL. Public health surveillance in the United States. *Epidemiol Rev.* 1988;10:164–190.

50. Green LW, George MA, Daniel M, et al. *Review and Recommendations for the Development of Participatory Research in Health Promotion in Canada.* Vancouver, British Columbia: The Royal Society of Canada; 1995.

51. Israel BA, Schulz AJ, Parker EA, Becker AB. Review of community-based research: assessing partnership approaches to improve public health. *Annual Review of Public Health.* 1998;19:173–202.

52. Cargo M, Mercer SL. The value and challenges of participatory research: Strengthening its practice. *Annu Rev Public Health.* Apr 21 2008; 29:325–350.

53. Minkler M, Salvatore A. Participatory approaches for study design and analysis in dissemination and implementation research. In: Brownson R, Colditz G, Proctor E, eds. *Dissemination and Implementation Research in Health: Translating Science to Practice*. New York, NY: Oxford University Press; 2012:192–212.

54. Haire-Joshu D, McBride T, eds. *Transdisciplinary Public Health: Research, Education, and Practice*. San Francisco, CA: Jossey-Bass Publishers; 2013.

55. Harper GW, Neubauer LC, Bangi AK, Francisco VT. Transdisciplinary research and evaluation for community health initiatives. *Health Promot Pract*. Oct 2008;9(4):328–337.

56. Stokols D. Toward a science of transdisciplinary action research. *Am J Community Psychol*. Sep 2006;38(1–2):63–77.

57. Hall KL, Vogel AL, Stipelman B, Stokols D, Morgan G, Gehlert S. A four-phase model of transdisciplinary team-based research: goals, team processes, and strategies. *Transl Behav Med*. Dec 1 2013;2(4):415–430.

58. Byrne S, Wake M, Blumberg D, Dibley M. Identifying priority areas for longitudinal research in childhood obesity: Delphi technique survey. *Int J Pediatr Obes*. 2008;3(2):120–122.

59. Russell-Mayhew S, Scott C, Stewart M. The Canadian Obesity Network and interprofessional practice: members' views. *J Interprof Care*. Mar 2008;22(2):149–165.

60. Brownson RC, Reis RS, Allen P, et al. Understanding administrative evidence-based practices: findings from a survey of local health department leaders. *Am J Prev Med*. Jan 2013;46(1):49–57.

61. Bekemeier B, Grembowski D, Yang Y, Herting JR. Leadership matters: local health department clinician leaders and their relationship to decreasing health disparities. *J Public Health Manag Pract*. Mar 2012;18(2):E1–E10.

62. Jacob R, Allen P, Ahrendt L, Brownson R. Learning about and using research evidence among public health practitioners. *Am J Prev Med*. 2017;52(3S3):S304–S308.

63. International Medical Volunteers Association. The Major International Health Organizations. http://www.imva.org/pages/orgfrm.htm. Accessed November 23, 2016.

64. Centers for Disease Control and Prevention. *Modernizing the Workforce for the Public's Health: Shifting the Balance. Public Health Workforce Summit Report* Atlanta, GA: CDC; 2013.

65. Maylahn C, Bohn C, Hammer M, Waltz E. Strengthening epidemiologic competencies among local health professionals in New York: teaching evidence-based public health. *Public Health Rep*. 2008;123(Suppl 1):35–43.

66. Yarber L, Brownson CA, Jacob RR, et al. Evaluating a train-the-trainer approach for improving capacity for evidence-based decision making in public health. *BMC Health Serv Res*. 2015;15(1):547.

67. Linkov F, LaPorte R, Lovalekar M, Dodani S. Web quality control for lectures: Supercourse and Amazon.com. *Croat Med J*. Dec 2005;46(6):875–878.

68. Maxwell ML, Adily A, Ward JE. Promoting evidence-based practice in population health at the local level: a case study in workforce capacity development. *Aust Health Rev*. Aug 2007;31(3):422–429.

69. Brownson RC, Ballew P, Brown KL, et al. The effect of disseminating evidence-based interventions that promote physical activity to health departments. *Am J Public Health*. Oct 2007;97(10):1900–1907.

70. Proctor EK. Leverage points for the implementation of evidence-based practice. *Brief Treatment and Crisis Intervention*. Sep 2004;4(3):227–242.

71. Chambers LW. The new public health: do local public health agencies need a booster (or organizational "fix") to combat the diseases of disarray? *Can J Public Health*. Sep-Oct 1992;83(5):326–328.

72. St Leger L. Schools, health literacy and public health: possibilities and challenges. *Health Promot Int*. Jun 2001;16(2):197–205.

73. Erwin PC, Harris J, Wong R, Plepys CM, Brownson RC. The Academic Health Department: academic-practice partnerships among accredited U.S. schools and programs of public health, 2015. *Public Health Rep*. Jul-Aug 2016;131(4):630–636.

74. Brownson RC, Diez Roux AV, Swartz K. Commentary: generating rigorous evidence for public health: the need for new thinking to improve research and practice. *Annu Rev Public Health*. 2014;35:1–7.

75. Bender K, Halverson PK. Quality improvement and accreditation: what might it look like? *J Public Health Manag Pract*. Jan-Feb 2010;16(1):79–82.

76. Public Health Accreditation Board. Public Health Accreditation Board Standards and Measures, version 1.5. 2013. http://www.phaboard.org/wp-content/uploads/SM-Version-1.5-Board-adopted-FINAL-01-24-2014.docx.pdf. Accessed November 20, 2016.

77. Kronstadt J, Meit M, Siegfried A, Nicolaus T, Bender K, Corso L. Evaluating the Impact of National Public Health Department Accreditation— United States, 2016. *MMWR Morb Mortal Wkly Rep*. Aug 12 2016;65(31):803–806.

78. McGinnis JM. Does proof matter? why strong evidence sometimes yields weak action. *Am J Health Promot*. May-Jun 2001;15(5):391–396.

79. Brownson RC, Bright FS. Chronic disease control in public health practice: looking back and moving forward. *Public Health Rep*. May-Jun 2004;119(3):230–238.

80. Balas EA. From appropriate care to evidence-based medicine. *Pediatr Ann*. Sep 1998;27(9):581–584.

81. Green LW, Ottoson JM, Garcia C, Hiatt RA. Diffusion theory, and knowledge dissemination, utilization, and integration in public health. *Annu Rev Public Health*. Jan 15 2009;30:151–174.

82. Westfall JM, Mold J, Fagnan L. Practice-based research—"blue highways" on the NIH roadmap. *JAMA*. Jan 24 2007;297(4):403–406.

GLOSSARY

Action planning: Planning for a specific program or policy with specific, time-dependent outcomes.

Adaptation: The degree to which an evidence-based intervention is changed or modified by a user during adoption and implementation to suit the needs of the setting or to improve the fit to local conditions.

Adjusted rates: Rate in which the crude (unadjusted) rate has been standardized to some external reference population (e.g., an age-adjusted rate of lung cancer). An adjusted rate is often useful when comparing rates over time or for populations (e.g., by age, gender, race) in different geographic areas.

Advocacy: Set of skills that can be used to create a shift in public opinion and mobilize the necessary resources and forces to support an issue. Advocacy blends science and politics in a social-justice value orientation with the goal of making the system work better, particularly for individuals and populations with the least resources.

Analytic epidemiology: Study designed to examine associations, commonly putative or hypothesized causal relationships. An analytic study is usually concerned with identifying or measuring the effects of risk factors or is concerned with the health effects of specific exposures.

Analytic framework: (causal framework, logic model) Diagram that depicts the inter relationships among population characteristics, intervention components, shorter-term intervention outcomes, and longer-term public health outcomes. Its purpose is to map out the linkages on which to base conclusions about intervention effectiveness. Similar frameworks are also used in program planning to assist in designing, implementing, and evaluating effective interventions.

Basic priority rating (BPR): A method of prioritizing health issues based on the size of the problem, the seriousness of the problem, the effectiveness of intervention, and its propriety, economics, acceptability, resources, and legality (known as PEARL).

Capacity building: The intentional, coordinated and mission-driven efforts aimed at strengthening the management and governance of public health agencies to improve their performance and impact.

Case-control study: Method of study in which persons with the disease (or other condition) of interest are compared with a suitable control group of persons without the disease. The relationship of an attribute to the disease is examined by comparing the diseased and nondiseased with regard to how frequently the attribute is present. Risk is estimated by the odds ratio.

Category-specific rates: Rates that characterize patterns of disease by person, place, or time for a defined population.

Causality: Relationship of causes to the effects they produce. A cause is termed "necessary" when it must always precede an effect (e.g., HIV exposure is necessary for AIDS to occur). This effect need not be the sole result of the one cause. A cause is termed "sufficient" when it inevitably initiates or produces an effect. A disease may have more than one sufficient cause (e.g., smoking, asbestos exposure, and aging may be sufficient causes for lung cancer). Any given causal factor may be necessary, sufficient, neither, or both.

Causal framework: See Analytic framework, logic model.

Changeability: Likelihood that a risk factor or behavior can be altered by a public health program or policy.

Coalition: Group of individuals and/or organizations that join together for a common purpose.

Cohort study: Method of study in which subsets of a defined population can be identified by those who are, have been, or in the future may be exposed or not exposed, or exposed in different degrees, to a factor or factors hypothesized to influence the probability of occurrence of a given disease or other outcome. The main feature of a cohort study is observation of large numbers over a long period (commonly years) with comparison of incidence rates in groups that differ in exposure levels. Risk is estimated by the relative risk.

Community: Group of people with diverse characteristics who are linked by social ties, share common perspectives, and engage in joint action in geographical locations or settings.

Confounding bias: An error that distorts the estimated effect of an exposure on an outcome, caused by the presence of an extraneous factor associated with both the exposure and the outcome.

Consensus conference: Mechanism commonly used to review epidemiologic evidence in which expert panels convene to develop recommendations, usually within a period of a few days.

Context or setting: Surroundings within which a health issue occurs, including assessment of the social, cultural, economic, political, and physical environment.

Cost-benefit analysis: Economic analysis that converts effects into the same monetary terms as the costs and compares them, yielding a measure of net benefits or a cost-benefit ratio. Lower cost-benefit ratios and higher net benefits are desirable.

Cost-effectiveness analysis: An economic analysis in which the total costs of an intervention are measured in monetary terms and then compared with the health outcomes (such as lives saved or cases detected) achieved by the intervention to yield a cost-effectiveness ratio. Lower ratios are preferred.

Cost-minimization analysis: Economic analysis in which the costs of different programs with equivalent benefits are compared, to determine the least costly alternative. The requirement of equal benefits among the programs compared severely limits its usefulness.

Cost-utility analysis: Economic analysis that converts benefits into a preference-based measure of health-related quality of life and compares this to the costs of the program to determine a cost-utility ratio, such as cost per additional quality-adjusted life-year. Lower ratios are preferred. Cost-utility analysis is sometimes considered a subset of cost-effectiveness analysis.

Cross-sectional studies: Method of study in which the presence or absence of a disease and the presence or absence of other variables are determined in each member of the study population or in a representative sample at one particular time.

Crude (unadjusted) rate: Rate that represents the actual frequency of disease in a defined population for a specified period.

Decision analysis: Technique used under conditions of uncertainty for systematically representing and examining all the relevant information for a decision and the uncertainty around that information. The available choices are plotted on a decision tree. At each branch, or decision node, each outcome and its probability of occurrence are listed.

Delphi method: Iterative circulation to a panel of experts of questions and responses that are progressively refined in light of responses to each round of questions; preferably, participants' identities should not be revealed to each other. The aim is to reduce the number of viable options or solutions, perhaps to arrive at a consensus judgment on an issue or problem, or a set of issues or problems, without allowing anyone to dominate the process. The method was originally developed at the RAND Corporation.

Descriptive epidemiology: Study of the occurrence of disease or other health-related characteristics in human populations. General observations are often made concerning the relationship of disease to basic characteristics such as age, sex, race, social class, geographic location, or time. The major characteristics in descriptive epidemiology can be classified under the headings of person, place, and time.

Determinant of health: Factor associated with or which influences a health outcome. Determinants include social, cultural, environmental, economic, behavioral, biological, and other factors.

Direct costs: All costs necessary to directly conduct an intervention or program. Include supplies, overhead, and labor costs, often measured by the number of full-time equivalent employees (FTEs) and their wages and fringe benefits.

Discounting: Conversion of amounts (usually currency) received over different periods to a common value in the current period, with the goal of determining the current payments that would be equal in value to distant payments.

Dissemination: Process of communicating either the procedures or the lessons learned from a study or program evaluation to relevant audiences in a timely, unbiased, and consistent fashion.

Distal outcomes: Long-term changes in morbidity and mortality.

Ecological framework: Model relating individual, interpersonal, organizational, community (including social and economic factors), and health policy factors to individual behavior change and their direct effect on health.

Economic evaluation: Analysis of the costs and benefits of a program or intervention, using existing or prospective data to determine the additional cost per additional unit of benefit.

Environmental assessment: Analysis of the political, economic, social, and technological contexts as part of the strategic planning process.

Epidemiology: Study of the health and illness of populations and the application of findings to improve community health.

Evaluation: Process that attempts to systematically and objectively determine the relevance, effectiveness, and impact of activities in the light of their objectives.

Evaluation designs: The qualitative and quantitative methods used to evaluate a program that may include both experimental and quasi-experimental studies.

Evidence-based medicine: Conscientious, explicit, and judicious use of current best evidence in making decisions about the care of individual patients. The practice of evidence-based medicine means integrating individual clinical expertise with the best available external clinical evidence from systematic research.

Evidence-based public health: The process of integrating science-based interventions with community preferences to improve the health of populations.

Evidence-informed decision making: The process of distilling and disseminating the best available evidence from research, practice and experience and using that evidence to inform and improve public health policy and practice.

Experimental study design: Study in which the investigator has full control over the allocations and/or timing of the interventions. The ability to allocate individuals or groups randomly is a common requirement of an experimental study.

Expert panel: Group of individuals who provide scientific peer review of the quality of the science and scientific interpretations that underlie public health recommendations, regulations, and policy decisions.

External validity: Study is externally valid, or generalizable, if it can produce unbiased inferences regarding a target population (beyond the subjects in the study). This aspect of validity is only meaningful with regard to a specified external target population.

Formative evaluation: Type of evaluation conducted in the early stages of an intervention to determine whether an element of a program or policy (e.g., materials, messages) is feasible, appropriate, and meaningful for the target population.

"Fugitive" literature ("grey" literature): Government reports, book chapters, the proceedings of conferences, and published dissertations that are therefore difficult to retrieve.

Guide to Clinical Preventive Services: Set of guidelines, published by the U.S. Preventive Services Task Force, that document the effectiveness of a variety of clinic-based interventions in public health through systematic review and evaluation of scientific evidence.

Guide to Community Preventive Services: Systematic Reviews and Evidence-Based Recommendations (the Community Guide): Set of guidelines, published by the Task Force on Community Preventive Services and supported by the Centers for Disease Control and Prevention (CDC), that summarize what is known about the effectiveness and cost-effectiveness of population-based interventions designed to promote health and prevent disease, injury, disability, and premature death, as well as to reduce exposure to environmental hazards.

Guidelines: Standardized set of information based on scientific evidence of the effectiveness and efficiency of the best practices for addressing health problems commonly encountered in public health or clinical practice. Where such evidence is lacking, guidelines are sometimes based on the consensus opinions of experts.

Health Belief Model: Value expectancy theory stating that individuals will take action to ward off, screen for, or control an ill-health condition if they regard themselves as susceptible to the condition, believe it to have potentially serious consequences, believe that a course of action available to them would be beneficial in reducing either their susceptibility to or the severity of the condition, and believe that the anticipated barriers to (or costs of) taking the action are outweighed by its benefits.

Health disparities: Inequalities in health indicators (such as infant mortality rates and life expectancy) that are observed among subpopulations. Health disparities often correlate with socioeconomic status.

Health equity: Exists when individuals have equal opportunities to be health; often associated with social determinants, race, ethnicity, gender, sexual identity.

Health impact assessment: Type of analysis requiring screening, scoping, appraisal, reporting, and monitoring to measure the effect of a nonhealth intervention on the health of a community.

Health indicator: Variable, susceptible to direct measurement, that reflects the state of health of persons in a community. Examples include infant mortality rates, incidence rates based on notifiable cases of disease, and disability days.

Impact evaluation: Assessment of whether intermediate objectives of an intervention have been achieved. Indicators may include changes in knowledge, attitudes, behavior, or risk-factor prevalence.

Incidence: Number of new cases of a disease.

Incidence rate: Occurrence of new cases of disease in a specific time period over the person-time for the population; reflects the true rate of disease occurrence.

Indirect costs: Expenses that are not directly linked to an intervention but are incurred by providers, participants, or other parties. In cost-utility analysis, these include time and travel costs to participants, averted treatment costs (future treatment costs that will be saved as a result of the intervention), and costs of treating side effects.

Information bias: Systematic error in measuring exposures or outcomes that affects the accuracy of information between study groups.

Intermediate measure ("upstream" measure): Short-term outcome most directly associated with an intervention, often measured in terms of knowledge, attitudes, or behavior change.

Internal validity: Degree to which the inference drawn from a study is warranted when account is taken of the study methods, the representativeness of the study sample, and the nature of the population from which it is drawn. Index and comparison groups are selected and compared in such a manner that the observed differences between them on the dependent variables under study may, apart from sampling error, be attributed only to the hypothesized effect under investigation.

Logic model: See Analytic framework, causal model.

Management: Process of constructing, implementing, and monitoring organized responses to a health problem or a series of interrelated health problems.

MATCH (the Multilevel Approach to Community Health): Conceptual and practical intervention planning model. MATCH consists of five phases: health goals selection, intervention planning, development, implementation, and evaluation.

Media advocacy: Advocacy that involves strategic use of the mass media in reaching policy, program, or educational goals.

Member validation: Process by which the preliminary results and interpretations are presented back to those who provided the evaluation data.

Meta-analysis: Systematic, quantitative method for combining information from multiple studies in order to derive a meaningful answer to a specific question.

Mixed methods evaluation: An approach for colleting, analyzing, and mixing both quantitative and qualitative data in a single study or series of studies to understand an evaluation problem.

Multiple linear regression: Mathematical modeling technique that finds the best linear model that relates given data on a dependent variable y to one or several independent variables x_1, x_2, etc. Other common regression models in epidemiology are the logistic and proportional hazards models.

Natural experiment: Study or evaluation design that generally takes the form of an observational study in which the researcher cannot control or withhold the allocation of an intervention to particular areas or communities but where natural or predetermined variation in allocation occurs. A common natural experiment would study the effects of the enactment of a policy on health status.

Needs assessment: Systematic procedure that makes use of epidemiologic, sociodemographic, and qualitative methods to determine the nature and extent of health problems, experienced by a specified population, and their environmental, social, economic, and behavioral determinants. The aim is to identify unmet health care needs and preventive opportunities.

Nominal group technique: Structured, small-group process designed to achieve consensus. Individuals respond to questions and then are asked to prioritize ideas as they are presented.

Objectivity: Ability to be unaffected by personal biases, politics, history, or other external factors.

Observational study design: Study that does not involve any intervention, experimental or otherwise. Such a study may be one in which nature is allowed to take its course, with changes in one characteristic being studied in relation to development of disease or other health condition. Examples of observational studies include the cohort study or the case-control study.

Odds ratio: Ratio of the odds of an event in the exposed group to the odds of an event in the control (unexposed) group. Commonly used in the case-control method to estimate the relative risk. The prevalence odds ratio is often calculated for cross-sectional data.

Original research article: Paper written by the author(s) who conducted the research.

Outcome evaluation: Long-term measure of effects such as changes in morbidity, mortality, and/or quality of life.

Paradigm: Pattern of thought or conceptualization; an overall way of regarding phenomena within which scientists normally work.

Participatory approaches: Collaborative, community-based research method, designed to actively involve community members in research and intervention projects

PATCH (the Planned Approach to Community Health): Community health planning model that relies heavily on local data to set priorities, design interventions, and evaluate progress. The goal of PATCH is to increase the capacity of communities to plan, implement, and evaluate comprehensive, community-based interventions.

Peer review: Process of reviewing research proposals, manuscripts submitted for publication, and abstracts submitted for presentation at scientific meetings, whereby they are judged for scientific and technical merit by other scientists in the same field.

Person-time: Sum of the amount of time that each at-risk person in a given population is free from disease (often measured in person-years)

PERT: The Program Evaluation and Review Technique involves a graphically displayed timeline for the tasks necessary in the development and implementation of public health programs.

Policy: Laws, regulations, and formal and informal rules and understandings that are adopted on a collective basis to guide individual and collective behavior.

Pooled analysis: Use of data from multiple studies where the data are analyzed at the level of the individual participant with the goal of obtaining a quantitative estimate of effect.

Population attributable risk (PAR): Incidence of a disease in a population that is associated with or attributable to exposure to the risk factor.

Population-based process: Administrative strategy that seeks to maximize expected health and well-being across an entire community or population, rather than maximizing outputs and outcomes within specific programs and organizations.

Power (statistical power): The likelihood that a study will detect an effect when there is an effect there to be detected.

PRECEDE-PROCEED: Systematic planning framework developed to enhance the quality of health education interventions. The acronym PRECEDE stands for Predisposing, Reinforcing, and Enabling Constructs in Educational Diagnosis and Evaluation. The model is based on the premise that, just as medical diagnosis precedes a treatment plan, so should educational diagnosis precede an intervention plan. The acronym PROCEED stands for Policy, Regulatory, and Organizational Constructs in Educational and Environmental Development. This part of the model is based on recognition of the need for health promotion interventions that go beyond traditional educational approaches to changing unhealthy behaviors.

Precision: Quality of being sharply defined or stated. In statistics, precision is defined as the inverse of the variance of a measurement or an estimate.

Prevalence rate: Number of existing cases of disease among surviving members of the population.

Preventable burden (preventability; prevented fraction): Proportion of an adverse health outcome that potentially can be eliminated as a result of a prevention strategy.

Primary data: New evidence collected for a particular study or program through methods such as community surveys, interviews, and focus groups. The process of primary data collection usually occurs over a relatively long period of time.

Process evaluation: Analysis of inputs and implementation experiences to track changes as a result of a program or policy. This occurs at the earliest stages of public health intervention and often is helpful in determining midcourse corrections.

Program: Organized public health action, such as direct service interventions, community mobilization efforts, policy development and implementation, outbreak investigations, health communication campaigns, health promotion programs, and applied research initiatives.

Program objectives: Statements of short-term, measurable, specific activities having a specific time limit or timeline for completion. Program objectives must be measurable and are designed to reach goals.

Public health surveillance: The ongoing systematic collection and timely analysis, interpretation, and communication of health information for the purpose of disease prevention and control.

Publication bias: Bias in the published literature where the publication of research depends on the nature and direction of the study results. Studies in which an intervention is not found to be effective are sometimes not published or submitted for publication. Therefore, systematic reviews that fail to include unpublished studies may overestimate the true effect of an intervention or a risk factor.

Quality-adjusted life-years (QALYs): Frequently used outcome measure in cost-utility analysis that incorporates the quality or desirability of a health state with the duration of survival. Each year of life is weighted on a scale from 0 (death) to 1 (perfect health), with weights derived from patient or population surveys.

Quality of the evidence: Quality refers to the appropriateness and integrity of the information obtained. High-quality data are reliable, valid, and informative for their intended use.

Qualitative data: Nonnumerical observations, using approved methods such as participant observation, group interviews, or focus groups. Qualitative data can enrich understanding of complex problems and help to explain why things happen.

Quantitative data: Data that are expressed in numerical quantities, such as continuous measurements or counts.

Quasi-experimental designs: Study in which the investigator lacks full control over the allocation and/or timing of intervention but nonetheless conducts the study as if it were an experiment, allocating subjects to groups. Inability to allocate subjects randomly is a common situation that may be best studied as a quasi-experiment.

Randomized controlled trials: Experiment in which subjects in a population are randomly allocated to two groups, usually called study and control groups, to receive or not receive an experimental preventive or therapeutic procedure, maneuver, or intervention. The scientifically rigorous nature of RCTs increases the internal validity while limiting the external validity, and the use of RCTs is often determined by the availability of resources as well as the research question at hand.

Rate: Rate is a measure of the frequency of occurrence of a phenomenon (e.g., a disease or risk factor) for a defined population during a specified period.

RE-AIM: Framework for consistent reporting of research results that takes account of Reach to the target population; Effectiveness or Efficacy; Adoption by target settings or institutions; Implementation of consistency of delivery of intervention; and Maintenance of intervention effects in individuals and settings over time.

Registries: Regularly updated listings of information containing all identified disease or health problem cases. Active registries seek data and use follow-up to obtain more reliable and complete information. Passive registries accept and merge reports but do not update or confirm information.

Relative risk (rate ratio, risk ratio): Ratio of the rate of disease or death among the exposed to the rate among the unexposed; synonymous with rate ratio or risk ratio.

Relative standard error: Standard error (i.e., the standard deviation of an estimate) as a percentage of the measure itself. A relative standard error of 50 % means the standard error is half the size of the rate.

Reliability: Degree of stability exhibited when a measurement is repeated under identical conditions. Reliability refers to the degree to which the results obtained by a measurement procedure can be replicated. Lack of reliability may arise from divergences between observers or instruments or instability of the attribute being measured.

Reportable diseases: Selected diseases for which data are collected, as mandated by law and/or regulation at national, state, and local levels.

Resource-based decision making: In the resource-based planning cycle, the spiral of increased resources and increased demand for resources helps to drive the cost of health care services continually higher, even as the health status for some populations decline. This is one among several theories of why health care costs increase.

Review articles: Summary of what is known on a particular topic through review of original research articles.

Risk assessment: Qualitative and quantitative estimation of the likelihood of adverse effects that may result from exposure to specified health hazards or from the absence of beneficial influences. Includes four steps: hazard identification, risk characterization, exposure assessment, and risk estimation.

Scientific literature: Theoretical and research publications in scientific journals, reference books, textbooks, government reports, policy statements, and other materials about the theory, practice, and results of scientific inquiry.

Secondary data: Evidence routinely collected by others, usually at a local, state, or national level. The availability of secondary data from government, university, and nonprofit agencies saves time and money.

Selection bias: Bias (error) due to systematic differences in characteristics between those who take part in the study and those who do not.

Sensitivity: Ability of a screening test to correctly identify presence of a disease.

Sensitivity analysis: Evaluation to assess how robust the results of a study or systematic review are to changes in how it was done. Assumptions about the data are systematically varied and the analysis repeated to determine the stability of the results.

Small area analysis: Investigation containing fewer than twenty cases of the disease of interest; often requires special considerations and statistical tests to deal with the low incidence of events.

Specificity: Ability of a screening test to correctly identify absence of a disease

Stakeholder: Individual or organization with an interest in an intervention, health policy, or health outcome.

Strategic planning: Process of identifying objectives and essential actions (preventive and therapeutic) believed sufficient to control a health problem.

Survey: Systematic (but not experimental) method of data collection that often consists of questionnaires or interviews. Survey data differ from surveillance data in that they are not ongoing but rather sporadic.

Sustainability: The extent to which an evidence-based intervention can deliver its intended benefits over an extended period of time after external support from the donor agency is terminated.

Systematic review: Review of a clearly formulated question that uses systematic and explicit methods to identify, select, and critically appraise relevant research and to collect and analyze data from the studies that are included in the review, the goal of which is an unbiased assessment of a particular topic Statistical methods (meta-analysis) may or may not be used to analyze and summarize the results of the included studies.

Time-series analyses: Quasi-experimental research design in which measurements are made at several different times, thereby allowing trends to be detected.

TOWS analysis: TOWS analysis takes into account the external Threats and Opportunities that face an organization in light of the Weaknesses and Strengths within the organization.

Transferability: Degree to which the results of a study or systematic review can be extrapolated to other circumstances, in particular to routine health care situations.

Transtheoretical model: Theory of health behavior change. It suggests that people move through one of five stages (precontemplation, contemplation, preparation, action, maintenance) and that health behavior change is an evolving process that can be more effectively achieved if the intervention processes match the stage of readiness to change behavior.

Triangulation: Triangulation generally involves the use of multiple methods of data collection and/or analysis to determine points of commonality or disagreement. It often involves a combination of qualitative and quantitative data.

Type 1 evidence: Data that show the importance of a particular health condition and its link with some preventable risk factor. For example, a large body of epidemiologic evidence shows that smoking causes lung cancer.

Type 2 evidence: Data that focus on the relative effectiveness of specific interventions to address a particular health condition. For example, a substantial body of evidence shows that several interventions are effective in preventing the uptake (initiation) of smoking in youth.

Type 3 evidence: Data that document the context under which an intervention is appropriate. For example, the approaches for changing the community (built) environment will differ for rural versus urban areas.

Unit of analysis: Unit of assignment in an intervention study. Most commonly, the unit will be an individual person but, in some studies, people will be assigned in groups to one or another of the interventions. This is done either to avoid contamination or for convenience, and the units might be schools, hospitals, or communities.

Vital statistics: Data compiled by state health agencies concerning events such as births, deaths, marriages, divorces, and abortions.

REFERENCES

Some definitions are adapted from the following sources:

Brownson RC, Baker EA, Leet TL, Gillespie KN, True WR. Evidence-Based Public Health. 2nd ed. New York: Oxford University Press; 2011.

Centers for Disease Control and Prevention. Framework for program evaluation in public health. Morbidity and Mortality Weekly Report 1999;48(RR-11):1–40.

Ginter PM, Duncan WJ, Swayne LM. Strategic Management of Health Care Organizations. 7th ed. West Sussex, UK: John Wiley & Sons Ltd; 2013.

Glanz K, Rimer B, Viswanath K, editors. Health Behavior and Health Education. 5th ed. San Francisco, CA: Jossey-Bass Publishers; 2015.

Green LW, Kreuter MW. *Health Promotion Planning: An Educational and Ecological Approach*. 4th ed. New York, NY: McGraw Hill; 2005.

Haddix AC, Teutsch SM, Corso PS. *Prevention Effectiveness. A Guide to Decision Analysis and Economic Evaluation*. 2nd ed. New York: Oxford University Press; 2002.

Kohatsu ND, Robinson JG, Torner JC. Evidence-based public health: an evolving concept. *Am J Prev Med*. Dec 2004;27(5):417–421.

Last JM. *A Dictionary of Public Health*. New York: Oxford University Press; 2007.

Porta M, editor. A Dictionary of Epidemiology. 6th ed. New York: Oxford University Press; 2014.

Novick LF, Morrow CB, Mays GP, eds. Public Health Administration. Principles for Population-Based Management. Second Edition. Sudbury, MA: Jones and Bartlett Publishers; 2008.

Petticrew M, Cummins S, Ferrell C, et al. Natural experiments: an underused tool for public health? *Public Health*. Sep 2005;119(9):751–757.

Rabin B, Brownson R. Developing the terminology for dissemination and implementation research. In: Brownson R, Colditz G, Proctor E, editors. Dissemination and Implementation Research in Health: Translating Science to Practice. New York: Oxford University Press; 2012. p. 23–51

Straus SE, Richardson WS, Glasziou P, Haynes R. Evidence-Based Medicine. How to Practice and Teach EBM. 4th ed. Edinburgh, UK: Churchill Livingston; 2011.

Witkin BR, Altschuld JW. Conducting and Planning Needs Assessments. A Practical Guide. Thousand Oaks, CA: Sage Publications, 1995.

INDEX